Falk Symposium 168

March 27 and 28, 2009, Madrid

IBD in Different Age Groups

Editors

G. Rogler, Zurich
M. Gassul, Badalona
A. Levine, Holon
A. López San Román, Madrid

13 figures and 34 tables, 2009

Basel · Freiburg · Paris · London · New York · Bangalore ·
Bangkok · Shanghai · Singapore · Tokyo · Sydney

Reprint of **Digestive Diseases** (ISSN 0257–2753)
Vol. 27, No. 3, 2009

Library of Congress Cataloging-in-Publication Data

Falk Symposium (168th : 2009 : Madrid, Spain)
  IBD in different age groups : Falk Symposium 168, March 27 and 28, 2009,
Madrid / editors, G. Rogler ... [et al.].
     p. ; cm. -- (Falk symposium series ; 168)
  "Reprint of Digestive diseases (ISSN 0257-2753) vol. 27, no. 3,
2009--Prelim."
  Includes bibliographical references and indexes.
  ISBN 978-3-8055-9273-4 (hardcover : alk. paper)
  1. Inflammatory bowel diseases--Congresses. I. Rogler, G. (Gerhard) II.
Digestive diseases. III. Title. IV. Series: Falk symposium ; 168.
  [DNLM: 1. Inflammatory Bowel Diseases--Congresses. WI 420 F191ida 2009]
  RC862.I53F35 2009
  616.3'44--dc22

                                                    2009036632

S. Karger
Medical and Scientific Publishers
Basel · Freiburg · Paris · London ·
New York · Bangalore · Bangkok ·
Shanghai · Singapore · Tokyo · Sydney

Disclaimer
The statements, opinions and data contained in this publication are solely those of the individual authors and contributors and not of the publisher and the editor(s). The appearance of advertisements in the journal is not a warranty, endorsement, or approval of the products or services advertised or of their effectiveness, quality or safety. The publisher and the editor(s) disclaim responsibility for any injury to persons or property resulting from any ideas, methods, instructions or products referred to in the content or advertisements.

Drug Dosage
The authors and the publisher have exerted every effort to ensure that drug selection and dosage set forth in this text are in accord with current recommendations and practice at the time of publication. However, in view of ongoing research, changes in government regulations, and the constant flow of information relating to drug therapy and drug reactions, the reader is urged to check the package insert for each drug for any change in indications and dosage and for added warnings and precautions. This is particularly important when the recommended agent is a new and/or infrequently employed drug.

KARGER

Fax +41 61 306 12 34
E-Mail karger@karger.ch
www.karger.com

Contents

KARGER

Fax +41 61 306 12 34
E-Mail karger@karger.ch
www.karger.com

© 2009 S. Karger AG, Basel

Access to full text and tables of contents,
including tentative ones for forthcoming issues:
www.karger.com/ddi_issues

Contents

Dig Dis 2009;27:205
DOI: 10.1159/000235585

Preface

The Falk Symposium No 168 which took place in Madrid from March 27th to March 28th was entitled 'IBD in Different Age Groups'. It was the first meeting of its kind that was planned to bring together adult and pediatric gastroenterologists that are interested in the field of inflammatory bowel diseases. The success of the meeting was overwhelming; the number of attending physicians was one of the highest in the history of the Falk meetings.

During the meeting, we learned that the incidence in children is not rising more as compared with adults; however, the total number of children with IBD is increasing. Subsequently, more young patients will have to make the transition from a pediatric to an adult gastroenterologist. Therefore, the need for an improvement of the interaction of both disciplines is evident.

The increasing number of very young patients is associated with all problems inherent to physical and mental development. We face a situation where risk factors and response to therapy may be different as the life of these patients goes by. Therefore, it was important that for the first time an IBD symposium took into account not only the potential differences in phenotypes and clinical evolution in IBD along life, but also the changes in environmental factors and the possible differences in the response of the host to them.

In fact, there were a lot of issues in which both adults and pediatric gastroenterologists learned from each other. The scientific committee tried to put together a number of specialists able to explain the differences in the pathogenesis, clinical manifestations and evolution and therapeutic approaches in order to obtain the greatest benefits, the lowest rate of unwanted effects and the best quality of life for these patients.

The presentations held at the 168th Falk meeting have been summarized in the papers collected in this issue. The scientific committee and the organizers hope that all readers will benefit as much as the audience during the meeting.

Gerhard Rogler
for the members of the Scientific Committee

KARGER

Fax +41 61 306 12 34
E-Mail karger@karger.ch
www.karger.com

© 2009 S. Karger AG, Basel
0257–2753/09/0273–0205$26.00/0

Accessible online at:
www.karger.com/ddi

Dig Dis 2009;27:206–211
DOI: 10.1159/000228551

Disease Behavior in Adult Patients: Are There Predictors for Stricture or Fistula Formation?

Iris Dotan

IBD Center, Department of Gastroenterology and Liver Diseases, Tel Aviv Sourasky Medical Center, Tel Aviv, Israel

Key Words

Serologic markers · Glycans · Prognosis

Abstract

In the current era, in inflammatory bowel disease step-up vs. top-down therapeutic approaches for the treatment of Crohn's disease (CD) are evaluated. As a consequence, we need to be able to differentiate between patients who will have more aggressive phenotypes to those with potentially more benign CD course. The former would require closer follow-up; however, more important might be the subgroup of patients to whom we want to offer biologic and immuno-modulator therapy early on. This strategy is the only one supposed to prevent hospitalization and surgical intervention, specifically in patients with fistulae. Patients with expected fibrostenotic disease phenotype require early identification as well. The data regarding primary prevention of fibrostenosis are scarce; however, the association of biologic therapy with fewer surgeries might suggest that at least a subgroup of these patients would benefit from early, step-up therapeutic strategy. They might also benefit more from early immunomodulator therapy, as this was shown to have a secondary (though modest) preventive effect. The patients with fibrostenotic phenotype are also candidates for the most needed but still practically nonexistent anti-fibrotic therapies. In any case where patients are identified as having a higher chance to develop the more aggressive phenotypes, fibrostenotic and perforating, recommendation to avoid triggers/accelerators of disease progression (smoking, NSAIDS use) should be kept rigorously. Until recently, we based our attempts to predict disease phenotype mainly on clinical characteristics. As would be the case with many clinical features, some of them are not even predictors, but already manifestations of the condition we are trying to predict. Intervention at this stage might be too late for this patient. In addition to known demographic and clinical predictors reported, more recently sophisticated predictors shall be described. These predictors belong to three major groups: serologic markers, genetic markers, mucosal disease/healing. The major serologic markers used: anti-*Saccharomyces cerevisiae* antibodies (ASCA), anti-neutrophil cytoplasmic antibodies (ANCA), outer membrane porin C (OmpC), CBir1-flagellin, antibodies against I2 protein and the anti-glycan antibodies: anti-laminaribioside carbohydrate (ALCA), anti-chitobioside carbohydrate (ACCA) and anti-mannobioside carbohydrate (AMCA) and their associations with penetrating and fibrostenotic disease shall be discussed. The associations of genetic polymorphisms such as CARD15 and TLR4 variants and more aggressive disease phenotype will be described as well. Finally, the data supporting the relationship between inflamed, in contrast to healed intestinal mucosa and more aggressive disease course will be illustrated. These predictors may be used in clinical practice and/or research in order to better stratify CD prognosis. Thus they may be significant in our therapeutic decisions. Models for using these predictors would be presented.

Copyright © 2009 S. Karger AG, Basel

KARGER

Fax +41 61 306 12 34
E-Mail karger@karger.ch
www.karger.com

© 2009 S. Karger AG, Basel
0257–2753/09/0273–0206$26.00/0

Accessible online at:
www.karger.com/ddi

Iris Dotan, MD
IBD Center, Department of Gastroenterology and Liver Diseases
Tel Aviv Sourasky Medical Center, 6 Weizmann Street
Tel Aviv 64239 (Israel)
Tel. +972 3 694 7305, Fax +972 3 697 4622, E-Mail irisd@tasmc.health.gov.il

Crohn's Disease Phenotype and Behavior: Not All Patients Are the Same

Crohn's disease (CD) is an inflammatory disorder with heterogeneous manifestations and complications. The notion that it is probably a syndrome or several diseases with intestinal manifestations piled into one sack lends support from its many phenotypes, and the recently reported many possible genotypes [1]. Thus, there are repeated attempts to stratify CD into more homogeneous groups. Examples are the Vienna and the Montreal classifications (table 1) [2, 3]. This paper will focus on disease behavior (B section of both classifications). The most common presentation of CD is the inflammatory type, manifested mainly as diarrhea, abdominal cramps, possible fever and extraintestinal manifestations such as arthralgia, but no fibrostenotic or perforating (fistulizing) complications. However, disease behavior is not a constant given. Rather, more than 70% of CD patients would develop the more aggressive disease behaviors (fibrostenotic and perforating) within 10 years. This was shown by Cosnes et al. retrospectively assessing well-characterized CD patients in one center, as well as by the EC-IBD collaboration [4, 5].

This change in behavior with time is specifically striking as disease location (section L in the Vienna and Montreal classifications) does not tend to similarly change with time [6]. The implications of developing a more aggressive disease behavior type are significant. These phenotypes are associated with more surgical interventions, more hospital admissions and a greater personal and economic burden [7]. Moreover, stricture (i.e. the fibrostenotic disease behavior type) or fistula (i.e. the penetrating disease behavior phenotype) are not only manifestations of aggressive disease, they also predict a more aggressive disease, whether defined as the need for surgery or more hospitalizations and the use of steroids, as shown in both adult and pediatric populations [8, 9]. Having mentioned the need for surgery it is important to point out the well-known diagrams of timing to first surgery in CD patients. While several studies show that 50–70% of CD patients would require surgery within 10 years of diagnosis, Veloso et al. [10] have shown that the major contribution for this increased risk is on account of the aggressive phenotypes: fibrostenotic and penetrating. In a recent population-based study, Romberg-Camps et al. [11] showed that stricturing and penetrating phenotypes at diagnosis were important predictors for surgery, and stricturing phenotype, together with a young age <40 years and small bowel disease location, was a predictor of disease recurrence.

Table 1. Vienna and Montreal classifications of Crohn's disease

Vienna	Montreal
Age at diagnosis (A)	*Age at diagnosis (A)*
A1 <40 years	A1 <17 years
A2 >40 years	A2 17–40 years
	A3 >40 years
Location (L)	*Location (L)*
L1 terminal ileum	L1 ileal
L2 colonic	L2 colonic
L3 ileocolonic	L3 ileocolonic
L4 upper gastrointestinal	L4 isolated upper
Behavior (B)	*Behavior (B)*
B1 nonstricturing-nonpenetrating	B1 nonstricturing-nonpenetrating
B2 stricturing	B2 stricturing
B3 penetrating	B3 penetrating
	P perianal disease

All these observations stress the point that the stricturing-fibrostenotic and penetrating-fistulizing phenotypes are not only aggressive phenotypes per se, but they also predict an aggressive course.

Disease Phenotype Predictors: Why Are They Required?

As intuition and data support the notion that stricture and fistula represent and predict aggressive disease behavior and course, one might ask why we need predictors for such disease behavior. There are several important reasons for that in addition to our wish and need to better understand the disease pathophysiology. The main reasons for the need to have predictors for disease behavior are:

(1) Patient information: Upon diagnosis patients wish to know what their disease course will be.

(2) Closer follow-up of patients with worse prognosis: Knowing which patient might have a worse disease course would enable to put that patient under closer follow-up and to intervene earlier in case symptoms worsen.

(3) Modifying disease course: In the last decade traditional step-up vs. top-down therapeutic approaches for the treatment of CD are being evaluated. It has been shown by several authors, in both adult and pediatric populations, that top-down therapy, i.e. earlier use of biologic and immunomodulator therapies, might modify disease course, decrease hospitalizations, prevent surgeries and decrease the need for steroid treatment [9, 12].

These potent treatments might, however, be associated with significant side effects, specifically serious infections and the risk of malignancies. In addition, they might not be needed for the subgroup of patients destined to have a benign course. Their high cost also justifies optimal treatment-to-patient adjustment.

As a consequence, we need to be able to differentiate between patients who will have more aggressive phenotypes to those with potentially more benign CD course. The former would require closer follow-up, but, more importantly, is the subgroup of patients to whom we would offer biologic and immunomodulator therapy early on. As mentioned, this strategy is the only one currently known to prevent hospitalization and surgical intervention, specifically in patients with fistulae [13].

Patients with expected fibrostenotic disease phenotype require early identification as well. The data regarding primary prevention of fibrostenosis are scarce; however, the association of biologic therapy with fewer surgeries might suggest that at least a subgroup of these patients would benefit from early, step-up therapeutic strategy. They might also benefit more from early immunomodulator therapy as this was shown to have a secondary (though modest) preventive effect on postoperative disease recurrence [14]. The patients with fibrostenotic phenotype are also candidates for the most needed but still practically non-existent antifibrotic therapies.

In any case where patients are identified as having a higher chance to develop the more aggressive phenotypes (fibrostenotic and perforating), it is recommended to avoid triggers/accelerators of disease exacerbation and progression (e.g. smoking, NSAIDS use).

What Are the Current and Near-Future Tools for Disease Phenotype Prediction?

Three major factors might assist in predicting CD behavior: clinical, serologic and genetic.

Until recently, we based our attempts to predict disease phenotype mainly on clinical characteristics. As would be the case with many clinical features, some of them are not even predictors but already manifestations of the condition we are trying to predict. Intervention at this stage might be too late for this patient. Still, important observations made through the years might and should be used to stratify patients into subgroups. When Cosnes et al. [4] retrospectively assessed a cohort of CD patients in a single center and asked the question we are

asking, i.e. what clinical factors might predict stricture formation, they identified several factors that intuitively make sense: jejunal involvement and ileal involvement had HRs of 3.2 [2.2–4.7] and 2.5 [1.9–3.3], and no colonic involvement had a HR of 2.0 [1.6–2.4]. No anoperineal disease and a recent diagnosis had a modest association with stricture formation (HRs 1.4 [1.1–1.8] and 1.3 [1–1.6], respectively). Predicting fistula formation was even harder, as only anoperineal disease, now considered an inherent part of the perforating phenotype, predicted fistula formation (HR 2.6 [2.3–3]) [4], while age <40, non-Caucasian origin and no upper gastrointestinal tract involvement had only modest effects (HR ~1.3). As specifically and directly addressing the question of stricture or fistula formation was usually part of larger-scale studies assessing different predictors of disease outcome, we might use data from studies looking at predictors for complicated/disabling disease. While the definition of 'complicated/disabling disease' is not unanimous amongst authors, it usually includes the use of steroids, hospital admission and surgery. As mentioned, stricture or fistula are often associated with this disease course. Interestingly, independent studies from several centers observed that >50% of CD patients would have a disabling disease course within 5 years [8, 15]. Beaugerie et al. [15] found that having 2 or more of the factors age <40 years, steroid treatment or perianal lesions had a ~90% positive predictive value for disabling disease. Thus, these might be used as indirect predictors also for stricture or fistula formation. As described, several clinical factors might be used to stratify CD patients into a 'higher-risk' group to develop stricture or fistula. However, most data come from retrospective studies, and are mainly associations, expressed as hazard ratios. Thus, stronger, more sophisticated predictors are required in order to 'fine-tune' our predictions. Here, attention should be given to the reports connecting mucosal healing or non-healing to CD postoperative recurrence, chances of surgery and disabling disease. While not specifically assessing stricture or fistula formation, these might be important predictors of the more aggressive disease phenotypes and course [16, 17]. They may specifically aid in the prediction (and thus potential prevention) of strictures, as the finding of significantly diseased mucosa in the small bowel equals small bowel disease, already associated with an increased risk for strictures.

Comment: Smoking, an important risk factor for postoperative CD recurrence and a negative prognostic factor in CD, was not addressed in this section as few studies

Table 2. Serologic markers and prognostic associations

Antibody	Directed against	Sensitivity/specificity (%)	
pANCA	neutrophil cytoplasm (colonic bacteria?)	60–70 in UC	
ASCA	mannans, *Saccharomyces cerevisiae*	60–70 (can be as low as 35) 95	young diagnosis age
OmpC	outer membrane porin C, *Escherichia coli*	31–55	IP disease, need for surgery
Anti-I2	I2 protein, *Pseudomonas fluorescens*		FS disease, need for surgery
CBir1	flagellin of commensal bacteria (clostridium?)		SB IP FS
gASCA	covalently bound mannan	50–56	young diagnosis age shorter duration
ALCA	laminaribioside	15–27	young diagnosis age FS/IP
ACCA	chitobioside	11–20	longer duration (high levels) noninflammatory behavior
AMCA	mannobioside	11–28	NOD2 association

See references 9, 18, 19, 21, 25 and 30–37.

directly assessed and reported on its association with stricture or fistula formation. However, its relation to worse-prognosis CD in general should be acknowledged.

Serologic Markers as Predictors for Stricture or Fistula Formation

In addition to known demographic and clinical predictors, more sophisticated predictors might be used to aid in stratifying CD patients. One such group of markers is the serologic one, gaining increasing support as important prognostic markers in CD.

The major serologic markers available are: anti-*Saccharomyces cerevisiae* antibodies (ASCA), anti-neutrophil cytoplasmic antibodies (ANCA), outer membrane porin C (OmpC), CBir1-flagellin, antibodies against I2 protein and the recently described anti-glycan antibodies: anti-laminaribioside carbohydrate (ALCA), anti-chitobioside carbohydrate (ACCA) and anti-mannobioside carbohydrate (AMCA). Table 2 shows these serologic markers and some of the reported prognostic associations reported for each one. As seen, several serologic markers that are associated with CD were associated with small bowel location, need for surgery, fibrostenotic, penetrating disease or a noninflammatory phenotype. Consistent associations reported by >1 groups

include ASCA and gASCA, OmpC, I2, CBir1-flagellin, ALCA and ACCA. The serologic markers associated with both stricturing and penetrating behavior are ASCA and gASCA, CBir 1-flagellin, ALCA and ACCA (noninflammatory behavior). Importantly, it is not only the qualitative serologic response that counts but the quantitative one, i.e. higher titers and several seroreactivities pose an increased risk. Thus, higher titers or cumulative seroreactivities were associated with stricturing or penetrating disease behavior in adult and pediatric populations, small bowel location, need for surgery, and a relapsing course of pediatric CD [18–25]. Different serologic panels were thus tested in pediatric and adult populations. Ferrante et al. [19] showed that gASCA, ACCA, AMCA and OmpC were independently associated with non-inflammatory behavior (stricture or fistula) and Dubinsky et al. [20] showed that the frequency of structuring/penetrating disease increased with increasing numbers of immune responses against OmpC, CBir1-flagellin and ASCA.

Interestingly, seroreactivities determined not only an increased risk for stricture or fistula formation. Pediatric patients having multiple seroreactivities progressed to stricturing or penetrating disease sooner after diagnosis as compared to seronegative patients [20].

Genetic Markers as Predictors for Stricture or Fistula Formation

Several genetic variants were reported as predictors of CD phenotypes. Specifically, NOD2 variants were associated with strictures in the adult population [26], and synergism between NOD2 genotype and seroreactivity predicted fistulizing disease as well [27].

A study in the pediatric population has reported that variants of the OCTN and DLG genes were associated with fistulizing disease [28].

Not surprisingly, a genotype-serotype-dosage effect existed. gASCA, AMCA, ALCA and ASCA combinations were positively associated with NOD2/CARD15 genotype. Moreover, seropositivity increased with increasing positive NOD2/CARD15 variants [23–25].

As more genetic variants are identified in CD patients, more genotype-phenotype associations are reported. Thus, Weersma et al. [29] assessed known risk allele for CD in 1,684 patients from The Netherlands. In addition to adding support to the notion that more risk alleles were associated with stricturing or penetrating disease, they added that the autophagy gene ATG16L1 had an independent significant association with stricturing and perianal disease.

Summary and Conclusions

Complicated disease behavior manifested as stricturing, fibrostenotic disease or fistulizing penetrating disease is common in CD patients and increases in prevalence in parallel to disease duration. Attempts to predict complicated disease behavior are important for informing patients regarding their potential prognosis, closer follow-up of patients at risk and, more importantly, trying to modify disease course, using the powerful tools currently available such as biologic treatments. Adopting a 'risk-stratified approach' in the treatment of CD patients is recommended. Such a tailored approach would combine clinical, serologic and genetic markers so that high-risk patients could be identified before significant complications occur. Then, at an early disease stage, therapeutic interventions are expected to be most efficacious and optimally administered. Such an approach should be prospectively evaluated in large independent well-characterized patient cohorts. This way, the true-positive predictive value of clinical, serologic and genetic panels (as it is clear that single predictors are of little value) could be evaluated. As several of the potential predictors, specifically recently identified genes, are not widely available, and as time from prediction to complication (or avoiding it) might be protracted, acquiring the data is expected to be a lengthy process. Yet, its significance for CD patients and their physicians is invaluable, as it will enable evidence-based, high-quality predictions and interventions that might change the disease course of the patients.

Disclosure Statement

The author declares that Glycomids Ltd., Lod, Israel supplies IBDx® kits for serologic research at TASMC.

References

1 Barrett JC, Hansoul S, Nicolae DL, et al: Genome-wide association defines more than 30 distinct susceptibility loci for Crohn's disease. Nat Genet 2008;40:955–962.

2 Gasche C, Scholmerich J, Brynskov J, et al: A simple classification of Crohn's disease: report of the Working Party for the World Congresses of Gastroenterology, Vienna 1998. Inflamm Bowel Dis 2000;6:8–15.

3 Silverberg MS, Satsangi J, Ahmad T, et al: Toward an integrated clinical, molecular and serological classification of inflammatory bowel disease: Report of a Working Party of the 2005 Montreal World Congress of Gastroenterology. Can J Gastroenterol 2005; 9(suppl A):5–36.

4 Cosnes J, Cattan S, Blain A, et al: Long-term evolution of disease behavior of Crohn's disease. Inflamm Bowel Dis 2002;8:244–250.

5 Wolters FL, Russel MG, Sijbrandij J, et al: Phenotype at diagnosis predicts recurrence rates in Crohn's disease. Gut 2006;55:1124–1130.

6 Louis E, Collard A, Oger AF, et al: Behaviour of Crohn's disease according to the Vienna classification: changing pattern over the course of the disease. Gut 2001;49:777–782.

7 Odes S, Vardi H, Friger M, et al: Effect of phenotype on health care costs in Crohn's disease: a European study using the Montreal classification. J Crohn Colitis 2007;1:87–96.

8 Loly C, Belaiche J, Louis E: Predictors of severe Crohn's disease. Scand J Gastroenterol 2008;43:948–954.

9 Gupta N, Cohen SA, Bostrom AG, et al: Risk factors for initial surgery in pediatric patients with Crohn's disease. Gastroenterology 2006;130:1069–1077.

10 Veloso FT, Ferreira JT, Barros L, et al: Clinical outcome of Crohn's disease: analysis according to the Vienna classification and clinical activity. Inflamm Bowel Dis 2001;7:306–313.

11 Romberg-Camps MJL, Dagnelie PC, Kester AD, et al: Influence of phenotype at diagnosis and of other potential prognostic factors on the course of inflammatory bowel disease. Am J Gastroenterol 2009;104:371–383.

12 Baert F, Caprilli R, Angelucci E: Medical therapy for Crohn's disease: top-down or step-up? Dig Dis 2007;25:260–266.

13 Lichtenstein GR, Yan S, Bala M, et al: Infliximab maintenance treatment reduces hospitalizations, surgeries, and procedures in fistulizing Crohn's disease. Gastroenterology 2005;128:862–869.

14 Ardizonne S, Macconi G, Sampietro GM, et al: Azathioprine and mesalamine for prevention of relapse after conservative surgery for Crohn's disease. Gastroenterology 2004; 127:730–740.

15 Beaugerie L, Seksik P, Nion-Larmurier I, et al: Predictors of Crohn's disease. Gastroenterology 2006;130:650–656.

16 Allez M, Lemann M, Bonnet J, et al: Long term outcome of patients with active Crohn's disease exhibiting extensive and deep ulcerations at colonoscopy. Am J Gastroenterol 2002;97:947–953.

17 Froslie KF, Jahnsen J, Moum BA, et al: Mucosal healing in inflammatory bowel disease: results from a Norwegian population-based cohort. Gastroenterology 2007;133: 412–422.

18 Dotan I, Fishman S, Dgani Y, et al: Antibodies against laminaribioside and chitobioside are novel serologic markers in Crohn's disease. Gastroenterology 2006;131:366–378.

19 Ferrante M, Henckaerts L, Joosens M, et al: New serological markers in inflammatory bowel disease are associated with complicated disease behavior. Gut 2007;56:1394–1403.

20 Dubinsky MC, Lin YC, Dutridge D, et al: Serum immune responses predict rapid disease progression among children with Crohn's disease: immune responses predict disease progression. Am J Gastroenterol 2006;101: 360–367.

21 Forcione DG, Rosen MJ, Kisiel JB, et al: Anti-Saccharomyces cerevisiae antibody (ASCA) positivity is associated with increased risk for early surgery in Crohn's disease. Gut 2004;53:1117–1122.

22 Desir B, Amre DK, Lu SE, et al: Utility of serum antibodies in determining clinical course in pediatric Crohn's disease. Clin Gastroenterol Hepatol 2004;2:139–146.

23 Henckaerts L, Pierik M, Josens M, et al: Mutations in pattern recognition receptor genes modulate seroreactivity to microbial antigens in patients with inflammatory bowel disease. Gut 2007;56:1536–1542.

24 Dassopoulos T, Frangakis C, Cruz-Correa M, et al: Antibodies to Saccharomyces cerevisiae in Crohn's disease: higher titers are associated with a greater frequency of mutant NOD2/CARD15 alleles and with a higher probability of complicated disease. Inflamm Bowel Dis 2007;13:143–151.

25 Papp M, Altorjay I, Dotan N, et al: New serological markers for inflammatory bowel disease are associated with earlier age at onset, complicated disease behavior, risk for surgery, and NOD2/CARD15 genotype in a Hungarian IBD cohort. Am J Gastroenterol 2008;103:665–681.

26 Abreu MT, Tayloe KD, Lin YC, et al: Mutations in NOD2 are associated with fibrostenosing disease in patients with Crohn's disease. Gastroenterology 2002;123:679–688.

27 Ippoliti AF, Devlin S, Yang H, et al: The relationship between abnormal innate and adaptive immune function and fibrostenosis in Crohn's disease patients Gastroenterology 2006;130:A127.

28 Cucchiara S, Latiano A, Palmieri O, et al: Role of CARD15, DLG5 and OCTN genes polymorphisms in children with inflammatory bowel diseases. World J Gastroenterol 2007;13:1221–1229.

29 Weersma RK, Stokkers PC, van Bodegraven AA, et al: Molecular prediction of disease risk and severity in a large Dutch Crohn's disease cohort. Gut 2009;58:388–395.

30 Rump JA, Scholmerich J, Gross V, et al: A new type of perinuclear anti-neutrophil cytoplasmic antibody (p-ANCA) in active ulcerative colitis but not in Crohn's disease. Immunobiology 1990;181:406–413.

31 Duerr RH, Targan SR, Landers CJ, et al: Anti-neutrophil cytoplasmic antibodies in ulcerative colitis: comparison with other colitides/diarrheal illnesses. Gastroenterology 1991;100:1590–1596.

32 Sendid B, Colombel JF, Jacquinot PM, et al: Specific antibody response to oligomannosidic epitopes in Crohn's disease. Clin Diagn Lab Immunol 1996;3:219–226.

33 Vermeire S, Joosens S, Peeters M, et al: Comparative study of ASCA (anti-Saccharomyces cerevisiae antibody) assays in inflammatory bowel disease. Gastroenterology 2001;120: 827–833.

34 Cohavy O, Harth G, Horwiz M, et al: Identification of a novel mycobacterial histone H1 homologue (HupB) as an antigenic target of pANCA monoclonal antibody and serum immunoglobulin A from patients with Crohn's disease. Infect Immun 1999;67:6510–6517.

35 Landers CJ, Cohavy O, Misra R, et al: Selected loss of tolerance evidenced by Crohn's disease-associated immune responses to auto- and microbial antigens. Gastroenterology 2002;123:689–699.

36 Lodes MJ, Cong Y, Elson CO, et al: Bacterial flagellin is a dominant antigen in Crohn disease. J Clin Invest 2004;113:1296–1306.

37 Amre DK, Lu SE, Costea F, et al: Utility of serological markers in predicting the early occurrence of complications and surgery in pediatric Crohn's disease patients. Am J Gastroenterol 2006;101:645–652.

Insights from Epidemiology

Dig Dis 2009;27:212–214
DOI: 10.1159/000228552

Pediatric Inflammatory Bowel Disease: Is It Different?

Arie Levine

Pediatric Gastroenterology and Nutrition Unit, Wolfson Medical Center, Tel Aviv University, Tel Aviv, Israel

Key Words

Ulcerative colitis · Crohn's disease · Behavior, stricture

Abstract

The clinical manifestations of Crohn's disease (CD) and ulcerative colitis (UC) are highly variable, with significant diversity in phenotypes of the diseases. This diversity may manifest as a difference in age of onset. Pediatric-onset disease may present differently and have a different natural history, with ramifications for disease management. Clear evidence exists at present that pediatric-onset UC may be different than adult-onset UC. The primary difference in disease phenotype is extent of disease. Approximately 60–70% of patients with pediatric-onset UC present with pancolitis, as opposed to approximately 20–30% in adults. Patients are more likely to have severe disease and become steroid-dependent. CD may be affected by an age gradient. There is an inverse linear relationship between age and colonic CD, the younger the patient, the more likely is the patient to have colonic CD. This inverse relationship is true through age 10. In addition, pediatric patients are more likely to have upper gastrointestinal involvement than their adult peers. Comparing adult and pediatric phenotypes is fraught with methodological obstacles. Disease behavior, with the exception of growth failure, seems to parallel disease behavior in adults. Patients with growth retardation are a high risk group for complications and should be managed as such.

Copyright © 2009 S. Karger AG, Basel

Introduction

The clinical manifestations of Crohn's disease (CD) and ulcerative colitis (UC) are highly variable, with significant diversity in phenotypes of the diseases. This diversity in adults is manifested by differences in the location and distribution of the diseases, the natural history and outcomes. Patients with IBD may also differ by age of onset, and this in turn raises the question if age of onset dictates any difference in disease phenotype or outcome.

Like adults, children and adolescents are prone to the same diverse array of complications stemming from the disease and its therapy. However, recent evidence indicated that pediatric onset of the disease may be associated with different presentations or behavior of the disease. The purpose of this article is to review what is presently known about disease behavior in children, and subsequently to evaluate if the disease behavior is similar to that of adult-onset disease, and if not, explore the ramifications.

Ulcerative Colitis

UC in adults usually starts in the rectum and may extend proximally. Most studies in adult populations have shown a spectrum of disease extension, with approximately 40–50% of adult patients exhibiting disease initially confined to the rectum or sigmoid colon. In contrast, 25–35% of patients will have a more severe phenotype characterized by extensive disease (pancolitis) [1]. In

Arie Levine
Pediatric Gastroenterology and Nutrition Unit
Wolfson Medical Center, Tel Aviv University
Tel Aviv 58100 (Israel)
Tel. +972 3 502 8808, Fax +972 3 502 8807, E-Mail alevine@wolfson.health.gov.il

addition, about 1/3 of patients with adult-onset UC will never have a relapse of the disease.

Clear evidence exists at present that pediatric-onset UC may be different from adult-onset UC. The primary difference in disease phenotype is extent of the disease. Approximately 60–70% of patients with pediatric-onset UC present with pancolitis, as opposed to approximately 20–30% in adults [2, 3]. Proctitis is an unusual manifestation of the disease in pediatric patients. This finding has been replicated in large North American (Inflammatory Bowel Collaborative Group, Pediatric Inflammatory Bowel Disease Consortium) and European registries (Porto group and EPIMAD French registries) that included over 800 patients. Pancolitis at presentation occurred in 60–80% of pediatric patients, while in one study, proctitis occurred in only 12% of patients [2]. Rectal sparing also appears to be more common in pediatric-onset disease than in adult-onset UC [4].

Clear evidence about the natural history of UC in children is problematic, and interpretation of the natural history is complicated by the fact that it was collected recently during the era of biologics use in UC. However, a recent study from a North American Registry demonstrated that about 80% of pediatric UC at onset had pancolitis, 80% had moderate-to-severe colitis, and 80% patients receive corticosteroids within 30 days of diagnosis. Of those receiving steroids, 45% were steroid dependent at 1 year [3]. Colectomy was performed in 5% of patients within a year of diagnosis. These numbers are clearly different from UC seen in adults, indicating that pediatric UC not only presents with more extensive disease, but also with more severe and refractory disease.

Crohn's Disease

Evidence exists that manifestations of CD may be affected by age. However, as opposed to a pediatric versus adult cutoff seen in UC, the phenotype of CD may be affected by an age gradient. There are two clear characteristics of disease location that appear to be true for pediatric CD. There is an inverse linear relationship between age and colonic CD: the younger the patient, the more likely the patient is to have colonic CD and the more likely they are to have isolated colitis [2, 5]. This inverse relationship is true through age 10, and is especially true for patients without NOD2 mutations [5]. For patients with NOD2 mutations, the vast majority of pediatric CD patients will manifest with ileo-colitis. Isolated involvement of the terminal ileum is significantly less common in pediatric disease.

In addition, pediatric patients are more likely to have upper gastrointestinal involvement than their adult peers. Several studies have found involvement proximal to the ileum in 16–51% of patients [5, 7–9]. However, the true prevalence of upper intestinal disease in childhood varies considerably between studies, primarily because of differences in methodology. There are two unresolved methodological flaws that may make comparison of pediatric and adult studies difficult. The first is the difference in routine workup. Pediatric gastroenterologists consider a gastroscopy + colonoscopy + radiology as part of the routine evaluation for CD, while many adult gastroenterologists confine themselves to a colonoscopy + radiology. This may lead to more detection of proximal involvement in pediatric-onset disease. The second confounding factor has to do with definitions of disease involvement using the Montreal or Vienna classifications in the original Vienna classification scheme, involvement required ulcerations or aphthous ulcers [10, 11]. The Montreal classification further clarified the definition of extent, without changing the macroscopic criteria. Furthermore, in recent years, several pediatric groups have started using microscopic involvement as diagnostic criteria, without any consensus or validation. There is no consensus at present as to what constitutes proof of involvement in duodenal or gastric biopsies, with the exception of the presence of granulomas. Thus, many nonspecific findings (nonspecific inflammation, etc.) on gastroduodenal biopsies may be interpreted as evidence of disease involvement in this region. Therefore, it may very well be that the differences in upper intestinal disease noted between pediatric studies and adult studies may reflect two extremes; overdiagnosis by pediatricians and underdiagnosis by adult gastroenterologists. Further confusion has been shown when the cecum is the only part of the colon involved. Though this was clearly defined as part of ileal disease when the ileum is involved, many investigators will define exclusive involvement of the ileum and cecum as ileo-colonic disease.

The Montreal classification has divided disease behavior into 3 broad categories [11]. These are inflammatory disease (without evidence of strictures or fistulae), stricturing disease and fistulizing disease. The most important variable found to determine disease behavior over time to date has been duration of disease. Thus, comparison of disease behavior requires collecting data from cohorts with extended follow-up.

Three recent studies [7–9] have looked at disease behavior and two compared pediatric-onset to adult-onset disease. These studies have shown that disease location and behavior change over time, but are similar to adult disease behavior. The prevalence of stricturing and fistulizing disease at 5 years was almost identical in pediatric and adult cohorts.

Perianal disease has been reported to commonly occur in both pediatric-onset and adult-onset CD. Again, differences in methodology plague efforts to compare these cohorts. Adult studies have confined perianal disease to fistula or abscess, while pediatric studies may define disease as the above plus fissures or tags. A recent study from a North American registry of new-onset CD, using the inclusive criteria, found perianal disease in 24% of patients; however, using the more restrictive classification yielded a prevalence of 10% at disease onset [14]. A recently published evaluation of perianal disease throughout follow-up is particularly useful for comparing adult and pediatric data. This study defined perianal disease in a uniform manner, and included both pediatric and adult cohorts. The investigators found that age of onset was not a determinant of perianal disease, rather location of disease was the preliminary determinant [15].

Growth retardation and growth failure is a type of disease behavior that is specific for pediatric-onset disease. It is considered a complication of the disease and, if not rectified, can lead to short stature that may become irreversible [16, 17]. Growth failure, defined as linear growth at or below 2 SD below the mean for age, or decreased growth velocity, can occur in 15–20% of children with CD. While it is beyond the scope of this study to review growth failure, it has implications as both a complication and as a marker. Approximately 30% of patients may manifest at presentation with growth retardation. Patients with low BMI have been shown to be at a higher risk for perianal fistulizing disease [14], while patients with growth failure at presentation were more likely to become steroid dependent and require surgery early in the disease [6].

In conclusion, pediatric-onset disease is not identical to adult-onset disease. Patients with pediatric-onset UC are more likely to have pancolitis, severe colitis and become steroid-dependent than adult patients. Pediatric-onset CD may differ with regard to disease location and extent. Younger children (similar to older adults) are more likely to have colonic disease, while children in general may have more upper intestinal involvement. Characterization of disease location continues to be plagued by methodological problems. Regarding disease behavior as defined by the Montreal classification, children with CD seem to have the same disease behavior patterns, which depend primarily on duration and site of the disease, independent of age of onset. Lastly, growth retardation is a peculiar disease behavior confined to pediatric-onset CD, requires special management, and may be a marker for more severe disease.

Disclosure Statement

The author declares that no financial or other conflict of interest exists in relation to the content of the article.

References

1 Henriksen M, Jahnsen J, Lygren I, Sauar J, Kjellevold Ø, Schulz T, Vatn MH, Moum B, IBSEN Study Group: Ulcerative colitis and clinical course: results of a 5-year population-based follow-up study (the IBSEN study). Inflamm Bowel Dis 2006;12:543–550.
2 Heyman MB, Kirschner BS, Gold BD, et al: Children with early-onset inflammatory bowel disease (IBD): analysis of a pediatric IBD consortium registry. J Pediatr 2005;146:35–40.
3 Hyams J, Markowitz J, Lerer T, et al: The natural history of corticosteroid therapy for ulcerative colitis in children. Clin Gastroenterol Hepatol 2006;4:1118–1123.
4 Glickman JN, Bousverous A, Farraye FA, et al: Pediatric patients with untreated ulcerative colitis may present initially with unusual morphologic findings. Am J Surg Pathol 2004; 28:190–197.
5 Levine A, Kugathasan S, Annese V, et al: Pediatric onset Crohn's colitis is characterized by genotype-dependent age-related susceptibility. Inflamm Bowel Dis 2007;13:1509–1515.
6 Markowitz J, Hyams J, Mack D, et al: Corticosteroid therapy in the age of infliximab: acute

and 1-year outcomes in newly diagnosed children with Crohn's disease. Clin Gastroenterol Hepatol 2006;4:1124–1129.
7 Van Limbergen J, Russel RK, Drummond HE, et al: Definition of phenotypic characteristics of childhood-onset inflammatory bowel disease. Gastroenterology 2008;135:1114–1122.
8 Shaoul R, Karban A, Reif S, et al: Disease behavior in children with Crohn's disease: the effect of disease duration, ethnicity, genotype and phenotype. Dis Dig Sci 2008;54:142–150.
9 Vernier-Massouille G, Balde M, Salleron J, et al: Natural history of pediatric Crohn's disease: a population-based cohort study. Gastroenterology 2008;135:1106–1113.
10 Gasche C, Scholmerich J, Brynskov J, et al: A simple classification of Crohn's disease: report of the Working Party for the World Congresses of Gastroenterology, Vienna 1998. Inflamm Bowel Dis 2000;6:8–15.
11 Silverberg MS, Satsangi J, Ahmad T, et al: Toward an integrated clinical, molecular and serological classification of inflammatory bowel disease: Report of a Working Party of the 2005 Montreal World Congress of Gastroenterolo

gy. Can J Gastroenterol 2005;19(suppl A):5–36.
12 Cosnes J, Cattan S, Blain A, et al: Long-term evolution of disease behavior of Crohn's disease. Inflamm Bowel Dis 2002;8:244–250.
13 Louis E, Collard A, Oger AF, et al: Behavior of Crohn's disease according to the Vienna classification: changing pattern over the course of the disease. Gut 2001;49:777–782.
14 Keljo DJ, Markowitz J, Langton C, et al: Course and treatment of perianal disease in children newly diagnosed with Crohn's disease. Inflamm Bowel Dis 2009;15:383–387.
15 Karban A, Iati M, Davidovich O, et al: Risk factors for perianal Crohn's disease: the role of genotype, phenotype and ethnicity. Am J Gastroenterol 2007;102:1702–1708.
16 Shamir R, Philip M, Levine A: Growth retardation in pediatric Crohn's disease: pathogenesis and management. Inflamm Bowel Dis 2007;13: 620–628.
17 Hildebrand H, Karlberg J, Kristiansson B: Longitudinal growth in children and adolescents with inflammatory bowel disease. J Pediatr Gastroenterol Nutr 1994;18:165–173.

Dig Dis 2009;27:215–225
DOI: 10.1159/000228553

Environmental Factors Affecting Inflammatory Bowel Disease: Have We Made Progress?

Peter Laszlo Lakatos

1st Department of Medicine, Semmelweis University, Budapest, Hungary

Key Words

Inflammatory bowel disease · Ulcerative colitis · Crohn's disease · Environmental factors · Smoking · Gut flora

Abstract

The pathogenesis of inflammatory bowel disease (IBD) is only partially understood; various environmental and host (e.g. genetic, epithelial, immune, and nonimmune) factors are involved. The critical role for environmental factors is strongly supported by recent worldwide trends in IBD epidemiology. One important environmental factor is smoking. A meta-analysis partially confirms previous findings that smoking was found to be protective against ulcerative colitis and, after the onset of the disease, might improve its course, decreasing the need for colectomy. In contrast, smoking increases the risk of developing Crohn's disease and aggravates its course. The history of IBD is dotted by cyclic reports on the isolation of specific infectious agents responsible for Crohn's disease or ulcerative colitis. The more recently published cold chain hypothesis is providing an even broader platform by linking dietary factors and microbial agents. An additional, recent theory has suggested a breakdown in the balance between putative species of 'protective' versus 'harmful' intestinal bacteria – this concept has been termed *dysbiosis* resulting in decreased bacterial diversity. Other factors such as oral contraceptive use, appendectomy, dietary factors (e.g. refined sugar, fat, and fast food), perinatal events, and childhood infections have also been associated with both diseases, but their role is more controversial. Nonetheless, there is no doubt that economic development, leading to improved hygiene and other changes in lifestyle ('westernized lifestyle') may play a role in the increase in IBD. This review article focuses on the role of environmental factors in the pathogenesis and progression of IBDs.

Copyright © 2009 S. Karger AG, Basel

Introduction

The pathogenesis of ulcerative colitis (UC) and Crohn's disease (CD) has only been partly understood. Inflammatory bowel disease (IBD) is a multifactorial disease with probable genetic heterogeneity [1]. In addition, several environmental risk factors (e.g. diet, smoking, measles or appendectomy) may contribute to its pathogenesis. During the past decades, the incidence pattern of both forms of IBD has changed significantly [2], showing some common but also quite distinct characteristics for the two disorders. Differences in geographic distribution, and particularly changes in incidence over time within one area, may provide insight into possible etiological factors. It is very unlikely, however, that these rapid changes can be attributed to variations in the genetic fac-

Peter Laszlo Lakatos, MD, PhD
1st Department of Medicine, Semmelweis University
Koranyi str. 2/A
HU–1083 Budapest (Hungary)
Tel. +36 1 210 0278 ext. 1500, 1520, Fax +36 1 313 0250, E-Mail kislakpet@bel1.sote.hu

tors. On the contrary, environmental factors are likely to play an important role. Diet, as a luminal antigen, was thought to be an important factor in the pathogenesis of IBD [1, 3]. In the past two decades, there has been a shift in the lifestyle in Eastern Europe, Asia, and Central America, as the lifestyle, including the diet, became more 'westernized'. This possibility is further supported by the differences in incidence and prevalence found within one region.

Additional important environmental factors, which have been extensively studied in both diseases, include smoking and dysbiosis of the gut flora. The link between smoking and IBD was first noted in 1982 when Harries et al. [4] noticed that a low proportion of UC patients were smokers. Two years later, a case-control study by Somerville et al. [5] reported that the relative risk of developing CD was 4.8 in those who smoked before disease onset, and 3.5 for those with a current smoking habit.

The normal intestine encounters a high concentration of foreign antigens, bacteria, and food. In the stomach and proximal small intestine, acid secretion, secretion of bile and phasic 'housekeeping' motility patterns hinder colonization. However, the number of bacteria dramatically increases in the distal small intestine to an estimated 10^{10} to 10^{12} bacterial cells/g content in the colon, which contributes to 60% of the fecal mass [6] Assumingly, more than 400–500 species of bacteria are represented, belonging to 30 genera (however, the exact number so far is impossible to determine). Despite the separation of this antigenic load from the largest complement of lymphocytes in the body (gut-associated lymphoid tissue; GALT) by only a single layer of polarized intestinal epithelium, most people do not mount an immune response to foreign antigens, and the interaction between the mucosal immune system and the fecal bacterial mass regulates physiologic bowel functions. The mucosal immune system has evolved to balance the need to respond to pathogens while maintaining active tolerance for commensal bacteria and food antigens. In IBD, this tolerance is disturbed and inflammation supervenes, driven by the intestinal microbial flora. The exact mechanism by which the intestinal mucosa loses tolerance for its bacterial neighbors remains elusive. The role of host genetic regulation of the innate immune response in the pathogenesis of CD has been brought to sharp focus through the identification of the NOD2 mutations and it is now undisputed that enteric bacterial flora plays a key role in the pathogenesis of IBD, both in UC and CD; however, an infectious origin for IBD has not been confirmed.

In addition, factors such as oral contraceptive use, appendectomy, dietary factors (e.g. refined sugar, fat, and fast food), perinatal events, and childhood infections have also been found to be associated with both diseases, but their role is more controversial. Knowledge of this heterogeneity has led to the re-examination of environmental influences on IBD (fig. 1). This review article focuses on the role of environmental factors in the pathogenesis and progression of IBDs.

Smoking in IBD: Friend or Foe?

The Effect of Smoking Cessation and Smoking on the Risk of Developing Inflammatory Bowel Disease

The percentage of current smokers in a group of patients with CD is significantly higher than that observed in a control population matched for sex and age (45–55% vs. 30–40%) [7]. Accordingly, an increased life-time risk was reported in current smokers when compared to nonsmokers by both Calkins [8] (OR 2.0; 95% CI 1.65–2.47) and in the more recent meta-analysis by Mahid et al. [9] (OR 1.76; 95% CI 1.40–2.22).

Compared to patients who never smoked, former smokers were reported to be an increased risk for developing CD [8]. This risk decreased only after four years of smoking cessation. In a recent population-based study by Bernstein et al. [10], similar data were reported, with both, current smoking (OR 1.96) and never-smoked (OR 1.78) were associated with an increased risk for developing CD. This latter association could not be replicated in the recent meta-analysis by Mahid et al. [9], though a trend was observed (p = 0.08). The effect of passive smoking remains controversial [11]. In one recent prospective study [12], CD patients were more likely than controls to have prenatal smoke exposure (OR 1.72; 95% CI 1.1–2.71). In addition, passive smoke exposure during childhood, with parents or other household members being smokers (OR 2.04; 95% CI 1.28–3.31) was also associated with increased risk, in concordance with previous data by Lashner et al. [13].

In contrast, UC affects predominantly non-smokers and former smokers. The percentage of current smokers (smoking more than seven cigarettes per week) in a group of patients with UC is about 10–15% [14, 15]. These percentages are significantly lower than those observed in a control population matched for gender and age (25–40%). The meta-analysis by Calkins [8], conducted more than 15 years ago, yielded a pooled odds ratio of 0.41 (0.34–0.48) for current smokers compared with lifetime nonsmokers. The effect of smoking seems to only postpone the event, as the relative risk of UC was also higher in former smokers (OR 1.64; 95% CI 1.36–1.98). In a recent meta-analysis by Mahid et al. [9], comparable values were reported, which also included new available data. Current smoking decreased the risk for UC (OR 0.58; 95% CI 0.45–0.75), while former smoking was associated with a greater risk (OR 1.79; 95% CI 1.37–2.34). Interestingly, in patients who stopped smoking, UC developed in 52% of patients in the first 3 years after cessation, as reported by Motley et al. [16], in concordance with other studies [17]. On the contrary, active smoking in early childhood was associated with a gradually increasing risk for developing UC (OR for starting to smoke at an age <10 years: 7.02 and <15 years: 3.46) [12]. The same trend was observed for passive smoking by the mother (OR 1.53; 95% CI 0.93–2.49).

The relationship between smoking and UC has also been examined at the population level. The prevalence of UC was increased fivefold in patients from the Mormon Church in Britain and Ireland, where smoking is strongly discouraged, compared with that of the general population. In contrast, CD was equally as common [18]. Somewhat contradictory, in a recent population-based case-control study [10], among others, never having smoked was also associated with an increased risk (OR 1.66; 95% CI 1.17–2.35).

Effect of Smoking and Its Cessation on Disease Phenotype and Course

In CD, smoking is associated with disease location: most, but not all, studies report a higher prevalence of ileal disease and a lower prevalence of colonic involvement in smokers [19, 20, 21]. A recent review [21] and previous data have demonstrated that smoking, when measured up to the time point of disease behavior classification, was associated more frequently with complicated disease, penetrating intestinal complications [19, 22, 23], and greater likelihood to progress to complicated disease, as defined by the development of strictures or fistulae [21], and a higher relapse rate [24]. Of note, the previously noted disease severity, as assessed from the therapeutic needs, was found to be similar in young patients who started smoking and in their matched controls [25]. The need for steroids and immunosuppressant's was increased in smokers compared to nonsmokers [20]. Whether the daily smoking habits (e.g. more than 15 cigarettes per day) or the total pack-years smoked is more impor-

tant in the above-mentioned associations remains questionable.

The effect of smoking is to some extent different between male and female patients. In CD, women are affected more drastically by smoking. The relative risk associated with smoking for women may be greater than for men; one study demonstrated a threefold difference [11]. This was already demonstrated by Sutherland et al. [26] in 1990, who reported that in a group of 174 patients, who required surgery for CD, smokers had a 29% greater risk than nonsmokers, over 10 years. However, the increased risk was more marked in females than males (OR 4.2; 95% CI 2.0–4.2 in females, and OR 1.5; 95% CI 0.8–0.6 in males).

In most studies, the risk of surgery as well as the risk for further resections during the course of disease is also higher in smokers [19, 26, 27]. In addition, in a recent French publication [28], light smokers had higher resection rates compared to non-smokers in CD, suggesting that complete smoking cessation should be advised to all smokers with CD. These findings were reinforced by Cottone et al. [29], who have shown that macroscopic lesions on the ileal site of the anastomosis were observed one year after surgery in 70% of smokers, versus 35% of nonsmokers and 27% of ex-smokers. The risk for symptomatic postoperative recurrence was more marked in heavy smokers than in mild smokers [29].

The disease activity in ex-smokers is not different from that of nonsmokers, and is less marked than in current smokers [24]. The beneficial effect of smoking cessation might be seen within a year following cessation. A large prospective intervention study by Cosnes et al. [30] performed in a selected group of 59 patients who stopped smoking following a smoking cessation intervention, examined the disease course from one year following smoking cessation onwards. The flare-up rate, therapeutic needs, and disease severity were similar in patients who had never smoked and in those who stopped smoking, with both displaying a better course than current smokers. Quitters had a 65% lower risk of flare-up compared to continuing smokers. The need for corticosteroids, immunosuppressive therapy, or a dose increase of immunosuppressants was also lower. Interestingly, after quitting, some patients developed UC-like lesions of the distal colon, whereas previously they displayed typical CD. The harmful effect of smoking on the course of CD is, however, not a universal finding. Studies in patients from Israel have not found differences in the need for surgery or for immunosuppressants between smokers and nonsmokers [31, 32]. Finally, the development and severity of perineal complications do not seem to be influenced by the smoking status [24].

In a recent paper by Aldhous et al. [33], using the Montreal classification, the harmful effect of smoking was only partially confirmed. Although current smoking was associated with less colonic disease, the smoking habits at the time of diagnosis were not associated with time to development of stricturing disease, internal penetrating disease, perianal penetrating disease, or time to first surgery. Age at diagnosis was also similar in current smokers and non-smokers and was only delayed in ex-smokers.

In UC, disease extent at the time of diagnosis is not affected by smoking, but the disease course is usually milder in smokers compared to non-smokers. Flare-up, hospitalization rates [17], the need for oral steroids [34], and colectomy rates [34, 35] are reported to be lower, while age at onset is older in smokers compared to non-smokers, though not in all studies. Relapse rates are lower in patients who began smoking after the diagnosis of UC [36]. In concordance, in a recent Europe-wide population-based cohort [37], the relapse rate was lower (hazard ratio 0.8; 95% CI 0.6–0.9) in smokers compared to nonsmokers, while being higher in women. In a retrospective analysis of a large patient series with UC, current smoking was found to decrease the 10-year cumulative colectomy risk from 0.42 to 0.32 [34]. Accordingly, a meta-analysis of several large series with a total of 1,489 UC patients also found the risk for colectomy to be lower (OR 0.57; 95% CI 0.38–0.85) in current smokers compared to non-smokers [38].

Interestingly, some studies also reported a gender association; when compared to non-smokers, male UC patients who smoked ran a more benign disease course as assessed by the decreased need for immunosuppressive therapy (8 vs. 26%), whereas this difference was not observed in females [8]. Additionally, smoking delayed the onset of disease, yet only in males.

In addition, in smokers with distal UC at diagnosis, the proximal extension of the disease is less frequent [34, 39], while primary sclerosing cholangitis is observed almost exclusively in nonsmokers [40]. Disease regression [41] was also more likely to occur in smokers compared to nonsmokers or ex-smokers, 5 years (30 vs. 5 vs. 8%) but not 10 years after the diagnosis. Also, those with extensive disease were the lightest smokers, whereas those with healthy colons were the heaviest smokers.

In contrast, intriguing new data by Aldhous et al. [41] showed that current and nonsmokers had an almost identical age at onset (31.1 vs. 29.4 years) and this was delayed only in ex-smokers (46.5 years). Colectomy rates did not differ. This group, however, had a greater exposure to smoking compared to the group of current smokers.

A link between smoking habits and the course of UC has also been reported. In intermittent smokers, many patients note symptomatic exacerbation when they stop smoking, followed by symptom relief when they smoke again [16]. Moreover, smokers with UC who quit experience an increase in disease activity, hospital admissions, and the need for major medical therapy (oral steroids, immunosuppressants), within the first years following the cessation of smoking [42]. However, the risk of colectomy in the short-term did not increase compared to matched nonsmokers and continuing smokers.

Pathogenic Microbes

A large part of research has traditionally been devoted to finding a causative biological source to any disease. This has also been the case in IBD; however, to date, there is no compelling evidence of an etiological role for any single pathogenic microorganism. Several microorganisms, such as *Mycobacterium paratuberculosis, Listeria monocytogenes, Chlamydia trachomatis, Escherichia coli, Cytomegalovirus, Saccharomyces cerevisiae,* and many more, have been proposed as having a potential etiological role.

The suggested etiologic role of *M. paratuberculosis* in CD also became controversial. This bacterium is the causative agent of Johne's disease, a chronic granulomatous ileitis in ruminants, which closely resembles CD. *M. paratuberculosis* was initially isolated from CD tissues some 20 years ago [43] and follow-up studies tried to culture *M. paratuberculosis*, testing for specific DNA sequences in intestinal tissues, or measuring serum antibodies against *M. paratuberculosis*. These studies yielded conflicting or inconclusive results [44, 45]. More recently, *M. paratuberculosis* has been identified by in situ hybridization to the *M. paratuberculosis*-specific *IS900* gene in tissue specimens of CD [46], as well as in 40% of CD granuloma isolated from surgical specimens by laser capture microdissection [47]. Others, using PCR technology, have localized *M. paratuberculosis* to macrophages and myofibroblasts within the lamina propria [48]. However, the possibility of an association between *M. paratuberculosis* and CD remains inconclusive. A recent 2-year clinical trial [49] using clarithromycin, rifabutin, and clofazimine also failed to identify a sustained benefit from antibiotic treatment in CD. Of note, however, the used doses were lower than those usually administered in everyday practice and the short-term benefit of the combination therapy was significantly more effective at week 16 than placebo (p = 0.02).

A fascinating hypothesis termed the cold chain hypothesis was published in the Lancet in 2003 [50]: an association between refrigeration and CD. Some so-called psychrotrophic bacteria are capable of growing at low temperatures and at a reduced rate. Common pathogens include *Yersinia enterocolitica*, *Listeria monocytogenes*, and *Clostridium botulinum* [51]. Several studies have demonstrated the presence of various *Yersinia* species in intestinal mucosal samples from CD patients. The specific pathogens detected were either *Y. enterocolitica* or *Y. pseudotuberculosis*, and sometimes even both [52, 53]. There are numerous aspects of yersiniosis that resemble the inflammatory reaction seen in CD, making these two conditions differential diagnoses, including ileitis or ileocolitis, mesenteric lymphadenitis, reactive arthritis, and erythema nodosum. Additionally, granuloma may be observed in histological samples [52].

Recent data have also demonstrated a role for the presence of mucosa-associated and intramucosal bacteria in the pathogenesis of IBD as well as colorectal cancer. In the study by Martin et al. [54], mucosa-associated or intramucosal *E. coli* (adherent-invasive *E. coli*; AIEC) were present in 43 and 29% in CD versus 17 and 9% in controls, respectively. Similarly, in another study [55], the prevalence of *Clostridium* spp., *Ruminococcus torques* and *Escherichia coli* was significantly higher in ileocolonic mucosa samples from CD patients. This supports a role for mucosa-adherent bacteria in the pathogenesis of CD.

Finally, a viral etiology has also been proposed as the cause of IBD, particularly for CD. An early measles infection during the perinatal period notably increases the risk of CD [56]. The finding of paramixovirus-like particles in CD endothelial granulomas suggests an association between perinatal measles and predisposition to CD based on some epidemiological and serologic data [57]; however, these preliminary findings were not confirmed by later studies [58]. Importantly, the progressive decline of measles virus infection in the last decades with the concomitant rise of CD during the same period of time speaks against an etiologic role for the measles in CD. The hypothesis that measles vaccination, rather than the measles infection, might be a risk factor for CD was also raised, yet again, results of additional studies failed to confirm this association [59]. In contrast, a role for cytomegalovirus infection was proposed in UC [60].

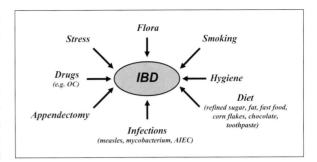

Fig. 1. Environmental factors in IBD. OC = Oral contraceptives; AIEC = adherent-invasive *E. coli*.

Nonpathogenic Intestinal Flora

In the last decade, the focus of interest for a microbial etiology behind IBD has shifted from infectious to commensal agents. Based on fairly solid data, a substantial body of evidence has accumulated suggesting that the normal enteric flora is the one playing a key role in the development of IBD [61]. This was even more evident after the discovery of the genetic factors (e.g. NOD2/CARD15, TLR4, and CD14) responsible for alterations in bacterial perception [1]. The beneficial effect of antibiotics in the treatment of CD, and to a lesser extent UC, has been appreciated for years. Diversion of the faecal stream from inflamed bowel loops has also been known to induce symptomatic improvement in CD patients, while re-emergence of inflammation often occurs upon restoration of intestinal continuity [62].

Changes in the normal flora of IBD patients have already been observed with dysbacteriosis being commonly reported. It was proposed, based on the clinical picture of IBD, that the intestinal flora might play a role in the initiation and perpetuation of the inflammatory reaction. Fabia et al. [63] demonstrated a radical decrease in the concentration of anaerobic bacteria as well as *Lactobacillus* in active IBD patients. On the contrary, patients with inactive IBD showed no such decrease. Swidsinski et al. [64] compared over 300 IBD patients with a mere 40 control individuals. Using various laboratory techniques, they also demonstrated abnormalities in the flora. In addition, a much greater number and concentration of bacteria are found in the biofilms covering the epithelium that is involved by IBD than that of healthy subjects. Furthermore, a direct association was also reported between bacterial concentration and disease severity.

The phenomenon of decreased bacterial diversity of the intestinal microflora obtained from stool samples in IBD patients has also been suggested, based on culture-dependent microbiological techniques [65]. Recently, a German group reported on the relative lack of the *Bacteroides* group (usually accounting 50–90% of the anaerobic faecal microflora) by utilizing 16sDNA-based single-strand conformation polymorphism (SSCP) fingerprint, cloning experiments and real-time PCR. Moreover, the bacterial profiles were stable, at least for the observed period of 6 weeks. This was in concordance with previous findings, suggesting that the mucosa-associated microflora contained only a small number of bacteria of the *Bacteroides/Prevotella* group [66]. However, in a recent study comparing the fecal microflora of healthy controls and CD patients, no differences were noted between patients and healthy controls [66]. This lack of significant difference may, at least partially, be explained by the differences in mucosal and fecal microflora.

The most convincing evidence comes from experimental data. In the majority of IBD animal models, intestinal inflammation fails to develop when the animals are kept in a germfree environment. This critical observation has led to the widely accepted paradigm 'no bacteria, no colitis'. However, once normal flora was introduced into their environment, the mutant-strain mice quickly developed colitis [67, 68].

It is worth mentioning that bacterial superinfection (most commonly *Clostridium difficile*, but also *Entamoeba histolytica, Campylobacter* spp., and so on) is also able to elicit a relapse of IBD. In the study by Mylonaki et al. [69], 10.5% of all relapses were associated with enteric infections, while in another study [70], 20% of all relapses were correlated to *C. difficile* positivity.

In a recent report from Germany [71], the authors were able to discriminate CD from UC based on the biostructure of the fecal flora and leukocyte count in the fecalmucus transition zone. Most prominent was the depletion of *Faecalibacterium prausnitzii* (Fprau <1×10^9/ml) with a normal leukocyte count in CD, especially during active disease. The density of this species was closely associated with the probability and duration of the remission. If confirmed, this or similar microbial changes in combination with other possible noninvasive markers could be very useful for predicting disease activity and short- or long-term disease course.

Finally, modern-day absence of exposure to intestinal helminths appears to be an important environmental factor contributing to development of these illnesses. Helminths interact with both host innate and adoptive immunity to stimulate immune regulatory circuitry and to reduce effector pathways that drive aberrant inflammation. In a recent German study [72], helminth infection was associated with a decreased risk (OR 0.34) for CD. In addition, preliminary results have shown beneficial effects of worm therapies in both UC and CD [73].

Hygiene Factors

The hygiene hypothesis as a potential explanation for IBD comes from observations that the rise in the incidence of IBD, both in developed and developing countries, has coincided with improvements in hygiene over the 20th century. The 'IBD hygiene hypothesis' states that raising children in extremely hygienic environments negatively affects immune development, which predisposes them to immunological diseases like IBD later in life. Many factors can be merged under the umbrella of hygiene factors including access to clean water, a hot water tap, a smaller family size, perinatal and early life events-infections-vaccinations, noncontaminated food, fast food, chewing gum toothpaste use, refrigeration (cold chain hypothesis, see above), oral contraceptive use, appendectomy are all part of today's modern life. Moreover, several studies report that the incidence of IBD is higher in urban as opposed to rural areas [7].

Perinatal factors; in a recent paper by Sonntag et al. [74] preterm birth (OR 1.5, 95% CI 1.1–2.0 for CD; OR 1.3, 95% CI 0.9–1.9 for UC), mother's disease during pregnancy (CD: OR 1.9, 95% CI 1.3–2.9; UC: OR 1.6, 95% CI 1.0–2.4), and disease in the first year of life (CD: OR 2.2, 95% CI 1.6–2.9; UC: OR 1.7, 95% CI 1.3–2.3) were associated with the development of IBD in later life, while no significant associations were found for the mode of delivery and breast-feeding. The majority of the evidence, however, supports a protective effect of breast-feeding in UC and CD [75]. A recent study based on an Italian population of 819 IBD patients suggested lack of breast-feeding to be associated with an increased risk of both CD and UC [76].

A further possible factor highly investigated is childhood vaccination. Childhood vaccinations have the ability to alter the maturation of the intestinal and systemic immune system and as such have been implicated in IBD. The hypothesis that measles vaccination, rather than the measles infection, might be a risk factor for CD was also raised. Thompson et al. [77] were the first to raise the possibility of a link between measles vaccination and IBD. In a cohort analysis of 3,545 individuals in the UK, they showed that individuals with a history of exposure to measles vaccination were 3-fold and 2.5-fold more likely to develop CD and UC, respectively, compared with unvaccinated controls, but additional studies failed to confirm this association [78]. Similar conflictive findings were reported for MMR and BCG vaccinations [79]. Of note however, these and also many other studies investigating the effect of different hygiene factors suffered from severe methodological shortcoming such as patient and control selection, different follow-up in the cohort and controls, recall bias, retrospective design, etc.

Family size and birth order as a potential marker for the hygiene hypothesis in IBD have been examined in several studies with inconsistent results. For example, Hampe et al. [80] found birth later in the sibling order was significantly associated with a lower risk for IBD. In contrast, in a recent study by Klement et al. [81], small number of siblings in the family (for 1 sibling vs. 5 or more, OR 2.63, 95% CI 1.49–4.62), and higher birth order (for birth order of 5 or higher vs. 1, OR 2.35, 95% CI 1.47–3.77) were associated with an increased risk. Similarly, bedroom sharing was associated with an increased risk for UC [81].

Finally, parameters of socioeconomic status and domestic hygiene have been investigated in relation to IBD. Earlier studies cited socioeconomic status as an important factor in the development of IBD, in that a higher socioeconomic status was more prevalent in IBD patients. However, the confounding effect of less household crowding and better domestic hygiene (e.g. hot tap) cannot be excluded. Gent et al. [82] found CD to be fivefold more common in IBD patients whose first house had a hot water tap and a separate bathroom, but no association was reported for mains drainage or access to a flush toilet. Moreover, domestic hygiene variables were not associated with UC. A similar finding was reported by Duggan et al. [83] who found availability of hot water before age 11 to be significantly associated with CD but not UC. Pet ownership and animal exposure during childhood [84] have been associated with an increased risk for CD, but results are again inconsistent [85].

Stress

In the 1950s, IBD was classified as a psychosomatic disorder [86] with many early studies finding an association between IBD and psychiatric diagnoses. Since then, there is a long but inconsistent history of observations suggesting that psychologic stress contributes to the course of UC and CD. In a literature review, Maunder [87] has reported prospective studies support a role for psychologic stress in the course of UC and for depressive symptoms in the course of CD. RCTs did not support the benefit of stress reduction for unselected patients with CD. In contrast, in a recent relatively large (n = 101) prospective follow-up study [88], patients under conditions of low stress and who scored low on avoidance coping (i.e., did not engage in social diversion or distraction) were least likely to relapse, supporting a biopsychosocial model of CD exacerbation, and for the first time it suggests that the way that patients cope may impact on relapse rate in CD.

Similarly, over the years there have been many case studies which have suggested that adverse life events can be a causal factor in relapse in IBD. However, although suggestive, these retrospective studies are frequently flawed by recall bias. Well designed prospective investigations of life events as causative factors for relapse in IBD are difficult to perform. Nonetheless, in a relatively recent 2-year prospective trial in 163 IBD patients in remission, using multivariate Cox regression analysis with time-dependent variables, life events were not associated with the rate of relapse after adjustment for significant covariates on the subsequent month (hazard ratio = 0.88, 95% CI = 0.68–1.13, p = 0.33) or in the time-lagged analysis [89]. In addition, life events occurring within 6 months of the onset of the IBD were also not associated with an increased risk for developing IBD in a questionnaire-based French study [90].

Diet

Low-fiber, high-sugar, high-animal-fat westernized diets have been proposed as a risk factor for the development of IBD [91]. The increasing incidence of CD in Eastern Europe and Asia, for example, has been proposed to correlate with changes towards more westernized diets [2].

In the literature, there are many reports of possible associations between diet and IBD with a range of foods being implicated, such as refined sugar, fast foods, margarine, corn flakes, microparticles and certain dairy products. While many studies offer interesting links between diet and IBD, there is, as yet, no conclusive evidence that any specific food or dietary factor directly contributes to the pathogenesis of either CD or UC. Most studies reviewed were subject to methodological limitations, which could have biased the results (e.g. most studies have investigated post-illness diet). Moreover, Russel et al. [92] suggested that while these nutritional factors may be true risk factors for IBD, they may also be just an expression of a 'modern lifestyle' also involving other risk factors for the development of IBD.

Somewhat in contrast, in children, there is stronger evidence for the use of enteral diet as a primary therapy in CD. A more recent Cochrane review [93] highlighted the role of enteral nutrition in promoting growth in children. In addition, in a relatively recent prospective cohort study from the UK [94], UC patients in remission were followed up for 12 months to determine the effect of habitual diet on relapse. Consumption of meat (OR 3.2; 95% CI 1.3–7.8), particularly red and processed meat (OR 5.19; 95% CI 2.1–12.9), protein (OR 3.00; 95% CI 1.25–7.19), and alcohol (OR 2.71; 95% CI 1.1–6.67) in the top tertile of intake increased the likelihood of relapse compared with the bottom tertile of intake, suggesting that modifiable dietary factors might be associated with disease course and short-term relapse at least in UC.

Oral Contraceptive Use

Similarly, oral contraceptives are a recent exposure, in this case from the beginning of the 1960s. The increase in incidence, especially of CD, has been hypothesized to be causally related to the exposure of oral contraceptives. Of note however, the increase in incidence in CD in some populations started early in the 1950s – before the introduction of oral contraceptives – and there was already a female predominance. The observational studies have not yielded entirely consistent results; therefore, it is of interest that two meta-analyses (from 1995 and 2008) [95, 96] demonstrated an elevated risk both for UC and CD (RR for CD = 1.46, 95% CI 1.26–1.70; RR for UC = 1.28, 95% CI 1.06–1.54 adjusted for smoking). The authors

conclude that the associations are weak and that a non-causal explanation (confounding) cannot be ruled out. It is therefore also of interest that the use of oral contraceptives does not seem to affect the recurrence rate or the severity of the disease after diagnosis.

Appendectomy

It might seem strange that appendectomy is grouped under the heading 'hygienic factors'. It is, however, natural because appendicitis is a modern disease that emerged as an epidemic during the first part of the 20th century.

Very little is known about the etiology of appendicitis, especially in the ages with highest incidence (late childhood and adolescence), although hygienic factors early in life have been proposed. Findings from a registry-based study in Sweden indicate that it is appendicitis, and not the appendicectomy as such, that is associated with a decreased risk of UC, giving further credence to such a hypothesis [97]. In addition, in a meta-analysis [98] from 2002, a pooled protective effect was reported for an appendectomy in UC in 17 case-control studies with an OR of 0.31 (95% CI 0.26–0.37). All these studies have suggested that alterations in mucosal immune responses leading to appendicitis or resulting from appendectomy may negatively affect the pathogenetic mechanisms of UC. Moreover, appendectomy decreased the risk for colectomy and immunosuppressant use in UC, while in CD it was associated with more proximal disease and has an increased risk of stricture and a lesser risk of anal fistulization [99, 100].

Disclosure Statement

The authors declare that no financial or other conflict of interest exists in relation to the content of the article.

References

1 Lakatos PL, Fischer S, Lakatos L, Gal I, Papp J: Current concept on the pathogenesis of IBD: crosstalk between genetic and microbial factors. Pathogenic bacteria, altered bacterial sensing or changes in mucosal integrity take 'toll'? World J Gastroenterol 2006; 12:1829–1840.

2 Lakatos PL: Recent trends in the epidemiology of inflammatory bowel diseases: up or down? World J Gastroenterol 2006;12:6102–6108.

3 Cashman KD, Shanahan F: Is nutrition an aetiological factor for inflammatory bowel disease? Eur J Gastroenterol Hepatol 2003; 15:607–613.

4 Harries AD, Baird A, Rhodes J: Non-smoking: a feature of ulcerative colitis. Br Med J (Clin Res Ed) 1982;284:706.

5 Somerville KW, Logan RF, Edmond M, Langman MJ: Smoking and Crohn's disease. Br Med J (Clin Res Ed) 1984;289:954–956.

6 Mahida YR, Rolfe VE: Host-bacterial interactions in inflammatory bowel disease. Clin Sci 2004;107:331–341.

7 Lakatos L, Mester G, Erdelyi Z, Balogh M, Szipocs I, Kamaras G, Lakatos PL: Striking elevation in incidence and prevalence of inflammatory bowel disease in a province of western Hungary between 1977–2001. World J Gastroenterol 2004;10:404–409.

8 Calkins BM: A meta-analysis of the role of smoking in inflammatory bowel disease. Dig Dis Sci 1989;34:1841–1854.

9 Mahid SS, Minor KS, Soto RE, Hornung CA, Galandiuk S: Smoking and inflammatory bowel disease: a meta-analysis. Mayo Clin Proc 2006;81:1462–1471.

10 Bernstein CN, Rawsthorne P, Cheang M, Blanchard JF: A population-based case control study of potential risk factors for IBD. Am J Gastroenterol 2006;101:993–1002.

11 Persson PG, Ahlbom A, Hellers G: Inflammatory bowel disease and tobacco smoke: a case-control study. Gut 1990;31:1377–1381.

12 Mahid SS, Minor KS, Stromberg AJ, Galandiuk S: Active and passive smoking in childhood is related to the development of inflammatory bowel disease. Inflamm Bowel Dis 2007;13:431–438.

13 Lashner BA, Shaheen NJ, Hanauer SB, Kirschner BS: Passive smoking is associated with an increased risk of developing inflammatory bowel disease in children. Am J Gastroenterol 1993;88:356–359.

14 Cosnes J, Nion-Larmurier I, Afchain P, Beaugerie L, Gendre JP: Gender differences in the response of colitis to smoking. Clin Gastroenterol Hepatol 2004;2:41–48.

15 Srivasta ED, Newcombe RG, Rhodes J, Avramidis P, Mayberry JF: Smoking and ulcerative colitis: a community study. Int J Colorectal Dis 1993;8:71–74.

16 Motley RJ, Rhodes J, Ford GA, Wilkinson SP, Chesner IM, Asquith P, Hellier MD, Mayberry JF: Time relationships between cessation of smoking and onset of ulcerative colitis. Digestion 1987;37:125–127.

17 Boyko EJ, Koepsell TD, Perera DR, Inui TS: Risk of ulcerative colitis among former and current cigarette smokers. N Engl J Med 1987;316:707–710.

18 Penny WJ, Penny E, Mayberry JF, Rhodes J: Prevalence of inflammatory bowel disease amongst Mormons in Britain and Ireland. Soc Sci Med 1985;21:287–290.

19 Lindberg E, Jarnerot G, Huitfeldt B: Smoking in Crohn's disease: effect on localisation and clinical course. Gut 1992;33:779–782.

20 Russel MG, Volovics A, Schoon EJ, van Wijlick EH, Logan RF, Shivananda S, Stockbrugger RW: Inflammatory bowel disease: is there any relation between smoking status and disease presentation? European Collaborative IBD Study Group. Inflamm Bowel Dis 1998;4:182–186.

21 Mahid SS, Minor KS, Stevens PL, Galandiuk S: The role of smoking in Crohn's disease as defined by clinical variables. Dig Dis Sci 2007;52:2897–2903.

22 Picco MF, Bayless TM: Tobacco consumption and disease duration are associated with fistulizing and stricturing behaviors in the first 8 years of Crohn's disease. Am J Gastroenterol 2003;98:363–368.

23 Louis E, Michel V, Hugot JP, Reenaers C, Fontaine F, Delforge M, El Yafi F, Colombel JF, Belaiche J: Early development of stricturing or penetrating pattern in Crohn's disease is influenced by disease location, number of flares, and smoking but not by NOD2/CARD15 genotype. Gut 2003;52:552–557.

24 Cosnes J, Carbonnel F, Carrat F, Beaugerie L, Cattan S, Gendre J: Effects of current and former cigarette smoking on the clinical course of Crohn's disease. Aliment Pharmacol Ther 1999;13:1403–1411.

25 Cosnes J, Carbonnel F, Beaugerie L, Le Quintrec Y, Gendre JP: Effects of cigarette smoking on the long-term course of Crohn's disease. Gastroenterology 1996;110:424–431.

26 Sutherland LR, Ramcharan S, Bryant H, Fick G: Effect of cigarette smoking on recurrence of Crohn's disease. Gastroenterology 1990; 98:1123–1128.

27 Breuer-Katschinski BD, Hollander N, Goebell H: Effect of cigarette smoking on the course of Crohn's disease. Eur J Gastroenterol Hepatol 1996;8:225–228.

28 Seksik P, Nion-Larmurier I, Sokol H, Beaugerie L, Cosnes J: Effects of light smoking consumption on the clinical course of Crohn's disease. Inflamm Bowel Dis 2009; 15:734—741.

29 Cottone M, Rosselli M, Orlando A, Oliva L, Puleo A, Cappello M, Traina M, Tonelli F, Pagliaro L: Smoking habits and recurrence in Crohn's disease. Gastroenterology 1994; 106:643–648.

30 Cosnes J, Beaugerie L, Carbonnel F, Gendre JP: Smoking cessation and the course of Crohn's disease: an intervention study. Gastroenterology 2001;120:1093–1099.

31 Odes HS, Fich A, Reif S, Halak A, Lavy A, Keter D, Eliakim R, Paz J, Broide E, Niv Y, Ron Y, Villa Y, Arber N, Gilat T: Effects of current cigarette smoking on clinical course of Crohn's disease and ulcerative colitis. Dig Dis Sci 2001;46:1717–1721.

32 Fidder HH, Avidan B, Lahav M, Bar-Meir S, Chowers Y: Clinical and demographic characterization of Jewish Crohn's disease patients in Israel. J Clin Gastroenterol 2003;36:8–12.

33 Aldhous MC, Drummond HE, Anderson N, Smith LA, Arnott ID, Satsangi J: Does cigarette smoking influence the phenotype of Crohn's disease? Analysis using the Montreal classification. Am J Gastroenterol 2007; 102:577–588.

34 Mokbel M, Carbonnel F, Beaugerie L, Gendre JP, Cosnes J: Effect of smoking on the long-term course of ulcerative colitis. Gastroenterol Clin Biol 1998;22:858–862.

35 Boyko EJ, Perera DR, Koepsell TD, Keane EM, Inui TS: Effects of cigarette smoking on the clinical course of ulcerative colitis. Scand J Gastroenterol 1988;23:1147–1152.

36 Fraga XF, Vergara M, Medina C, Casellas F, Bermejo B, Malagelada JR: Effects of smoking on the presentation and clinical course of inflammatory bowel disease. Eur J Gastroenterol 1997;9:683–687.

37 Hoie O, Wolters F, Riis L, Aamodt G, Solberg C, Bernklev T, Odes S, Mouzas IA, Beltrami M, Langholz E, Stockbrugger R, Vatn M, Moum B; on behalf of (EC-IBD): Ulcerative colitis: patient characteristics may predict 10-yr disease recurrence in a European-wide population-based cohort. Am J Gastroenterol 2007;102:1692–1701.

38 Cosnes J: Tobacco and IBD: relevance in the understanding of disease mechanisms and clinical practice. Best Pract Res Clin Gastroenterol 2004;18:481–496.

39 Samuelsson SM, Ekbom A, Zack M, Helmick CG, Adami HO: Risk factors for extensive ulcerative colitis and ulcerative proctitis: a population based case-control study. Gut 1991;32:1526–1530.

40 Loftus EV Jr, Sandborn WJ, Tremaine WJ, Mahoney DW, Zinsmeister AR, Offord KP, Melton LJ 3rd: Primary sclerosing cholangitis is associated with nonsmoking: a case-control study. Gastroenterology 1996;110: 1496–1502.

41 Aldhous MC, Drummond HE, Anderson N, Baneshi MR, Smith LA, Arnott ID, Satsangi J: Smoking habit and load influence age at diagnosis and disease extent in ulcerative colitis. Am J Gastroenterol 2007;102:589–597.

42 Beaugerie L, Massot N, Carbonnel F, Cattan F, Gendre JP, Cosnes J: Impact of cessation of smoking on the course of ulcerative colitis. Am J Gastroenterol 2001;96:2113–2116.

43 Chiodini RJ, Van Kruiningen HJ, Thayer WR, Merka RS, Coutu JA: Possible role of mycobacteria in inflammatory bowel disease: an unclassified Mycobacterium species isolated from patients with Crohn's disease. Dig Dis Sci 1984;29:1073–1079.

44 Wall S, Kunze ZM, Saboor S, Soufleri I, Seechurn P, Chiodini R, McFadden JJ: Identification of Spheroblast-like agents isolated from tissues of patients with Crohn's disease and control tissues by polymerase chain reaction. J Clin Microbiol 1993;31:1241–1245.

45 Bernstein CN, Blanchard JF, Rawsthorne P, Collins MT: Population-based case control study of seroprevalence of Mycobacterium paratuberculosis in patients with Crohn's disease and ulcerative colitis. J Clin Microbiol 2004;42:1129–1135.

46 Sechi LA, Mura M, Tanda F, Lissia A, Solinas A, Fadda G, Zanetti S, Manuela M, Francesco T, Amelia L, Antonello S, Giovanni F, Stefania Z: Identification of Mycobacterium avium subsp. Paratuberculosis in biopsy specimens from patients with Crohn's disease identified by in situ hybridization. J Clin Microbiol 2001;39:4514–4517.

Environment and Inflammatory Bowel Disease

47 Ryan P, Bennett MW, Aarons S, Lee G, Collins JK, O'Sullivan GC, O'Connell J, Shanahan F: PCR detection of *Mycobacterium paratuberculosis* in Crohn's disease granulomas isolated by laser capture microdissection. Gut 2002;51:665–670.

48 Hulten K, El-Zimaity HM, Karttunen TJ, Almashhrawi A, Schwartz MR, Graham DY, El-Zaatari FA: Detection of *Mycobacterium avium* subspecies paratuberculosis in Crohn's disease tissues by in-situ hybridization. Am J Gastroenterol 2001;96:1529–1535.

49 Selby W, Pavli P, Crotty B, Florin T, Radford-Smith G, Gibson P, Mitchell B, Connell W, Read R, Merrett M, Ee H, Hetzel D: Antibiotics in Crohn's Disease Study Group: two-year combination antibiotic therapy with clarithromycin, rifabutin, and clofazimine for Crohn's disease. Gastroenterology 2007;132: 2313–2319.

50 Hugot JP, Alberti C, Berrebi D, Bingen E, Cezard JP: Crohn's disease: the cold chain hypothesis. Lancet 2003;362:2012–2015.

51 Champagne CP, Laing RR, Roy D, Mafu AA, Griffiths MW: Psychrotrophs in dairy products: their effects and their control. Crit Rev Food Sci Nutr 1994;34:1–30.

52 Kallinowski F, Wassmer A, Hofmann MA, Harmsen D, Heesemann J, Karch H, Herfarth C, Buhr HJ: Prevalence of enteropathogenic bacteria in surgically treated chronic inflammatory bowel disease. Hepatogastroenterology 1998;45:1552–1558.

53 Lamps LW, Madhusudhan KT, Havens JM, Greenson JK, Bronner MP, Chiles MC, Dean PJ, Scott MA: Pathogenic Yersinia DNA is detected in bowel and mesenteric lymph nodes from patients with Crohn's disease. Am J Surg Pathol 2003;27:220–227.

54 Martin HM, Campbell BJ, Hart CA, Mpofu C, Nayar M, Singh R, Englyst H, Williams HF, Rhodes JM: Enhanced *Escherichia coli* adherence and invasion in Crohn's disease and colon cancer. Gastroenterology 2004; 127:685–693.

55 Martinez-Medina M, Aldeguer X, Gonzalez-Huix F, Acero D, Garcia-Gil LJ: Abnormal microbiota composition in the ileocolonic mucosa of Crohn's disease patients as revealed by polymerase chain reaction-denaturing gradient gel electrophoresis. Inflamm Bowel Dis 2006;12:1136–1145.

56 Ekbom A, Wakefield AJ, Zack M, Adami HO: Perinatal measles infection and subsequent Crohn's disease. Lancet 1994;344: 508–510.

57 Ekbom A, Daszak P, Kraaz W, Wakefield AJ: Crohn's disease after in-utero measles virus exposure. Lancet 1996;348:515–517.

58 Fisher NC, Yee L, Nightingale P, McEwan R, Gibson JA: Measles virus serology in Crohn's disease. Gut 1997;41:66–69.

59 Ghosh S, Armitage E, Wilson D, Minor PD, Afzal MA: Detection of persistent measles virus infection in Crohn's disease: current status of experimental work. Gut 2001;48: 748–752.

60 Hommes DW, Sterringa G, van Deventer SJ, Tytgat GN, Weel J: The pathogenicity of cytomegalovirus in inflammatory bowel disease: a systematic review and evidence-based recommendations for future research. Inflamm Bowel Dis 2004;10:245–250.

61 Guarner F, Malagelada JR: Gut flora in health and disease. Lancet 2003;361:512–519.

62 D'Haens GR, Geboes K, Peeters M, Baert F, Penninckx F, Rutgeerts P: Early lesions of recurrent Crohn's disease caused by infusion of intestinal contents in excluded ileum. Gastroenterology 1998;114:262–267.

63 Fabia R, Ar'Rajab A, Johansson ML, Andersson R, Willen R, Jeppsson B, Molin G, Bengmark S: Impairment of bacterial flora in human ulcerative colitis and experimental colitis in rats. Digestion 1993;54:248–255.

64 Swidsinski A, Ladhoff A, Pernthaler A, Swidsinski S, Loening-Baucke V, Ortner M, Weber J, Hoffmann U, Schreiber S, Dietel M, Lochs H: Mucosal flora in inflammatory bowel disease. Gastroenterology 2002;122: 44–54.

65 Sartor RB: Enteric microflora in IBD: pathogens or commensals? Inflamm Bowel Dis 1997;3:230–235.

66 Seksik P, Rigottier-Gois L, Gramet G, Sutren M, Pochart P, Marteau P, Jian R, Dore J: Alterations of dominant fecal bacterial groups in patients with Crohn's disease of the colon. Gut 2003;52:237–242.

67 Taurog JD, Richardson JA, Croft JT, Simmons WA, Zhou M, Fernandez-Sueiro JL, Balish E, Hammer RE: The germfree state prevents development of gut and joint inflammatory disease in HLA-B27 transgenic rats. J Exp Med 1994;180:2359–2364.

68 Rath HC, Schultz M, Freitag R, Dieleman LA, Li F, Linde HJ, Scholmerich J, Sartor RB: Different subsets of enteric bacteria induce and perpetuate experimental colitis in rats and mice. Infect Immun 2001;69:2277–2285.

69 Mylonaki M, Langmead L, Pantes A, Johnson F, Rampton DS: Enteric infection in relapse of inflammatory bowel disease: importance of microbiological examination of stool. Eur J Gastroenterol Hepatol 2004;16: 775–778.

70 Meyer AM, Ramzan NN, Loftus EV Jr, Heigh RI, Leighton JA: The diagnostic yield of stool pathogen studies during relapses of inflammatory bowel disease. J Clin Gastroenterol 2004;38:772–775.

71 Swidsinski A, Loening-Baucke V, Vaneechoutte M, Doerffel Y: Active Crohn's disease and ulcerative colitis can be specifically diagnosed and monitored based on the biostructure of the fecal flora. Inflamm Bowel Dis 2008;14:147–161.

72 Hafner S, Timmer A, Herfarth H, Rogler G, Scholmerich J, Schaffler A, Ehrenstein B, Jilg W, Ott C, Strauch UG, Obermeier F: The role of domestic hygiene in inflammatory bowel diseases: hepatitis A and worm infestations. Eur J Gastroenterol Hepatol 2008;20:561–566.

73 Summers RW, Elliott DE, Urban JF Jr, Thompson R, Weinstock JV: *Trichuris suis* therapy in Crohn's disease. Gut 2005;54:87–90.

74 Sonntag B, Stolze B, Heinecke A, Luegering A, Heidemann J, Lebiedz P, Rijcken E, Kiesel L, Domschke W, Kucharzik T, Maaser C: Preterm birth but not mode of delivery is associated with an increased risk of developing inflammatory bowel disease later in life. Inflamm Bowel Dis 2007;13:1385–1390.

75 Klement E, Cohen RV, Boxman J, Joseph A, Reif S: Breastfeeding and risk of inflammatory bowel disease: a systematic review with meta-analysis. Am J Clin Nutr 2004;80: 1342–1352.

76 Corrao G, Tragnone A, Caprilli R, Trallori G, Papi C, Andreoli A, Di Paolo M, Riegler G, Rigo GP, Ferrau O, Mansi C, Ingrosso M, Valpiani D: Risk of inflammatory bowel disease attributable to smoking, oral contraception and breastfeeding in Italy: a nationwide case-control study. Cooperative Investigators of the Italian Group for the Study of the Colon and the Rectum (GISC). Int J Epidemiol 1998;27:397–404.

77 Thompson NP, Montgomery SM, Pounder RE, Wakefield AJ: Is measles vaccination a risk factor for inflammatory bowel disease? Lancet 1995;345:1071–1074.

78 Ghosh S, Armitage E, Wilson D, Minor PD, Afzal MA: Detection of persistent measles virus infection in Crohn's disease: current status of experimental work. Gut 2001;48: 748–752.

79 Baron S, Turck D, Leplat C, Merle V, Gower-Rousseau C, Marti R, Yzet T, Lerebours E, Dupas JL, Debeugny S, Salomez JL, Cortot A, Colombel JF: Environmental risk factors in paediatric inflammatory bowel diseases: a population based case control study. Gut 2005;54:357–363.

80 Hampe J, Heymann K, Krawczak M, Schreiber S: Association of inflammatory bowel disease with indicators for childhood antigen and infection exposure. Int J Colorectal Dis 2003;18:413–417.

81 Klement E, Lysy J, Hoshen M, Avitan M, Goldin E, Israeli E: Childhood hygiene is associated with the risk for inflammatory bowel disease: a population-based study. Am J Gastroenterol 2008;103:1775–1782.

82 Gent AE, Hellier MD, Grace RH, Swarbrick ET, Coggon D: Inflammatory bowel disease and domestic hygiene in infancy. Lancet 1994;343:766–767.

83 Duggan AE, Usmani I, Neal KR, Logan RF: Appendicectomy, childhood hygiene, *Helicobacter pylori* status, and risk of inflammatory bowel disease: a case control study. Gut 1998;43:494–498.

84 Amre DK, Lambrette P, Law L, Krupoves A, Chotard V, Costea F, Grimard G, Israel D, Mack D, Seidman EG: Investigating the hygiene hypothesis as a risk factor in pediatric onset Crohn's disease: a case-control study. Am J Gastroenterol 2006;101:1005–1011.

85 Bernstein CN, Rawsthorne P, Cheang M, Blanchard JF: A population-based case control study of potential risk factors for IBD. Am J Gastroenterol 2006;101:993–1002.

86 Alexander T: An objective study of psychological factors in ulcerative colitis in children. Lancet 1965;85:22–24.

87 Maunder RG: Evidence that stress contributes to inflammatory bowel disease: evaluation, synthesis, and future directions. Inflamm Bowel Dis 2005;11:600–608.

88 Bitton A, Dobkin PL, Edwardes MD, Sewitch MJ, Meddings JB, Rawal S, Cohen A, Vermeire S, Dufresne L, Franchimont D, Wild GE: Predicting relapse in Crohn's disease: a biopsychosocial model. Gut 2008;57:1386–1392.

89 Vidal A, Gómez-Gil E, Sans M, Portella MJ, Salamero M, Piqué JM, Panés J: Life events and inflammatory bowel disease relapse: a prospective study of patients enrolled in remission. Am J Gastroenterol 2006;101:775–781.

90 Lerebours E, Gower-Rousseau C, Merle V, Brazier F, Debeugny S, Marti R, Salomez JL, Hellot MF, Dupas JL, Colombel JF, Cortot A, Benichou J: Stressful life events as a risk factor for inflammatory bowel disease onset: a population-based case-control study. Am J Gastroenterol 2007;102:122–131.

91 O'Sullivan M, O'Morain C: Nutrition in inflammatory bowel disease. Best Pract Res Clin Gastroenterol 2006;20:561–573.

92 Russel MGVM, Engels LG, Muris JW, Limonard CB, Volovics A, Brummer RJ, Stockbrugger RW: 'Modern life' in the epidemiology of inflammatory bowel disease: a case-control study with special emphasis on nutritional factors. Eur J Gastroenterol Hepatol 1998;10:243–249.

93 Akobeng AK, Thomas AG: Enteral nutrition for maintenance of remission in Crohn's disease. Cochrane Database Syst Rev 2007;18:CD005984.

94 Jowett SL, Seal CJ, Pearce MS, Phillips E, Gregory W, Barton JR, Welfare MR: Influence of dietary factors on the clinical course of ulcerative colitis: a prospective cohort study. Gut 2004;53:1479–1484.

95 Godet PG, May GR, Sutherland LR: Meta-analysis of the role of oral contraceptive agents in inflammatory bowel disease. Gut 1995;37:668–673.

96 Cornish JA, Tan E, Simillis C, Clark SK, Teare J, Tekkis PP: The risk of oral contraceptives in the etiology of inflammatory bowel disease: a meta-analysis. Am J Gastroenterol 2008;103:2394–2400.

97 Andersson RE, Olaison G, Tysk C, Ekbom A: Appendectomy and protection against ulcerative colitis. N Engl J Med 2001;344:808–814.

98 Koutroubakis IE, Vlachonikolis IG, Kouroumalis EA: Role of appendicitis and appendectomy in the pathogenesis of ulcerative colitis: a critical review. Inflamm Bowel Dis 2002;8:277–286.

99 Cosnes J, Carbonnel F, Beaugerie L, Blain A, Reijasse D, Gendre JP: Effects of appendicectomy on the course of ulcerative colitis. Gut 2002;51:803–807.

100 Cosnes J, Seksik P, Nion-Larmurier I, Beaugerie L, Gendre JP: Prior appendectomy and the phenotype and course of Crohn's disease. World J Gastroenterol 2006;12:1235–1242.

Insights from Epidemiology

Dig Dis 2009;27:226–235
DOI: 10.1159/000228554

Susceptibility Genes and Overall Pathogenesis of Inflammatory Bowel Disease: Where Do We Stand?

Claudio Fiocchi

Department of Pathobiology, Lerner Research Institute, and Department of Gastroenterology and Hepatology,
The Cleveland Clinic Foundation, Cleveland, Ohio, USA

Key Words

Inflammatory bowel disease · Crohn's disease · Ulcerative colitis

Abstract

The rapid accumulation of new knowledge on the genes, gene variations and genetic loci associated with both forms of inflammatory bowel disease (IBD), e.g. Crohn's disease (CD) and ulcerative colitis (UC), is shedding new light on the immunopathogenic mechanisms underlying these conditions. After the initial report of the association of *NOD2* mutations with ileal CD, a large number of additional genetic variants and loci has been found to be associated with both CD and UC, CD alone and, quite recently, UC-associated variants have also emerged. Much of this progress is due to the use of methods such as genome-wide associations (GWA) based on large numbers of reasonably well-characterized patient groups. Among several others, some of the most pathophysiologically relevant associations reported so far are with gene variants related to innate immunity, autophagy, apoptosis, Th1 and Th17 responses, T cell activation, and immunosuppression. Some of these associations have lent further support to previously construed disease mechanisms or disclosed brand new mechanisms, like in the case of the autophagy pathway. While this much progress is obviously welcome, it also brings new challenges. These include the fact that all the gene mutations uncovered so far only account for a minority of all IBD cases, the variable distribution of gene mutations among worldwide IBD populations, and the still unknown effects of gene-gene and gene-environment interactions. Nevertheless, there is no question that genetic information will be quickly utilized not only for a better understanding of IBD pathogenesis, but it will also soon be incorporated into the armamentarium of better diagnostic and therapeutic tools.

Copyright © 2009 S. Karger AG, Basel

Introduction

After half a century of continuous research the exact pathogenesis of inflammatory bowel disease (IBD) is still unclear, and one could rightfully ask the question of how long will it take to completely unravel its secrets [1]. One of the reasons explaining this disappointing state of affairs is that both forms of IBD, Crohn's disease (CD) and ulcerative colitis (UC), belong to the so-called group of 'complex diseases', indicating that numerous and diverse factors, conditions and mechanisms are reciprocally involved in highly complex biological networks underlying this class of disorders. Complex diseases affect a large portion of humanity and, although they are distinct and fall in many separate categories according to the organ or

Claudio Fiocchi, MD
Department of Pathobiology, Lerner Research Institute
Department of Gastroenterology and Hepatology, The Cleveland Clinic Foundation
Cleveland, Ohio 44195 (USA)
Tel. +1 216 445 0895, Fax +1 216 636 0104, E-Mail fiocchc@ccf.org

system affected, they often share common predisposing factors and analogous mechanisms of tissue damage. Among the former are a huge number of genes and genetic mutations, which often determine not only whether the disease will appear or not, but also whether it will be mild or severe, of short or long duration, and how well the patient will respond to therapy [2]. More and more this seems to be true for IBD, which is characterized by a vast and heterogeneous constellation of manifestations and different outcomes. This review will briefly appraise the various components of IBD pathogenesis, and then will attempt to elucidate how the major genetic variations currently associated with CD and UC might contribute to the mechanisms of gut inflammation.

Basic Components of IBD Pathogenesis

At present, the distinct components leading to CD and UC are fairly well defined, and there is general agreement that environmental, genetic, microbial and immune factors somehow interact closely with each other, the result of this interaction being a chronic inflammatory process that damages the gut and triggers symptoms [3–5]. The continuous increase in spreading of IBD worldwide leaves no doubts that environmental factors are at the root of the disease, but they alone cannot be blamed for directly causing gut inflammation [6]. Instead, it is far more likely that environmental factors, such as food, drugs, smoking, geography and social status, stress, and microbes in or outside the gut, act directly to skew the immune system towards pro-inflammatory responses, or do so indirectly by modulating genes that normally control the host's immune and intestinal homeostasis. The latter possibility appears increasingly viable and credible based on current developments and discoveries in the field in IBD genetics.

Genetics of IBD

All diseases are 'genetic', but the degree of contribution by any given gene or gene combination is extremely variable, and the expression of any disease is also highly dependent on the balance of genetic versus environmental influences [7]. Some autoimmune/chronic inflammatory conditions, such as psoriasis, are under strong genetic influence, while others, like multiple sclerosis, are at the other end of the spectrum, with weak genetic but strong environmental pressure. IBD is probably in the middle of the two extremes, with external and genetic factors both playing roughly equally important roles in disease pathogenesis.

Early investigation of IBD genetics focused on histocompatibility antigen (HLA) phenotypes, and reports of significantly increased or decreased HLA frequencies in UC and CD appeared in the literature [8]. About a decade later an association of HLA-DR2 with UC was reported in Japanese patients [9], followed by linkage analysis studies supporting an association between various HLAs and UC in European Caucasoid subjects [10]. At the same time, evidence of possible associations of immune genes with IBD started to emerge, such as an increased frequency of the allele 2 of the IL-1 receptor antagonist in patients with UC [11]. Although groundbreaking, these early studies were limited by the small number of subjects or families studied, a relative lack of patient homogeneity, and the intrinsic restrictions of a candidate gene approach. This situation has drastically changed with the realization that far larger and more homogenous populations need to be studied to obtain valid and interpretable results and with the advent of massive genome-wide association (GWA) screening approaches [12, 13]. When applied to IBD, these new methods wide opened the field of IBD genetics, and a large number of associations have so far been reported in CD and UC [14–18], as well as distinguishing genetic differences between these types of IBD [19, 20].

The First Gene: NOD2/CARD15

In 1996, a GWA on two consecutive and independent panels of families affected by CD identified a putative CD susceptibility locus on chromosome 16 [21], and 5 years later specific variations of the NOD2 gene on this chromosome were independently reported by two groups [22, 23]. These reports not only represented a milestone in IBD genetics, but also a lucky break. In fact, the product of the NOD2 (also named CARD15) gene, which officially belongs to a family of genes regulating apoptosis, is an intracellular sensor of bacterial products, including those from the commensal enteric flora which, at the same time of the gene discovery, was increasingly being scrutinized as the possible target of the abnormal immune response occurring in IBD patients and animal models of IBD [24]. This connection triggered a frantic search aiming at understanding the function of the NOD2-encoded receptor and the underlying effects relevant to IBD pathogenesis. The specific bacterial moiety recognized by NOD2 was

Table 1. Major IBD-associated genetic variations identified by genome-wide screens

Chromosome	Gene	Product function	CD	UC
1p31	*IL-23 receptor*	immune inflammatory response	+	+
5q33	*IL12b (p40)*	immune inflammatory response	+	+
9p24	*JAK2*	signaling	+	+
17q21	*STAT3*	transcription factor	+	+
18p11	*PTPN2*	T cell tyrosine phosphatase	+	–
9q32	*TNFS15*	immune inflammatory response	+	–
6q27	*CCR6*	chemokine receptor	+	–
3p21	*MST1*	macrophage chemotaxis	+	–
2q37	*ATG16L1*	autophagosome pathway	+	–
5q33	*IRGM*	autophagosome pathway	+	–
16q12	*NOD2/CARD15*	bacterial recognition	+	–
20q13	*TNFRSF6B*	inflammatory response, apoptosis	+	+
21q22	*PSMG1*	proteasome-related protein	+	+
12q12	*MUC19*	epithelial integrity	–	+
1q32	*IL-10*	immune inflammatory response	–	+

readily identified as muramyl dipeptide (MDP), a peptidoglycan component of the bacterial cell wall [25, 26]. Nevertheless, the consequences of recognizing MDP by products of a variant NOD2 receptor are still far from clear. In humans, CD-associated *NOD2* variants have been reported to cause a decreased pro-inflammatory cytokine response to lipopolysaccharide (LPS) and peptidoglycan by monocytes and dendritic cells [27–29], beside being clinically associated with the ileal and fibrostenosing phenotype of CD [30]. This paradoxical response immediately raised the question of how a reduced production of pro-inflammatory mediators could cause gut inflammation. A preliminary hypothesis has been put forward that perhaps gut inflammation represents an overzealous adaptive immune response trying to compensate a defective antibacterial innate immune response, but this is far from proven yet. In animal models lacking or having a defective *NOD2* gene, the situation is even less clear and a controversy is still raging on whether defective *NOD2* function represents a loss or gain of function [31].

The existing confusion on the consequences and outcome of *NOD2* defects in CD is actually very indicative of the difficulties awaiting IBD investigators aiming at understanding how any given gene defect leads to IBD. Considering the already substantial number of IBD genetic variants presently recorded, and the many more likely to be uncovered, this task appears overwhelming.

Innate Immunity IBD Candidate Genes

The increasingly appreciated role of the intestinal flora as a target of abnormal immunity in IBD has led to an expanded investigation of its composition, the ways that enteric bacteria communicate with the gut, the physiological effects of this interaction, and the possible pathophysiological consequences of when the crosstalk between gut microbiota and the host goes awry [32–35]. Microorganisms are recognized by pattern recognition receptors abundantly distributed on or inside cells of the innate immune system, particularly epithelial cells and cells of monocytic/macrophage lineage, which carry Toll-like receptors (TLR) and NOD-like receptors (NLR) [36]. In addition, a large number of other receptors, surface, signaling and secreted molecules also contribute to innate immunity [37, 38], with the ultimate goal of maintaining an effective but yet controlled immune response while avoiding inflammation [39]. Therefore, given its crucial role, it is not surprising that possible genetic defects in many innate immunity genes have been actively sought after, and several have been reported and claimed to be of pathogenic relevance (table 1) [16].

Evidence that innate immunity may be defective in IBD, particularly CD, has emerged [40], while potentially pathogenic bacteria continue to be proposed as specific etiological agents, like adhesive-invasive *E. coli* in ileal CD and *Mycobacterium paratuberculosis* [41, 42]. Because bacteria do utilize TLRs and NLRs to communicate with the host, it is reasonable to assume that genetic defects of these receptors may lead to abnormal recognition of microbial antigens and secondarily inflammation. For instance, *M. paratuberculosis* is recognized by TLR2, TLR4 and NOD2 [43], and gene mutations in *TLR2* and *TLR4* have been found to be linked to increased susceptibility to this microbe in cattle [44], raising the theoretical possibility that humans with mutations in the same *TLR* genes may also be more prone to acquire or abnormally respond to *M. paratuberculosis* infection. Genetic variants of *TLR4* have also been detected in CD patients [45], providing additional basis for a defective function of this key innate immune pathway in this condition. Defensins, natural antimicrobial peptides produced by Paneth cells, are molecules also involved in innate immunity, and the hypothesis has been put forward that Crohn's disease is α-defensin deficiency syndrome [46]. In fact, *NOD2* mutations are seemingly associated with diminished mucosal α-defensin expression in CD [47], and in ileal CD there is a selective reduction of α-defensin production only in those patients carrying the SNP10 mutation [48]. If so, mutations in the *HD-5*, *HD-6* and *HBD-2* genes on chromosome 8p23 could then be pathogenetically relevant. Along these lines, an extensive list of IBD candidate genes involved in innate immunity now waits to be investigated in greater detail (table 2).

Autophagy Genes

Autophagy is a cellular 'cleanup' and nutrient stress (starvation) response system with a variety of homeostatic and disease-related effects. As a result of GWA, genetic variants in two autophagy genes, the *ATG16L1* and *IRGM* genes, have been recently identified and linked to CD [49–51]. Mutations of *ATG16L1* gene in humans with CD or in mice leads to fewer granules or diffuse granular contents in Paneth cells, while loss of autophagy in macrophages from *ATGL16L1*-mutant mice results in aberrant IL-1β production [52]. Both findings potentially point to an altered interaction with the luminal flora and/or an exaggerated pro-inflammatory response. Other implications may also exist for defective autophagy in CD. *IRGM* induces autophagy to eliminate intracellular mycobacteria, and this could theoretically cause a putative *M. paratuberculosis* agent to persist in CD mucosa and cause inflammation [53]; moreover, autophagy in the thymic epithelium is essential to shape the T cell repertoire and establishment of tolerance, and defective autophagy early in life could lead to reactivity towards 'tissue-specific' self antigens [54]. Finally, autophagy and apoptosis are closely related processes [55], and they may mutually inhibit each other and eventually result in defective apoptosis, an abnormality well documented in CD [56].

Table 2. Innate immunity IBD candidate genes

Chromosome	Gene	Chromosome	Gene
7q22	*MUC3A*	11p15	*SIGIRR*
7q21	*MDR1*	16p13	*SOCS1*
3q13	*PXR/NR1I2*	11p15	*TOLLIP*
10q22	*DLG5*	16p13	*MEFV*
5q31	*OCTN1/2*	7p14	*NOD1/CARD4*
19p13	*Myosin IX B*	16q12	*NOD2/CARD15*
4q31	*TLR2*	19p13	*GRIM19*
4q35	*TLR3*	5q12	*Erbin*
9q33	*TLR4*	3p25	*TAK1/NR2C2*
1q42	*TLR5*	9q23	*HBD-5, -6*
4p14	*TLR6*	8q23	*HBD-2*
3p21	*TLR9*		

Apoptosis-Related Genes

In addition to a potential defect in apoptosis related to autophagy, genetic variations have been reported in some genes that directly influence apoptosis. GWA associations have revealed polymorphisms in the *TNFSF15* and *TNFRSF6B* genes, which encode for a TNF-like factor (TL1A) and a TNF decoy receptor (DC3), respectively, the first having the ability to induce apoptosis and the second the ability to prevent apoptosis [57, 58]. Intriguingly, TNFSF15/TL1A is one of the ligands for TNFRSF6B/DC3, perhaps creating a dual defect in the regulation of apoptosis. It remains to be established whether these two specific genetic variations are actually related to the defective apoptosis of mucosal T cells in CD [59, 60], but they certainly create a reasonable basis for such scenario.

Th1 and Th17 Response-Related Genes

Gene variants related to specific pathways of immune or inflammatory responses have also been reported in IBD. These genes include *IL-23R* and *IL12b*, which respectively encode for the IL-23 receptor (IL-23R) and the p40 (IL-12b) subunit belonging to the IL-12 family of cytokines [61, 62], and represent two of the most convincingly replicated gene associations in both CD and UC.

The biological relevance of these two gene products is very high because IL-23R and IL12b are essential for the development of T helper cells responses along the Th1 and Th17 pathways, whose end products are IFN-γ and IL-17, respectively [63–65]. IFN-γ and IL-17 are typically elevated in IBD, IFN-γ more so in CD while IL-17 production is elevated in both CD and UC [66, 67]. At the moment it is not known how the multiple variants of *IL-23R* and *IL12b* may impact on the excessive Th1 and Th17 responses seen in IBD, and this is an area where intense investigation is currently under way [68]. Also of interest is the fact that *IL-23R* mutations are found in other autoimmune/chronic inflammatory conditions including ankylosing spondylitis, multiple sclerosis and autoimmune thyroid disease [69], suggesting that mutations in the IL-12 family of cytokine genes may be dominant in several immune-mediated disorders with a common epidemiological background and shared inflammatory pathways of tissue injury.

T Cell Activation-Related Genes

Related to Th1 and Th17 responses are the JAK2 signaling molecule and the STAT3 transcription factor, which are involved in multiple activation pathways in a variety of cell types. Interestingly, variations in the *JAK2* and *STAT3* genes have been described and replicated in CD, UC, or both [70–72], another observation indicative of the possibility that major pathways of immune cell activation are genetically defective in IBD. Alternatively, a combination of genetic defects in cell activation, differentiation, regulation and effector function may be needed for full-blown clinical manifestations in IBD, or to determine the IBD subtype, the degree of disease severity, or response to therapy.

Immunosuppression-Related Genes

On the opposite side of immune activation genes are those whose products are proteins that directly suppress immunity by deactivating stimulatory signaling pathways or indirectly through the secretion of soluble immunosuppressive molecules. Variants in this class of immunosuppressive genes have also been detected by GWA in IBD patients, including the *PTPN2* and the *IL-10* genes [62, 71, 73]. PTPN2 is a tyrosine phosphatase expressed abundantly in T cells and its action is critical in counterbalancing the signals derived from the phos-

phorylation of several signaling molecules downstream of the T cell receptor activation pathway; IL-10 is a dominant immunosuppressive cytokine that counteracts the activation signals derived from a variety of immunostimulatory cytokines such as IL-2, IL-7, IL-15 and many others. Considering their foremost inhibitory function, it is easy to see how deficiencies in PTPN2 or IL-10 may lead to an overactive immune response and inflammation.

Genetic Associations in CD and UC: Commonalities and Dissimilarities

An aspect that is very revealing of the burgeoning fascination with IBD genetics and the fast pace with which this type of research is taking place is the quickness with which CD and UC are becoming gradually separated at the genetic and genomic levels. Initially, most reports were focused on CD due to its generally stronger genetic overtone, as exemplified by the early detection of *NOD2* mutations. Then, as the use of GWA was expanded to both CD and UC, a greater number of loci was found to be associated with CD than UC, but recently a series of studies have appeared in the literature claiming the identification of genetic loci or variants specifically associated with UC. Susceptibility loci for UC have been recently identified at the *ECM1* locus and on chromosomes 1p36 and 12q15 [74, 75], as well as variants for the *IL-10* and *IL-10R* genes [73, 76]. The latter two are particularly interesting because their products are involved in mediation of immunosuppressive functions. Overall, it seems clear that the study of IBD genetics will in the near future define genes or groups of genes that are selectively associated with either CD or UC, or both [72].

Limitations and Challenges of Current IBD Genetic Studies

While precipitous progress is occurring in the field of IBD genetics, the rapid accumulation of abundant but purely observational data is not accompanied by an equal rapid progress in understanding the biology of the newly discovered genes, variants and loci.

While it is possible to speculate and start investigating the prospective implications of the several gene variants linked to IBD, the sheer number of these associations is in itself an enormous obstacle to surmount. More than 30 distinct susceptibility loci have been defined for CD alone

Table 3. IBD candidate genes of uncertain significance

Chromosome	Gene	Name, function
5p13	PTGER4	prostaglandin E receptor 4 (G-protein-coupled receptor family member)
10q21	ZNF365	Zinc finger protein 365
10q24	NKX2-3	NK2 transcription factor related (NKX transcription family member)
1q22	ITLN1	intelectin 1 (galactofuranose binding)
6p22	CDKAL1	CDK5 regulatory subunit-associated protein 1-like 1
12q12	LRRK2	leucine-rich repeat kinase 2 (leucine-rich repeat kinase family member)
17q12	ORMDL5	ORM1-like 3 (S. cerevisiae)
2p23	GCK3	glucokinase (hexokinase 4) regulator
2p16	PUS10	pseudouridylate synthase 10
6p25	LYRM4	LYR motif containing 4
6p25	SLC22A23	solute carrier family 22, member 23 (transmembrane uniporter, symporter, antiporter family member for organic ions)
Plasmid Ip28-1	BafACA1_F30	(no official name/Borrelia afzelii ACA-1 strain)

[70], and at present around 40 IBD-associated genes and loci have been described. Although many of them, at least conceptually, make some sense based on current knowledge of IBD pathogenesis, it will take considerable time and resources to work out how each variation may impact on triggering or maintaining the disease. Additionally, there is a substantial number of other IBD candidate genes detected by GWA that do not readily make biological sense, and several are just listed in various gene databases without any information on their possible biological function (table 3).

Another important issue is the distribution and frequency of IBD genes in the population at large. While NOD2/CARD15 mutations appear to be equally distributed among patients with white, black and Hispanic background [77], the same mutations are not associated with CD patients in Japan or China [78, 79]. These observations are important because they indicate that other genes may predispose to IBD in various populations worldwide, and the mechanisms underlying gut inflammation may be distinct from one ethnic group to another.

One more challenge in interpreting the multiple IBD gene association comes from the complex interactions that normally occur among genes, very much like those that occur among cells, cytokines and signaling molecules. The phenomenon of gene-gene interaction, also called epistasis, can be investigated by using a variety of mathematical and statistical models, but these in turn have their own drawbacks: first, statistical analyses test hypotheses regarding quantities, not biological responses; second, statistical interactions do not imply biological interactions; third, the interactions of 2 (or more) genes cannot be inferred from the individual action of each gene [80]. For instance, one is spontaneously compelled to assume that the risk of IBD is further increased when a patient harbors two unrelated IBD genetic variations. This instinctive but naive assumption is based on the independent action of each gene per se, but one cannot necessarily expect the same effect when the two genes interact in vivo in the presence of other modifying genes and innumerous other factors derived from both the endogenous and exogenous environment [81].

Thus, at least for the time being, an answer to the investigation of the biological significance of the numerous IBD genetic variations must rely on the systematic investigation of each variation by traditional in vitro testing of relevant cells derived from patients carrying the mutation of interest, complemented by in vivo studies with animals deficient in the specific gene of interest (knock out), animals overexpressing the gene (transgenic), and animals where the human variant has been introduced (knock in). Considering the already sizeable number of genes of potential interest to IBD, the feasibility of such demanding approach becomes questionable. The Human Genome Project, which looks into global responses, may alleviate some the investigational burden, but we also have to learn how to discover and integrate global networks among the environmental, genetic, microbial and immune components of IBD pathogenesis, each one of them influencing the action of the others (fig. 1).

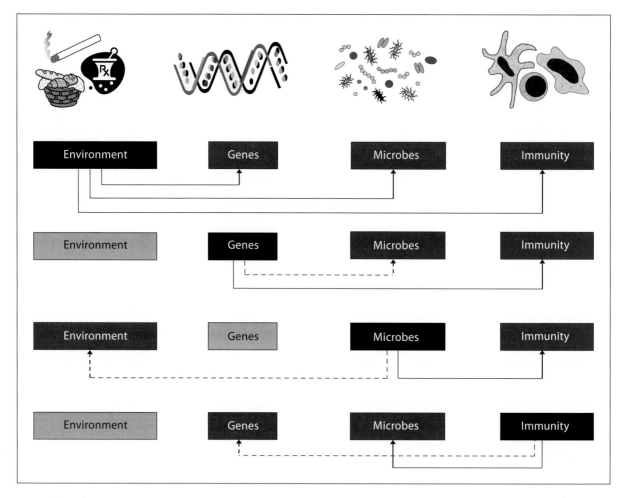

Fig. 1. Global networks among components of IBD pathogenesis.

Conclusions and Therapeutic Implications

Taking into consideration the large amount of new data on IBD genetics and the massive pre-existing information on IBD pathogenesis, both of which are constantly growing, how can we manage the IBD information overload? Obviously, novel and more effective approaches and systems are needed. Genomic analyses of differentially expressed genes in normal, CD and UC intestine will help [82, 83], particularly when integrated with the results of GWA studies. This combination of molecular classification and gene expression prognostic signatures may predict outcome and pave the way to improved therapeutic strategies, as it is currently postulated for breast

cancer [84]. Selection of therapeutic targets must also be improved by creating detailed genomic profiles in well-defined experimental systems to allow the identification of dominant genes and their regulatory elements by bioinformatics analysis, such as genes encoding central transcription factors. Pharmacogenomic studies must also be actively implemented in IBD, so that accurate drug targets, anticipated side effects, and optimal response to medications can be reliably predicted in selected groups of patients carrying precise IBD genetic patterns [85]. As the future unfolds, new solutions will certainly emerge.

The integration of knowledge derived from genetic and genomic analyses still seems out of reach to the clinician and patient alike, but in reality the incorporation of this new knowledge into clinical practice is much closer than it appears to be. If one considers that only a decade ago the intended use of biologicals was still completely novel and under a cloud of ignorance and suspicion, its current routine use and the desire for newer, better and more powerful biologicals is nothing short of remarkable, and represents a strong testimonial of how quickly innovation coming from the bench gets absorbed into day-to-day clinical practice. The very same phenomenon will inevitably happen with information coming from genetic and genomic analyses, which is already transforming our current thinking of IBD pathogenesis. At the end of the 19th century Sir William Osler stated that 'if were not for the great variability among individuals, medicine might as well be a science and not an art'. Today, at the beginning of the 21st century, it is perhaps time to time to modify this statement and propose that 'if were not for the great variability among genes, medicine might as well be an art and not a science'.

Disclosure Statement

The author declares that no financial or other conflict of interest exists in relation to the content of the article.

References

1 Editorial: Crohn's disease. Lancet 1976;ii: 1284–1285.
2 Lander ES, Schork NJ: Genetic dissection of complex traits. Science 1994;265:2037–2048.
3 Podolsky DK: Inflammatory bowel disease. N Engl J Med 2002;347:417–429.
4 Xavier RJ, Podolsky D: Unraveling the pathogenesis of inflammatory bowel disease. Nature 2007;448:427–434.
5 Scaldaferri F, Fiocchi C: Inflammatory bowel disease: progress and current concepts of etiopathogenesis. J Dig Dis 2007;8:171–178.
6 Danese S, Sans M, Fiocchi C: Inflammatory bowel disease: the role of environmental factors. Autoimmun Rev 2004;3:390–400.
7 Chakravarti A, Little P: Nature, nurture and human disease. Nature 2003;421:412–414.
8 Asquith P, Stokes PL, Mackintosh P, Holmes GKT, Cooke WT: Histocompatibility antigens in patients with inflammatory bowel disease. Lancet 1974;i:113–115.
9 Asakura H, Tsuchiya M, Aiso S, Watanabe M, Kokayashi K, Hibi T, Ando K, Takata H, Sekiguchi S: Association of the human lymphocyte-DR2 antigen with Japanese ulcerative colitis. Gastroenterology 1982;82:413–418.
10 Satsangi J, Welsh KI, Bunce M, Julier C, Farrant JM, Bell JI, Jewell DP: Contribution of genes of the major histocompatibility complex to susceptibility and disease phenotype in inflammatory bowel disease. Lancet 1996; 347:1212–1217.
11 Tountas NA, Casini-Raggi V, Yang H, Di Giovane FS, Vecchi M, Kam L, Melani L, Pizarro TT, Rotter JI, Cominelli F: Functional and ethnic association of allele 2 of the interleukin-1 receptor antagonist gene in ulcerative colitis. Gastroenterology 1999;117: 806–813.

12 Cardon LR: Delivering new disease genes. Science 2006;314:1403–1405.
13 Donnelly P: Progress and challenges in genome-wide association studies in humans. Nature 2008;456:728–731.
14 Cho JH, Weaver CT: The genetics of inflammatory bowel disease. Gastroenterology 2007;133:1327–1339.
15 Cho JH: The genetics and immunopathogenesis of inflammatory bowel disease. Nat Rev 2008;8:458–466.
16 Van Limbergen J, Russell RK, Nimmo ER, Ho G-T, Arnott ID, Wilson DC, Satsangi J: Genetics of the innate immune response in inflammatory bowel disease. Inflamm Bowel Dis 2007;13:338–355.
17 Duerr RH: Genome-wide association studies herald a new era of rapid discoveries in inflammatory bowel disease research. Gastroenterology 2007;132:2045–2062.
18 Massey D, Parkes M: Common pathways in Crohn's disease and other inflammatory diseases revealed by genomics. Gut 2007;56: 1489–1492.
19 Dubois PC, van Heel DA: New susceptibility genes for ulcerative colitis. Nat Genet 2008; 6:686–688.
20 Brant SR: Exposed: the genetic underpinnings of ulcerative colitis relative to Crohn's disease. Gastroenterology 2009;136:396–399.
21 Hugot JP, Laurent-Puig P, Gower-Rousseau C, Olson JM, Lee JC, Beaugerie L, Naom I, Dupas JL, Van Gossum A, Orholm M, Bonatti-Pellie C, Weissenbach J, Methew CG, Lennard-Jones JE, Cortot A, Colombel JF, Thomas G: Mapping of a susceptibility locus for Crohn's disease on chromosome 16. Nature 1996;379:821–823.

22 Hugot JP, Chamaiilard M, Zouali H, Lesage S, Cezard JP, Belaiche J, Almer S, Tysk C, O'Morain CA, Gassull M, Binder V, Finkel Y, Cortot A, Modigliani R, Laurent-Puig P, Gower-Rousseau C, Macry J, Colombel JF, Sahbatou M, Thomas G: Association of NOD2 leucine-rich repeat variants with susceptibility to Crohn's disease. Nature 2001;411:599–603.
23 Ogura Y, Inohara N, Benito A, Chen FF, Yamaoka S, Nunez G: Nod2, a Nod1-Apaf-1 family member that is restricted to monocytes and activates NF-κB. J Biol Chem 2001; 276:4812–4818.
24 Sartor RB: Intestinal microflora in human and experimental inflammatory bowel disease. Curr Opin Gastroenterol 2001;4:324–330.
25 Girardin SE, Boneca IG, Viala J, Chamaillard M, Labigne A, Thomas G, Philpott DJ, Sansonetti PJ: Nod2 is a general sensor of peptidoglycan through muramyl dipeptide (MDP) detection. J Biol Chem 2003;278: 8869–8872.
26 Inohara N, Ogura Y, Fontalba A, Gutierrez O, Pons F, Crespo J, Fukase K, Inamurai S, Kusumoto S, Hashimoto M, Foster SJ, Moran AP, Fernandez-Luna JL, Nunez G: Host recognition of bacterial muramyl dipeptide mediated through NOD2. J Biol Chem 2003; 278:5509–5512.
27 Bonen DK, Ogura Y, Nicolae DL, Inohara N, Saab L, Tanabe T, Chen FF, Foster SJ, Duerr RH, Brant SR, Cho JH, Nunez G: Crohn's disease-associated NOD2 variants share a signaling defect in response to lipopolysaccharide and peptidoglycan. Gastroenterology 2003; 124:140–146.
28 Li J, Moran T, Swanson E, Julian C, Harris J, Bonen DK, Hedi M, Nicolae DL, Abraham C, Cho JH: Regulation of IL-8 and IL-1β expression in Crohn's disease associated with NOD2/CARD15 mutations. Hum Mol Genet 2004;13:1715–1725.

29 Kramer M, Netea MG, de Jong DJ, Kullberg BJ, Adema GJ: Impaired dendritic cell function in Crohn's disease pateints with NOD2 3020insC mutation. J Leukoc Biol 2006;79: 860–866.

30 Abreu MT, Taylor KD, Ling YC, Hang T, Gaiennie J, Landers CJ, Vasiliauskas EA, Kam LY, Rojany M, Papadakis KA, Rotter JI, Targan SR, Yang H: Mutations in NOD2 are associated with fibrostenosing disease in patients with Crohn's disease. Gastroenterology 2002;123:679–688.

31 Eckmann L, Karin M: NOD2 and Crohn's disease: loss or gain of function? Immunity 2005;22:661–667.

32 Eckburg PB, Bik EM, Bernstein CN, Purdom E, Dethlefsen L, Sargent M, Gill SR, Nelson KE, Relman DA: Diversity of the human intestinal microbial flora. Science 2005;308: 1635–1638.

33 Turnbaugh PJ, Ley RE, Hamady M, Fraser-Liggett CM, Knoight R, Gordon JI: The human microbiome project. Nature 2007;449: 804–810.

34 Sartor RB: Microbial influences in inflammatory bowel disease. Gastroenterology 2008;134:577–594.

35 Neish AS: Microbes in gastrointestinal health and disease. Gastroenterology 2009; 136:65–80.

36 Medzhitov R: Recognition of microorganisms and activation of the immune response. Nature 2007;449:819–826.

37 Ouellette AJ: Paneth cells and innate immunity in the crypt microenvironment. Gastroenterology 1997;113:1779–1784.

38 Creagh EM, O'Neill LAJ: TLRs, NLRs and RLRs: a trinity of pathogen sensors that cooperate in innate immunity. Trends Immunol 2006;27:352–357.

39 Barton GM: A calculated response: control of inflammation by the innate immune system. J Clin Invest 2008;118:413–420.

40 Marks DJB, Hardbord MWN, MacAllister R, Rahman F, Young J, Al-Lazikani B, Lees W, Novelli M, Bloom S, Segal AW: Defective acute inflammation in Crohn's disease: a clinical investigation. Lancet 2006;367:668–678.

41 Darfeuille-Michaud A, Boudeau J, Bulois P, Neut C, Glasser AL, Barnich N, Bringer MA, Swidsinski A, Beaugerie L, Colombel JF: High prevalence of adherent-invasive *Escherichia coli* associated with ileal mucosa in Crohn's disease. Gastroenterology 2004; 127:412–421.

42 Prantera C: Mycobacteria and Crohn's disease: the endless story. Dig Liver Dis 2007;39: 452–454.

43 Ferwerda G, Kullberg BJ, de Jong DJ, Girardin SE, Langenberg DML, van Crevel R, Ottehoff THM, Van der Meer JWM, Netea MG: *Mycobacterium paratuberculosis* is recognized by Toll-like receptors and NOD2. J Leukoc Biol 2007;82:1011–1018.

44 Mucha R, Bhide MR, Chakurkar EB, Novak M, Mikula I: Toll-like receptors TLR1, TLR2 and TLR4 gene mutations and natural resistance to *Mycobacterium avium* subsp. *paratuberculosis* infection in cattle. Vet Immunol Immunopathol 2009;128:381–388.

45 De Jager PL, Franchimont D, Waliszewska A, et al: The role of the Toll receptor pathway in susceptibility to inflammatory bowel disease. Genes Immun 2007;8:387–397.

46 Fellermann K, Wehkamp J, Herrlinger KR, Stange EF: Crohn's disease: a defensin deficiency syndrome? Eur J Gastroenterol Hepatol 2003;15:627–634.

47 Wehkamp J, Harder J, Weichenthal M, Schwab M, Schaffeler E, Schlee M, Herrlinger KR, Stallmach A, Noack F, Fritz P, Schroder JM, Bevins CL, Fellermann K, Stange EF: NOD2(CARD15) mutations in Crohn's disease are associated with diminished mucosal α-defensin expression. Gut 2004;53:1658–1664.

48 Wehkamp J, Salzman NH, Porter E, Nuding S, Weichental M, Petras RE, Shen B, Schaffeler E, Schwab M, Linzmeier R, Feathers RW, Chu H, Lima H, Fellermann K, Ganz T, Stange EF, Bevins CL: Reduced Paneth cell α-defensins in ileal Crohn's disease. Proc Natl Acad Sci USA 2005;102:18129–18134.

49 Hampe H, Franke A, Rosenstiel P, et al: A genome-wide association scan of nonsynonymous SNPs identifies a susceptibility variant for Crohn disease in ATG16L1. Nat Genet 2007;39:207–211.

50 Rioux JD, Xavier RJ, Taylor KD, et al: Genome-wide association study identifies new susceptibility loci for Crohn disease and implicates autophagy in disease pathogenesis. Nat Genet 2007;39:596–604.

51 Parkes M, Barrett JC, Prescott NJ, et al: Sequence variants in the autophagy gene IRGM and multiple other replicating loci contribute to Crohn's disease susceptibility. Nat Genet 2007;39:830–832.

52 Yano T, Kurata S: An unexpected twist for autophagy in Crohn's disease. Nat Immunol 2009;10:134–136.

53 Singh SB, Davis AS, Taylor GA, Deretic V: Human IRGM induces autophagy to eliminate intracellular mycobacteria. Science 2006;313:1438–1441.

54 Nedjic J, Aichinger A, Emmerich J, Mizushima N, Klein L: Autophagy in thymic epithelium shapes the T-cell repertoire and is essential for tolerance. Nature 2008;455: 396–401.

55 Maiuri MC, Zalxkvar E, Kimchi A, Kroemer G: Self-eating and self-killing: crosstalk between autophagy and apoptosis. Nat Rev Mol Cell Biol 2007;8:741–752.

56 Sturm A, Fiocchi C: Life and death in the gut: more killing, less Crohn's. Gut 2002;50:148–149.

57 Yamazaki K, McGovern D, Ragoussis J: Single nucleotide polymorphisms in TNFSF15 confer susceptibility to Crohn's disease. Hum Mol Genet 2007;14:3499–3506.

58 Kugathasan S, Baldassano RN, Bradfield JP, et al: Loci on 20q13 and 21q22 are associated with pediatric-onset inflammatory bowel disease. Nat Genet 2008;40:1211–1215.

59 Boirivant M, Marini M, Di Felice G, Pronio AM, Montesani C, Tersigni R, Strober W: Lamina propria T cells in Crohn's disease and other gastrointestinal inflammation show defective CD2 pathway-induced apoptosis. Gastroenterology 1999;116:557–565.

60 Ina K, Itoh J, Fukushima K, et al: Resistance of Crohn's disease T-cells to multiple apoptotic stimuli is associated with a Bcl-2/Bax mucosal imbalance. J Immunol 1999;163: 1081–1090.

61 Duerr RH, Taylor KD, Brant SR, et al: A genome-wide association study identifies IL23R as an inflammatory bowel disease gene. Science 2006;314:1461–1463.

62 Wellcome Trust Case Control Consortium: Genome-wide association study of 14,000 cases of seven common diseases and 3,000 shared controls. Nature 2007;447:661–673.

63 Brombacher F, Kastelein RA, Alber G: Novel IL-12 family members shed light on the orchestration of Th1 responses. Trends Immunol 2003;24:207–212.

64 Iwakura Y, Ishigame H: The IL-23/IL-17 axis in inflammation. J Clin Invest 2006;116: 1218–1222.

65 McKenzie BS, Kastelein RA, Cua DJ: Understanding the IL-23/IL-17 immune pathway. Trends Immunol 2006;27:17–23.

66 Monteleone G, MacDonald TT, Wathen NC, Pallone F, Pender SLF: Enhancing lamina propria Th1 cell responses with interleukin 12 produces severe tissue injury. Gastroenterology 1999;117:1069–1077.

67 Fujino S, Andoh A, Bamba S, Ogawa A, Hata K, Araki Y, Fujiyama Y: Increased expression of interleukin 17 in inflammatory bowel disease. Gut 2003;52:65–70.

68 Abraham C, Cho JH: IL-23 and autoimmunity: new insights into the pathogenesis of inflammatory bowel disease. Annu Rev Med 2008, Epub ahead of print.

69 Wellcome Trust Case Control Consortium, Australo-Anglo-American Spondylitis Consortium: Association scan of 14,500 nonsynonymous SNPs in four diseases identifies autoimmune variants. Nat Genet 2007;39: 1329–1337.

70 Barrett JC, Hansoul S, Nicolae DL, et al: Genome-wide association defines more than 30 distinct susceptibility loci for Crohn's disease. Nat Genet 2008;40:955–962.

71 Franke A, Balschun T, Karlsen TH, et al: Replication of signals from recent studies of Crohn's disease identifies previously unknown disease loci for ulcerative colitis. Nat Genet 2008;40:713–715.

72 Anderson CA, Massey DCO, Barrett JC, et al: Investigation of Crohn's disease risk loci in ulcerative colitis further defines their molecular relationship. Gastroenterology 2009; 136:523–529.

73 Franke A, Balschun T, Karlsen TH, et al: Sequence variants in IL10, ARPC2 and multiple other loci contribute to ulcerative colitis susceptibility. Nat Genet 2008;40:1319–1323.

74 Fisher SA, Tremelling M, Anderson CA, et al: Genetic determinants of ulcerative colitis include the ECM1 locus and five loci implicated in Crohn's disease. Nat Genet 2008;40:710–712.

75 Silverberg MS, Cho JH, Rioux JD, et al: Ulcerative colitis-risk loci on chromosome 1p36 and 12q15 found by genome-wide association study. Nat Genet 2009;41:216–220.

76 Grundtner P, Gruber S, Murray SS, Vermeire S, Rutgeerts P, Decker T, Lakatos PL, Gasche C: The IL-10R1 S138G loss-of-function allele and ulcerative colitis. Genes Immun 2009;10:84–92.

77 Kugathasan S, Loizides A, Babusukumar U, McGuire E, Wang T, Hooper P, Nebel J, Kofman G, Noel R, Rudolph CD, Tolia V: Comparative phenotypic and CARD15 mutational analysis among African American, Hispanic, and white children with Crohn's disease. Inflamm Bowel Dis 2005;11:631–638.

78 Inoue N, Tamura K, Kinouchi Y, Fukuda Y, Ogura Y, Inohara N, Nuñez G, Kishi Y, Koike Y, Shimosegawa T, Shimoyama T, Hibi T: Lack of common NOD2 variants in Japanese patients with Crohn's disease. Gastroenterology 2002;123:86–91.

79 Leong RWL, Lau JY, Sung JYJ: The epidemiology and phenotype of Crohn's disease in the Chinese population. Inflamm Bowel Dis 2004;10:646–651.

80 Cordell HJ, Clayton DG: Genetic association studies. Lancet 2005;366:1121–1131.

81 Achkar JP, Fiocchi C: Gene-gene interactions in inflammatory bowel disease: biological and clinical implications. Am J Gastroenterol 2009, in press.

82 Lawrance IC, Fiocchi C, Chakravarti S: Ulcerative colitis and Crohn's disease: distinctive gene expression profiles and novel susceptibility candidate genes. Hum Mol Genet 2001;10:445–456.

83 Wu F, Chakravarti S: Differential expression of inflammatory and fibrogenic genes and their regulation by NF-κB inhibition in a mouse model of chronic colitis. J Immunol 2007;179:6988–7000.

84 Sotiriou C, Pusztai L: Molecular origins of cancer: gene-expression signatures n breast cancer. N Engl J Med 2009;360:790–800.

85 Evans WE, McLeod HL: Pharmacogenomics: drug disposition, drug targets, and side effects. N Engl J Med 2003;248:538–549.

Dig Dis 2009;27:236–239
DOI: 10.1159/000228555

Genetic Determinants of Pediatric Inflammatory Bowel Disease: Is Age of Onset Genetically Determined?

Rebecca Scherr[a]   Jonah Essers[b]   Hakon Hakonarson[c]   Subra Kugathasan[a]

[a]Department of Pediatrics, Emory University School of Medicine and Children's Health Care of Atlanta, Atlanta, Ga.,
[b]Division of Gastroenterology, Children's Hospital Boston, Boston, Mass., and [c]Center for Applied Genomics and
Division of Human Genetics, Department of Pediatrics, The Children's Hospital of Philadelphia, Philadelphia, Pa., USA

Key Words

Inflammatory bowel disease · Crohn's disease · Genome-wide association studies

0Abstract

Inflammatory bowel disease (IBD) is thought to develop as a result of dysregulation of the immune response to normal gut flora in a genetically susceptible host. Approximately 25% of incident cases of IBD occur during childhood and the rest occur throughout adulthood, peaking in the second and third decades of life. What determines the age of onset remains unexplained currently. Studying early-onset presentation of complex diseases such as IBD is appealing to geneticists and scientists alike because of the expectation that these efforts will increase the probability of finding novel risk variants. Genome-wide association studies (GWAS) have yielded more susceptible loci in IBD than in any other complex common disease studied. Using 35 confirmed Crohn's disease risk alleles from adult studies, a recent pediatric replication study detected no significant association between risk score and age of onset through age 30, indicating age of onset does not have any impact on increased disease development in IBD. The first GWAS study using an exclusively pediatric IBD cohort found 2 novel risk variants that were not previously reported in predominately adult GWAS studies. However, during the data-mining of adult GWAS, these 2 novel loci (TNFRSF6 and PSMG1) were found with nominal significance suggesting that these risk loci are not restricted to early-onset CD cases. These analyses illustrate that the genetic effects of established CD risk variants is similar in early- and late-onset CD. However, the quest to find early-onset IBD risk variants is continuing. As such, GWAS studies involving large pediatric-onset CD cohorts and early-onset ulcerative colitis presentations are presently underway. A future joint analysis of genome-wide association data of early- and late-onset cohorts will likely reveal more IBD risk variants since the power to detect small effects of genes increases.

Copyright © 2009 S. Karger AG, Basel

Genetic Basis of Inflammatory Bowel Disease

Crohn's disease (CD) and ulcerative colitis (UC) collectively known as inflammatory bowel disease (IBD) are chronic inflammatory disorders of the gastrointestinal tract that occur most commonly during the adolescent to young adult ages. Inflammatory bowel disease is characterized, respectively, by confluent inflammation of the colonic mucosa in UC and discontinuous transmural intestinal inflammation in CD. IBD is thought to develop as a result of dysregulation of the immune response to

KARGER

Fax +41 61 306 12 34
E-Mail karger@karger.ch
www.karger.com

© 2009 S. Karger AG, Basel
0257–2753/09/0273–0236$26.00/0

Accessible online at:
www.karger.com/ddi

Subra Kugathasan, MD
Emory University School of Medicine, Division of Pediatric Gastroenterology
Emory Children's Center, 2015, Uppergate Drive, Room 248
Atlanta, GA 30322 (USA)
Tel. +1 404 727 4542, Fax +1 404 727 4069, E-Mail subra.kugathasan@emory.edu

'normal' gut flora in a genetically susceptible host. IBD is highly heritable and this concept is strongly supported by family, twin, and phenotype concordance studies and is now confirmed by the discoveries of many susceptibility genes [1].

Age of Onset of IBD and Justification for Genetic Studies Using Pediatric-Onset IBD Subjects

IBDs are lifelong conditions with an onset that can occur at any age, but peaking in the late teens and early twenties, the age where childhood transcends from puberty into adulthood. One of the most compelling hypotheses is that pediatric-onset IBD is more likely to be influenced by genetics compared to late-adult onset as there is less time for environmental modifiers to have influenced the disease. Early-onset disease is frequently examined in genetic studies because it is presumed to contain a more severe subset of patients under a higher influence of genetic effects. While this question about differing age of onset among the chronic complex inflammatory disorders such as IBD encourages debate, a fundamental issue in IBD remains unanswered. Does early (pediatric)-onset IBD represent the same disease process occurring in adults but merely at an earlier age (i.e., age of onset is a random event) or does IBD in children have a very different etiology and pathogenesis (hence different natural history) but just with the same clinical presentation as in adults? Although no hard scientific evidence exists about differing etiology, pediatric-onset IBD does 'differ' from adult IBD in many aspects [2]. In fact, there is growing evidence from clinical observations as well as epidemiologic and natural history studies that pediatric-onset IBD represents a distinct disease with differences in disease type, disease location, disease behavior, gender preponderance and genetically attributable risk compared to its 'adult' counterpart [3]. Early-onset IBD demonstrates unique characteristics in phenotype such as colonic involvement, severity, and familiarity, all of which justify ascertaining children with IBD for genetic studies to potentially identify new IBD loci that may be exclusive to pediatric IBD [4]. Extensive anatomical involvement at presentation with early disease progression is now clearly established as a feature of both childhood CD as well as UC [5]. Recent data suggest that the age-of-onset approach may be effective in identifying genes contributing modest effect sizes to the pathogenesis of IBD despite access to relatively smaller cohorts [6].

Gene Discoveries in IBD (Adult Studies)

Initial family-based linkage studies of IBD implicated the NOD2 gene in CD and the MHC region on chromosome 6p in UC for increased susceptibility [7]. Recently, genome-wide association scans (GWAS), which employ high-density single-nucleotide polymorphism (SNP) array technology, have increased the possible genetic factors linked to IBD pathogenesis [8]. This method of broad, unbiased screening for the contribution of common genetic variation for disease susceptibility has provided strong evidence for many CD and UC susceptibility loci. GWAS has identified loci in both UC and CD that are already known to be involved in adaptive immunity: IL23R, IL12B, STAT3, loci on 3p21 (MST1) and 10q24 (NKX2–3). Variants in innate immunity genes, particularly those mediating autophagy and bacterial sensing (ATG16L1, IRGM and NOD2), have also been discovered through these methods in CD [9]. Loci on 5p13 (PTGER1), 10q21 (ZNF365) and 18p11 (PTPN2) have also been reported, exclusively with CD. The list of established CD loci has been increased after a recent meta-analysis on a dataset of 3,230 cases and 4,829 controls [10]. Twenty-one additional susceptibility loci were found, including CCR6, LRRK, CDKAL, ICOSLG, and ITLN1. Despite these advances, many other genetic variants remain unknown. Barrett et al.'s [10] recent projection estimates that the first 30 loci identified only account for approximately 20% of all the susceptibility loci in CD. To date, the majority of this genetic analysis in IBD has been done in adult cohorts, with adult-onset disease as the primary phenotype; therefore, even less is known about early-onset variants.

Gene Discoveries from IBD Cohorts with Early-Onset Disease

When studying early-onset presentations of disease, there is an assumption that these represent a more severe, more genetically influenced group of patients. It is appealing to geneticists to study these patients because of the increased chance of finding novel risk variants. Studies in other diseases have identified specific genes that predispose to early onset, and in other diseases which display enrichment of gene burden, general risk variants have been determined. For example, in Huntington's disease the discovery of the influence of CAG repeat length and additional genetic modifiers provided a basis for the idea that there is a genetic basis to age of onset phenotypes [11]. It has also been used to describe early-onset

Alzheimer's disease, breast and ovarian cancer, and myocardial infarction. Based on these findings, there is reason to believe that genetic variation can explain the different phenotypes seen in adult versus pediatric IBD, but this has yet to be determined.

Through the many genetic studies done to date it has now become possible to study the collective influence of many risk variants in CD pathogenesis. Several CD susceptibility alleles have been confirmed in both pediatric and adult populations. However, most of the genetic variation seen in adults has not been studied in children in a large cohort with adequate power. Two pediatric studies have been carried out recently attempting to replicate the effect of those adult-onset IBD loci in children. Peterson et al. [12] replicated 6 loci (including IL23R, ATG16L1 and IRGM) identified from adults GWAS studies. In a second study, Essers et al. [13] genotyped a pediatric-onset IBD cohort at all confirmed CD risk loci. Of the 34 SNPs, 15 were associated with pediatric-onset IBD and statistical analysis determined that this was unlikely to have occurred by chance. Six of the alleles had never been validated in pediatric studies previously. Additionally, CARD15, IL23R, and ATG16L1 alleles were replicated in this cohort. Their association with pediatric CD has been previously established, and replication in that cohort provides reassurance that samples are representative of pediatric CD in the larger population. In 28 of 34 SNPs tested, the OR 95% confidence bounds include the previously established value. Thirty of 34 ORs reflect effect sizes in the same direction as reported ORs. This data argues that there are similar genetic determinants, with similar effect sizes in pediatric- and later-onset CD. The OR was identical in both pediatric cohorts and adult studies indicating that there was no effect of age of onset on the loci discovered in the adult cohort. To test for single alleles that might exert a disproportionate influence on the age of onset of CD, they modeled age of onset, using all 30 alleles in the risk score acting as independent variables in a linear regression equation. They detected no single risk variant has any association on age of onset through age 30.

However, until a GWAS is performed in an exclusively pediatric-onset IBD cohort, it is very difficult to deny that additional pediatric-onset IBD susceptibility genes do not exist. The ideal way to discover unknown early-onset susceptibility loci is using GWAS on an adequately powered pediatric cohort. To that effect, we have recently performed the first pediatric GWAS IBD scan. Two novel loci, the TNFRSF6B and PSMG1 genes, were discovered using over 1,000 cases of pediatric IBD [14]. The gene TNFRS6B, which encodes a decoy receptor for the FasL pathway (DCR3), was found to increase the risk for pediatric-onset CD and UC. Our functional studies suggest that this variant regulates DCR3 protein abundance, lymphocyte JAK/STAT signaling, and serum cytokine levels. This effect is most pronounced in patients with pancolitis phenotypes of UC or colon-only CD, the two pediatric specific phenotypes that differ from adult-onset IBD. However, during the data-mining of adult GWAS, these 2 novel loci (TNFRSF6 and PSMG1) were found with nominal significance suggesting that these risk loci are not restricted to early-onset CD cases. Another larger pediatric GWAS scan involving nearly 3,000 pediatric onset IBD patients has been completed by us, and further new gene discoveries are awaiting publication.

Although unlikely, pediatric CD may represent a distinct disease entity from later-onset disease, with unique genetic risk factors – as is the case with early-onset Alzheimer's disease and breast cancer. On the other extreme, pediatric CD and later-onset disease could have identical genetic architecture, but with earlier-onset patients inheriting a larger dose of genetic risk factors. Another hypothesis is that environmental exposures, genetic variation outside the CD causal pathway, or rare variants in common risk loci modulate the age at which disease presents.

Discussion and Future Directions

Essers et al. [13] recently showed that the overall burden of confirmed risk alleles explains only 20% of the genetic variance of CD which at most is a minor factor in determining the age at which CD presents. Additionally, they report similar effect sizes of all confirmed CD risk alleles in a pediatric cohort and confidently validated six such alleles in children for the first time. Furthermore, most ORs agreed with published data, suggesting that the same adult CD alleles are active in pediatric CD when replicated in a pediatric-onset cohort. These findings suggest there is heritability, but other undiscovered factors are also important determinants in the early-onset presentation of CD. Rare but highly penetrant variation in known risk loci or differences in the timing of host-environment interactions are plausible mechanisms that deserve additional attention in light of these genetic findings. In addition, some of these studies have found differences in UC and CD risk scores. Essers et al. [13] observed that children with UC have a marked decrease in CD risk scores and their scores are similar to controls. Even without using UC-specific alleles, the calculated risk score showed there was a notable separation in the distributions between UC and CD patients.

This raises the possibility that with further investigations, by accounting for both CD- and UC-specific associations in the score, genotype-based approaches could be used in distinguishing IBD subtypes in clinically indeterminate cases. Also investigating the additive IBD risk in individuals carrying increasing numbers of variants may provide an opportunity to identify high-risk individuals.

All of these findings contribute to help in the better understanding of the pathogenesis of CD, and investigators will need to decide the most beneficial way to use a wealth of banked DNA and genotype data. Re-sequencing of risk loci and exploration of the role of the gut micro-biome in early-onset pathogenesis should be encouraged. It is unlikely that further discovery of common CD risk alleles will increase the ability to detect a major effect of 'overall genetic load' in age of onset since current known risk variants explain less than 10% of the variance in this phenotype. The fact that common variants that individually provide relatively small alteration of disease susceptibility can combine to have a dramatic influence on disease risk provides new insight and strategies in pursuing functional studies, molecular diagnostic development and targeted drug design, thereby laying the foundation for the development of personalized treatment algorithms. Thus, the molecular markers discovered in this and previous studies may have future potential to be incorporated into high-dimensional molecular panels that can be used in clinical diagnosis and management.

Although we have identified and replicated a number of novel and previously reported loci in this study, there are likely many more genetic loci to be discovered that modulate both early- and adult-onset IBD risk. Our genotyping platform captures only a subset of the common Caucasians genetic variation; therefore, it is quite plausible that numerous other common variants may be discovered using a platform with more complete coverage of Caucasian genetic diversity. Application of appropriate genotyping platforms to examine genetic variation in non-Caucasian IBD patients may also reveal novel loci not addressed by this or recent genome scans. Similarly, replication of early-onset IBD susceptibility loci in non-Caucasian populations is warranted to determine the ethnic heterogeneity of their effect. Loci discovered by our study likely represent surrogates of causal variants. Fine-mapping and re-sequencing of these regions may reveal haplotypes that confer more profound risk or protection from IBD. More detailed functional exploration of genes associated with susceptibility loci reported in this study will be instrumental in shedding light on their role in IBD pathogenesis. Taken together, our results substantially advance the current understanding of pediatric-onset IBD by highlighting key pathogenetic mechanisms, and allowing for the first time a comparison between genetic susceptibility in an exclusively pediatric cohort and the previously described populations with predominantly adult-onset disease.

Disclosure Statement

The authors declare that no financial or other conflict of interest exists in relation to the content of the article.

References

1 Biank V, Broeckel U, Kugathasan S: Pediatric inflammatory bowel disease: clinical and molecular genetics. Inflamm Bowel Dis 2007;13:1430–1438.

2 Kugathasan S, Cohen S: Searching for new clues in inflammatory bowel disease: tell tales from pediatric IBD natural history studies. Gastroenterology 2008;135:1038–1041.

3 Van Limbergen J, Russell RK, Drummond HE, et al: Definition of phenotypic characteristics of childhood-onset inflammatory bowel disease. Gastroenterology 2008;135:1114–1122.

4 Levine A, Kugathasan S, Annese V, et al: Pediatric onset Crohn's colitis is characterized by genotype-dependent age-related susceptibility. Inflamm Bowel Dis 2007;13:1509–1515.

5 Hyams J, Markowitz J, Lerer T, et al: The natural history of corticosteroid therapy for ulcerative colitis in children. Clin Gastroenterol Hepatol 2006;4:1118–1123.

6 Li JL, Hayden MR, Warby SC, et al: Genome-wide significance for a modifier of age at neurological onset in Huntington's disease at 6q23–24: the HD MAPS study. BMC Med Genet 2006;7:71.

7 Satsangi J: Gene discovery in IBD: a decade of progress. J Pediatr Gastroenterol Nutr 2008;46(suppl 1):E1–E2.

8 Duerr RH, Taylor KD, Brant SR, et al: A genome-wide association study identifies IL23R as an inflammatory bowel disease gene. Science 2006;314:1461–1463.

9 Rioux JD, Xavier RJ, Taylor KD, et al: Genome-wide association study identifies new susceptibility loci for Crohn disease and implicates autophagy in disease pathogenesis. Nat Genet 2007;39:596–604.

10 Barrett JC, Hansoul S, Nicolae DL, et al: Genome-wide association defines more than 30 distinct susceptibility loci for Crohn's disease. Nat Genet 2008;40:955–962.

11 Andrew SE, Goldberg YP, Kremer B, et al: The relationship between trinucleotide (CAG) repeat length and clinical features of Huntington's disease. Nat Genet 1993;4:398–403.

12 Peterson N, Guthery S, Denson L, et al: Genetic variants in the autophagy pathway contribute to paediatric Crohn's disease. Gut 2008;57:1336–1337; author reply 1337.

13 Essers JB, Lee JJ, Kugathasan S, et al: Established genetic risk factors do not distinguish early and later onset Crohn's disease. Inflamm Bowel Dis 2009, Epub ahead of print.

14 Kugathasan S, Baldassano RN, Bradfield JP, et al: Loci on 20q13 and 21q22 are associated with pediatric-onset inflammatory bowel disease. Nat Genet 2008;40:1211–1215.

Dig Dis 2009;27:240–245
DOI: 10.1159/000228556

The Intestinal Epithelial Barrier: Does It Become Impaired with Age?

Johannes Meier   Andreas Sturm

Medizinische Klinik m.S. Hepatologie, Gastroenterologie, Endokrinologie und Stoffwechsel, Charité-Universitätsmedizin Berlin, Campus Virchow-Klinikum, Berlin, Germany

Key Words
Inflammatory bowel disease · Epithelial barrier · Immunosenescence · Immune response

Abstract

The proportion of the population aged over 65 is increasing rapidly and malnutrition is a more common problem in elderly patients. The intestinal epithelium covers the surface of the digestive tract and consists of epithelial cells that constitute an efficient physical barrier between the dietary and enteric flora pathogens found in the intestinal lumen and the individuum, while at the same time allowing an exchange between nutrients and the systemic circulation. There is only a very limited amount of information available on whether and how age, with concomitant inflammation, influences the epithelial barrier. Although there is evidence that age does not correlate with the area of the duodenal surface epithelium or the number of intraepithelial lymphocytes, absorption of certain nutrients, e.g. lipids, does seem to be impaired in the elderly. However, impaired blood flow, ischemic changes and the increased use of NSAIDs naturally contribute to an impaired epithelial barrier in elderly patients.

Copyright © 2009 S. Karger AG, Basel

The Epithelial Barrier

The surface of the digestive tract is covered by epithelial cells that constitute an efficient physical barrier between the dietary and enteric flora pathogens found in the intestinal lumen and the individuum, but also allows an exchange between nutrients and the systemic circulation [1]. The epithelial defense mechanism can be categorized into three key components: preepithelial, epithelial and postepithelial, the latter being represented by the lamina propria [2]. The preepithelial mucus barrier is composed of mucin associated with other proteins and lipids and forms a continuous gel into which a bicarbonate-rich fluid is secreted, maintaining a neutralizing pH at the epithelial surface. Phosphatidylcholine is the predominant surface bioactive phospholipid found within the gastrointestinal tract [3]. Intestinal epithelial cells secrete mucins and glycocalyx, which contain membrane-anchored negatively charged mucin-like glycoproteins and hydrophobic phospholipids [4]. The tight adherence of mucin to the apical surfaces of epithelia is owed to the existence of the specific complex between mucin oligosaccharides and the mucin-binding protein of the apical mucosal membrane [5]. The hydrophobic lining of the luminal surface has an important functional role. It prevents microorganisms from getting into contact with and adhering to the plasma membrane. It furthermore protects the mucosal epithelium against chemical and me-

Dr. Andreas Sturm
Medizinische Klinik m.S. Hepatologie, Gastroenterologie,
Endokrinologie und Stoffwechsel, Charité-Universitätsmedizin Berlin
Campus Virchow-Klinikum, Augustenburger Platz 1, DE–13353 Berlin (Germany)
Tel. +49 30 450 565 206, Fax +49 30 450 553 929, E-Mail andreas.sturm@charite.de

chanical injuries [6]. Epithelial cells provide the second line of the mucosal defense system. Whereas in the upper digestive tract this layer consists of a stratified epithelium, the stomach and the small and large bowel are surfaced with a simple epithelial layer sealed by tight junctions [7]. When intact, the uptake of antigens, macro- and microorganisms through this layer is restricted by luminal cell-surface structures. The mucosal surface epithelial cells are rapidly proliferating with a complete turnover every 24–96 h [8]. The proliferative compartment of epithelial cells is localized in the crypt region and is segregated from a gradient of increasingly differentiated epithelial cells present along the vertical axis of the functional villus compartment [9, 10].

Restoring the Epithelial Barrier

Damage and impairment of the intestinal surface barrier are observed in the course of various diseases and may result in increased penetration and absorption of toxic and immunogenic factors into the body, leading to inflammation, uncontrolled immune response, and a dysequilibrium of the host homeostasis. Thus, rapid resealing of the epithelial surface barrier following injuries or physiological damage is essential in order to preserve normal homeostasis. Observations over the past several years have demonstrated the ability of the intestinal tract to rapidly reestablish the continuity of the surface epithelium after extensive destruction [11–14]. The continuity of the epithelial surface is reestablished by at least three distinct mechanisms. First, epithelial cells adjacent to the injured surface migrate into the wound to cover the denuded area. Those epithelial cells that migrate into the wound defect dedifferentiate, form pseudopodia-like structures, reorganize their cytoskeleton, and redifferentiate after closure of the wound defect. This process has been termed epithelial restitution and does not require cell proliferation [15]. Intestinal epithelial restitution occurs within minutes to hours both in vivo and in vitro. Secondly, epithelial cell proliferation is necessary to replenish the decreased cell pool. Third, maturation and differentiation of undifferentiated epithelial cells is needed to maintain the numerous functional activities of the mucosal epithelium. The separation of intestinal epithelial wound healing in three distinct processes is rather artificial and simplified. These three wound-healing processes overlap and distinct processes may not be observed in vivo where these processes overlap. The preservation of this barrier following injuries is regulated by a broad spectrum of structurally distinct regulatory factors, including cytokines, growth factors, adhesion molecules, neuropeptides and phospholipids [16–19]. However, this artificial and simplified model provides a tool to better understand the physiology and pathophysiology of intestinal epithelial wound healing. Moreover, deeper lesions or penetrating injuries will require additional repair mechanisms that involve inflammatory processes and non-epithelial cell populations. Inflammatory processes, in particular, may interfere with epithelial cell migration and proliferation and thus modulate intestinal epithelial healing.

Important Modulators of Intestinal Epithelial Cell Function

The epithelial cell populations of the intestinal mucosa are modulated by a number of factors that are present within the lumen, the epithelium itself or the underlying lamina propria. Although the full variety of regulatory factors that play a role in the control of intestinal epithelial and non-epithelial cell populations has not yet been fully defined, there is increasing appreciation of the diversity of these factors in general and the importance of several specific peptide and non-peptide factors produced or released within the intestine. The identification and characterization of numerous regulatory peptide and non-peptide factors has led to the recognition of a network of interrelated factors within the intestine. The constituents of this network generally possess multiple functional properties and exhibit pleiotropism in their cellular sources and targets. As a result, this network is highly redundant in several dimensions [20]. Regulatory peptides, in particular, seem to play a key role in intestinal epithelial wound repair. Various members of several distinct regulatory peptide families are known to modulate a broad spectrum of intestinal epithelial cell functions including cell migration, proliferation and/or differentiation. As outlined above, the latter epithelial cell functions are highly relevant for the modulation of intestinal epithelial wound repair.

Morphometric Changes in the Elderly Mucosa

Since small bowel malabsorption is an important cause of malnutrition and morbidity in the elderly, Lipski et al. [21] investigated the effect of ageing on small bowel morphology by examining distal duodenal biopsy specimens from adults across a wide age range without evidence of malabsorption or malnutrition. In their study, they coded duodenal architecture as either normal, partial villus atrophy, or subtotal villus atrophy. Enterocytes were described as either normal or megaloblastic; the brush border was either normal or indistinct, and Brunner glands were either normal or abnormal. In their study, they revealed that there is no significant correlation between age and areas of duodenal surface epithelium, crypts and lamina propria, height of villi and surface epithelium, depths of crypts, crypt to villus ratio, number of intraepithelial lymphocytes, duodenal architecture, enterocytes or brush borders.

Functional Changes in the Elderly Mucosa

As pointed out above, the epithelial defense mechanism can be categorized into three key components: preepithelial, epithelial and postepithelial, the latter being represented by the lamina propria. Within the preepithelial mucus barrier, phosphatidylcholine is a major protective factor. As studies investigating changes in the lipid components in the mucosa of elderly patients were lacking, Keelan et al. [22] investigated the effect of aging on choline and amine-phospholipid composition of rabbit brush border. As in weaning rabbits the choline-phospholipid contents were significantly lower than in young rabbits, their contents dropped in the jejunum, but not ileum, of mature rabbits. Interestingly, and in contrast to the choline contents, the amine-phospholipid contents increase in the jejunal and ileal mucosa with advancing age. However, since they are restricted to the rabbit mucosa, the data presented here are adaptable to the human mucosa only to a limited extent.

Changes in Permeability of Elderly Mucosa

Only a few studies have investigated changes in intestinal permeability in the elderly mucosa. Hollander and colleagues [23] demonstrated that intestinal permeability to medium-sized probes (mannitol, polyethylene glycol) increased in 29-month-old compared to 3-month-old rats. In humans, studies of intestinal permeability were performed measuring the intestinal absorption of different-sized molecules such as lactulose, mannitol, polyethylene glycol and EDTA. Although the overall uptake of lactulose and mannitol decreased slightly with age, no differences were found when the renal function of the probands was taken into account [24, 25]. Particularly the lactulose:mannitol ratio (LTM) did not differ between young and old subjects, indicating that intestinal permeability to these sugars does not change significantly with age in humans [26]. Altered intestinal permeability is a highly relevant issue in the context of oral drug absorption in the elderly patient; however, more conclusive studies are needed.

Changes in Nutritional Absorption in the Elderly Mucosa

Weight loss and malnutrition is a common problem in elderly patients. Lipids represent a major source of energy, but the question of whether and how lipid absorption is impaired in the elderly is not easily answered. In animals, reduced gastric lipase and bile acid secretion as well as decreasing lipid solubilisation were shown, leading to a decrease in the overall lipid absorption [27]. In humans, postprandial serum bile acid levels were reduced, but no correlation between age and 72-hour fecal fat excretion was found [28]. Absorption of fat may take longer in the elderly [29], and prolonged absorption of fats may induce postprandial satiety, thereby reducing overall nutritional intake in the elderly patient [30]. More recently, Woudstra et al. [31] demonstrated the reduced uptake of several fatty acids in 24-month-old compared to 1-month-old rats. These differences disappeared when the mucosal surface area was considered, suggesting that the observed age-related changes in lipid uptake are largely due to a nonspecific reduction in the intestinal surface area.

Concerning carbohydrates, a decreased absorption of D-xylose in ageing humans and an age-associated decline in D-glucose absorption in mice and rats has been demonstrated [32–35]. However, interpretation of these data is complex since D-xylose excretion is also dependent on renal function. When the results were stratified according to kidney function, the significance was lost in the different age groups. Ferraris et al. [36] explained the reduction of carbohydrate uptake with a reduced site density of the Na^+-dependent glucose transporter SGLT1 in the intestinal brush border membrane of aged mice. This observation was not confirmed by other studies showing normal amounts of essential glucose transport components such as SGLT1, GLUT2 and Na^+K^+-ATPase [37, 38].

With regard to amino acids, the absorption of tyrosine, arginine and aspartic acid declines in senescent rodents [39]. However, systematic human studies and data of structural differences are missing.

Changes in Immune Response in the Elderly Mucosa

The intestine is a major site of infectious challenge which has to be controlled by effective immune defense mechanisms. Aging is associated with a progressive decline in both the innate and adaptive immune response [40, 41], leading to higher mortality due to bacterial and viral infections, autoimmune phenomena and malignancies [42–45].

The adaptive immunity of the elderly is compromised by decreased T-cell memory function [46], altered T cell receptor (TCR) signal transduction [47], exhaustion of naive T cell population [41] and reduction in the population of antibody-producing B cells along with a smaller immunoglobulin diversity [48, 49].

Little is known about changes in mucosal immunity due to immunosenescence. Some studies measured normal or even increased amounts of intestinal IgA in old animals and elderly patients [50, 51]. Others report a decline in luminal IgA titers [52], which interestingly does not result from reduced antibody secretion of lamina propria plasma cells, but is presumably due to an impaired homing mechanism of immunoblasts to the mucosal layer [53]. The clinical implications of an alteration in mucosal adaptive immunity can be seen in the reduced antibody response and T-cell function following oral vaccination [54].

Age-related changes in the innate immune response are supported by cumulative evidence [for a review, see 55]. Impairment of multiple neutrophil functions, such as phagocytic capacity, chemotactic response to GM-CSF, synthesis of reactive oxygen and intracellular killing, is observed in the elderly [56, 57]. The amount of neutral killer cells (NK) and natural killer T cells (NKT) were shown to increase in the elderly [58, 59]. Reduced cytotoxicity was shown in NK cells of the elderly, whereas production of cytokines and antibody-dependent cell-mediated cytotoxicity was not impaired [60, 61]. Dendritic cells and macrophages are important components of the mucosa-associated lymphatic tissue (MALT). There is evidence of changes in their biological properties in advanced age, although multiple contradictory results have been published. Some studies have reported decreased chemotaxis and phagocytosis in aged mice and humans [62, 63], others did not [64]. Reduced capacity of antigen presentation was explained by altered expression of MHC class II molecules on aged macrophages [65]. There is general agreement that a decrease in cytokine production occurs in rodent macrophages and dendritic cells during aging. In human monocytes, discordant results were shown [for a review, see 66]. However, peripheral blood monocytes revealed defective TLR1/2-induced TNF-α and IL-6 production with advanced age, whereas cytokine production following ligation of TLR2/6, TLR4 and TLR5 remained unchanged [67].

In chronic inflammatory bowel disease (IBD), cytokine production as TNF-α, IL-6 and IL-13 and TLR-dependent signaling play a central role in the initiation and perpetuation of chronic inflammation. The incidence of IBD shows a continuous fall with advancing age [68]. This might in part be explained by altered cytotoxic efficiency and cytokine production of the ageing mucosal immune cells. As the elderly population is growing, more data gathered in experimental models and humans are needed to estimate the impact of aging on mucosal immunity and pathology.

Summary

Functional studies in elderly patients with a focus on the intestinal epithelial barrier and its function are lacking. Only in other organ systems dysfunction of the choroid plexuses and the blood-cerebrospinal fluid barrier [69] and impaired retinal angiogenesis [70] has +been clearly associated with the ageing process. However, from a clinical point of view, impaired blood flow, ischemic changes and the increased use of NSAIDs naturally contribute to an impaired epithelial barrier in elderly patients, leading to increased risk for ulcers in those patients. Following a period of stress caused by illness or injury, it has been shown that elderly patients continued to underfeed themselves for 10–15 days, while younger patients increased their energy intake [71]. Elderly patients may have decreased functional reserve of the intestine and may become undernourished more rapidly during acute hospitalizations, consequently requiring an extended period of intensive nutritional monitoring due to reduced adaptive responses.

Disclosure Statement

The authors declare that no financial or other conflict of interest exists in relation to the content of the article.

References

1 Madara JL, Nash S, Moore R, et al: Structure and function of the intestinal epithelial barrier in health and disease. Monogr Pathol 1990;31:306–324.

2 Scheiman JM: NSAIDs, gastrointestinal injury, and cytoprotection. Gastroenterol Clin North Am 1996;25:279–298.

3 Schmitz MG, Renooij W: Phospholipids from rat, human, and canine gastric mucosa: composition and metabolism of molecular classes of phosphatidylcholine. Gastroenterology 1990;99:1292–1296.

4 Maury J, Nicoletti C, Guzzo-Chambraud L, et al: The filamentous brush border glycocalyx, a mucin-like marker of enterocyte hyper-polarization. Eur J Biochem 1995;228:323–331.

5 Slomiany A, Grabska M, Slomiany BL: Essential components of antimicrobial gastrointestinal epithelial barrier: specific interaction of mucin with an integral apical membrane protein of gastric mucosa. Mol Med 2001;7:1–10.

6 Frey A, Giannasca KT, Weltzin R, et al: Role of the glycocalyx in regulating access of microparticles to apical plasma membranes of intestinal epithelial cells: implications for microbial attachment and oral vaccine targeting. J Exp Med 1996;184:1045–1059.

7 Kraehenbuhl JP, Pringault E, Neutra MR: Review article: Intestinal epithelia and barrier functions. Aliment Pharmacol Ther 1997;11(suppl 3):3–8; discussion 8–9.

8 Potten CS, Kellett M, Rew DA, et al: Proliferation in human gastrointestinal epithelium using bromodeoxyuridine in vivo: data for different sites, proximity to a tumour, and polyposis coli. Gut 1992;33:524–529.

9 Cheng H, Leblond CP: Origin, differentiation and renewal of the four main epithelial cell types in the mouse small intestine. III. Entero-endocrine cells. Am J Anat 1974;141:503–519.

10 Schmidt GH, Wilkinson MM, Ponder BA: Cell migration pathway in the intestinal epithelium: an in situ marker system using mouse aggregation chimeras. Cell 1985;40:425–429.

11 McCormack SA, Viar MJ, Johnson LR: Migration of IEC-6 cells: a model for mucosal healing. Am J Physiol 1992;263:G426–G435.

12 Nusrat A, Delp C, Madara JL: Intestinal epithelial restitution. Characterization of a cell culture model and mapping of cytoskeletal elements in migrating cells. J Clin Invest 1992;89:1501–1511.

13 Moore R, Carlson S, Madara JL: Rapid barrier restitution in an in vitro model of intestinal epithelial injury. Lab Invest 1989;60:237–244.

14 Feil W, Wenzl E, Vattay P, et al: Repair of rabbit duodenal mucosa after acid injury in vivo and in vitro. Gastroenterology 1987;92:1973–1986.

15 Taupin D, Podolsky DK: Trefoil factors: Initiators of mucosal healing. Nat Rev Mol Cell Biol 2003;4:721–732.

16 Fiocchi C: Inflammatory bowel disease: etiology and pathogenesis. Gastroenterology 1998;115:182–205.

17 Dignass AU, Sturm A, Podolsky D: Epithelial injury and restitution; in Domschke W, Stoll T, Brasitius TA, Kagnoff MF (eds): Intestinal Mucosa and Its Diseases. Dordrecht, Kluwer Academic Publisher, 1999, pp 293–299.

18 Okamoto R, Watanabe M: Cellular and molecular mechanisms of the epithelial repair in IBD. Dig Dis Sci 2005;50(suppl 1):S34–S38.

19 Okamoto R, Watanabe M: Molecular and clinical basis for the regeneration of human gastrointestinal epithelia. J Gastroenterol 2004;39:1–6.

20 Dignass AU, Sturm A: Peptide growth factors in the intestine. Eur J Gastroenterol Hepatol 2001;13:763–770.

21 Lipski PS, Bennett MK, Kelly PJ, et al: Ageing and duodenal morphometry. J Clin Pathol 1992;45:450–452.

22 Keelan M, Walker K, Thomson AB: Intestinal morphology, marker enzymes and lipid content of brush border membranes from rabbit jejunum and ileum: effect of aging. Mech Ageing Dev 1985;31:49–68.

23 Ma TY, Hollander D, Dadufalza V, et al: Effect of aging and caloric restriction on intestinal permeability. Exp Gerontol 1992;27:321–333.

24 Beaumont DM, Cobden I, Sheldon WL, et al: Passive and active carbohydrate absorption by the ageing gut. Age Ageing 1987;16:294–300.

25 Saweirs WM, Andrews DJ, Low-Beer TS: The double sugar test of intestinal permeability in the elderly. Age Ageing 1985;14:312–315.

26 Saltzman JR, Kowdley KV, Perrone G, et al: Changes in small-intestine permeability with aging. J Am Geriatr Soc 1995;43:160–164.

27 Holt PR, Balint JA: Effects of aging on intestinal lipid absorption. Am J Physiol 1993;264:G1–G6.

28 Arora S, Kassarjian Z, Krasinski SD, et al: Effect of age on tests of intestinal and hepatic function in healthy humans. Gastroenterology 1989;96:1560–1565.

29 Salemans JM, Nagengast FM, Tangerman A, et al: Effect of ageing on postprandial conjugated and unconjugated serum bile acid levels in healthy subjects. Eur J Clin Invest 1993;23:192–198.

30 Wisen O, Hellstrom PM: Gastrointestinal motility in obesity. J Intern Med 1995;237:411–418.

31 Woudstra TD, Drozdowski LA, Wild GE, et al: An isocaloric PUFA diet enhances lipid uptake and weight gain in aging rats. Lipids 2004;39:343–354.

32 Doubek WG, Armbrecht HJ: Changes in intestinal glucose transport over the lifespan of the rat. Mech Ageing Dev 1987;39:91–102.

33 Freeman HJ, Quamme GA: Age-related changes in sodium-dependent glucose transport in rat small intestine. Am J Physiol 1986;251:G208–G217.

34 Hosoda S: The gastrointestinal tract and nutrition in the aging process: an overview. Nutr Rev 1992;50:372–373.

35 Lindi C, Marciani P, Faelli A, et al: Intestinal sugar transport during ageing. Biochim Biophys Acta 1985;816:411–414.

36 Ferraris RP, Vinnakota RR: Regulation of intestinal nutrient transport is impaired in aged mice. J Nutr 1993;123:502–511.

37 Drozdowski L, Woudstra T, Wild G, et al: The age-associated decline in the intestinal uptake of glucose is not accompanied by changes in the mRNA or protein abundance of SGLT1. Mech Ageing Dev 2003;124:1035–1045.

38 Thompson JS, Crouse DA, Mann SL, et al: Intestinal glucose uptake is increased in aged mice. Mech Ageing Dev 1988;46:135–143.

39 Chen TS, Currier GJ, Wabner CL: Intestinal transport during the life span of the mouse. J Gerontol 1990;45:B129–B133.

40 Gomez CR, Boehmer ED, Kovacs EJ: The aging innate immune system. Curr Opin Immunol 2005;17:457–462.

41 Weng NP: Aging of the immune system: how much can the adaptive immune system adapt? Immunity 2006;24:495–499.

42 Katz JM, Plowden J, Renshaw-Hoelscher M, et al: Immunity to influenza: the challenges of protecting an aging population. Immunol Res 2004;29:113–124.

43 Boren E, Gershwin ME: Inflamm-aging: autoimmunity, and the immune-risk phenotype. Autoimmun Rev 2004;3:401–406.

44 Effros RB: Genetic alterations in the ageing immune system: impact on infection and cancer. Mech Ageing Dev 2003;124:71–77.

45 Prelog M: Aging of the immune system: a risk factor for autoimmunity? Autoimmun Rev 2006;5:136–139.

46 Min H, Montecino-Rodriguez E, Dorshkind K: Reduction in the developmental potential of intrathymic T cell progenitors with age. J Immunol 2004;173:245–250.

47 Garcia GG, Miller RA: Differential tyrosine phosphorylation of zeta chain dimers in mouse CD4 T lymphocytes: effect of age. Cell Immunol 1997;175:51–57.

48 Song H, Price PW, Cerny J: Age-related changes in antibody repertoire: contribution from T cells. Immunol Rev 1997;160:55–62.

49 Han S, Yang K, Ozen Z, et al: Enhanced differentiation of splenic plasma cells but diminished long-lived high-affinity bone marrow plasma cells in aged mice. J Immunol 2003;170:1267–1273.

50 Arranz E, O'Mahony S, Barton JR, et al: Immunosenescence and mucosal immunity: significant effects of old age on secretory IgA concentrations and intraepithelial lymphocyte counts. Gut 1992;33:882–886.

51 Ebersole JL, Smith DJ, Taubman MA: Secretory immune responses in ageing rats. I. Immunoglobulin levels. Immunology 1985;56: 345–350.

52 Schmucker DL, Thoreux K, Owen RL: Aging impairs intestinal immunity. Mech Ageing Dev 2001;122:1397–1411.

53 Schmucker DL, Owen RL, Outenreath R, et al: Basis for the age-related decline in intestinal mucosal immunity. Clin Dev Immunol 2003;10:167–172.

54 Fujihashi K, Koga T, McGhee JR: Mucosal vaccination and immune responses in the elderly. Vaccine 2000;18:1675–1680.

55 Gomez CR, Nomellini V, Faunce DE, et al: Innate immunity and aging. Exp Gerontol 2008;43:718–728.

56 Fulop T, Larbi A, Douziech N, et al: Signal transduction and functional changes in neutrophils with aging. Aging Cell 2004;3:217–226.

57 Tortorella C, Simone O, Piazzolla G, et al: Age-related impairment of GM-CSF-induced signalling in neutrophils: role of SHP-1 and SOCS proteins. Ageing Res Rev 2007; 6:81–93.

58 Ishimoto Y, Tomiyama-Miyaji C, Watanabe H, et al: Age-dependent variation in the proportion and number of intestinal lymphocyte subsets, especially natural killer T cells, double-positive CD4+ CD8+ cells and B220+ T cells, in mice. Immunology 2004;113:371–377.

59 Mariani E, Pulsatelli L, Meneghetti A, et al: Different IL-8 production by T and NK lymphocytes in elderly subjects. Mech Ageing Dev 2001;122:1383–1395.

60 Mocchegiani E, Malavolta M: NK and NKT cell functions in immunosenescence. Aging Cell 2004;3:177–184.

61 Peralbo E, Alonso C, Solana R: Invariant NKT and NKT-like lymphocytes: two different T cell subsets that are differentially affected by ageing. Exp Gerontol 2007;42:703–708.

62 Fietta A, Merlini C, De Bernardi PM, et al: Nonspecific immunity in aged healthy subjects and in patients with chronic bronchitis. Aging (Milano) 1993;5:357–361.

63 Plackett TP, Boehmer ED, Faunce DE, et al: Aging and innate immune cells. J Leukoc Biol 2004;76:291–299.

64 Corsini E, Di PR, Viviani B, et al: Increased carrageenan-induced acute lung inflammation in old rats. Immunology 2005;115:253–261.

65 Plowden J, Renshaw-Hoelscher M, Gangappa S, et al: Impaired antigen-induced CD8+ T cell clonal expansion in aging is due to defects in antigen presenting cell function. Cell Immunol 2004;229:86–92.

66 van Duin D, Shaw AC: Toll-like receptors in older adults. J Am Geriatr Soc 2007;55:1438–1444.

67 van Duin D, Mohanty S, Thomas V, et al: Age-associated defect in human TLR-1/2 function. J Immunol 2007;178:970–975.

68 Piront P, Louis E, Latour P, et al: Epidemiology of inflammatory bowel diseases in the elderly in the province of Liege. Gastroenterol Clin Biol 2002;26:157–161.

69 Redzic ZB, Preston JE, Duncan JA, et al: The choroid plexus-cerebrospinal fluid system: from development to aging. Curr Top Dev Biol 2005;71:1–52.

70 Kelly J, Ali KA, Yin J, et al: Senescence regulates macrophage activation and angiogenic fate at sites of tissue injury in mice. J Clin Invest 2007;117:3421–3426.

71 Woudstra T, Thomson AB: Nutrient absorption and intestinal adaptation with ageing. Best Pract Res Clin Gastroenterol 2002;16: 1–15.

Dig Dis 2009;27:246–251
DOI: 10.1159/000228557

Links between Autophagy, Innate Immunity, Inflammation and Crohn's Disease

Vojo Deretic

Department of Molecular Genetics and Microbiology, University of New Mexico School of Medicine,
Albuquerque, N. Mex., USA

Key Words

Autophagy · Innate immunity · Crohn's disease

Abstract

Autophagy is a fundamental biological process that endows eukaryotic cells with the ability to autodigest portions of their own cytoplasm. Autophagy plays roles in aging, development, neurodegeneration, cancer and immunity. The immunological role of autophagy was first recognized for the ability of autophagy to sanitize the cellular interior by killing intracellular microbes and, indirectly, by the adaptations that successful intracellular pathogens have evolved to protect themselves from autophagy. Since then, the repertoire of autophagy functions in immunity has been vastly expanded to include numerous intersections of regulatory and effector nature with innate and adaptive immunity. Autophagy acts both as an effector and a regulator of pattern recognition receptors, it supports MHC II presentation of cytosolic (self and microbial) antigens, it shapes central tolerance via thymic selection of the T cell repertoire, is an effector of Th1/Th2 polarization, affects homeostasis of T, B, and specialized immune cells such as Paneth cells, and – when defective – can be a contributing factor to chronic inflammatory conditions in human populations such as Crohn's disease.   Copyright © 2009 S. Karger AG, Basel

Introduction

The study of the immunological roles of autophagy has become a rapidly growing field taking on the role of a frontier in contemporary immunological research. Autophagy is the evolutionarily conserved, ubiquitous biological process of cleaning the eukaryotic cell's interior. During autophagy, large portions of the cytoplasm that can be as big as whole organelles (e.g. mitochondria) are captured by isolation membranes (phagophores) and sequestered into autophagosomes for degradation within the specialized lytic organelles termed autolysosomes [1–6]. The genes (*Atg*) involved in this pathway [7] have been identified in species from yeast to humans. Autophagy affects a wide range of immunological processes: (1) innate and adaptive immunity against intracellular pathogens, including bacteria (e.g. *Mycobacterium tuberculosis*), protozoa and viruses [3, 4, 8–18; see also Deretic V. (ed): Autophagy in Immunity and Infection: a Novel Immune Effector. Weinheim, Wiley-VCH, 2006]; (2) antigen presentation [18–21]; (3) homeostasis of immune cells [22–24], and (4) inflammatory disorders, such as Crohn's disease [25–29]. More broadly, autophagy affects cell death and survival, and is implicated in many human health and disease states such as cancer, aging and longevity [30–32]. We particularly stress the utility of autophagy as a cell-autonomous defense against intracellular pathogens. When induced, autophagy can eliminate notorious intracellular microbes [8, 9, 33]. In contrast to

Vojo Deretic, PhD
Department of Molecular Genetics and Microbiology
University of New Mexico Health Sciences Center
915 Camino de Salud, NE, Albuquerque, NM 87131-001 (USA)
Tel. +1 505 272 0291, Fax +1 505 272 5309, E-Mail vderetic@salud.unm.edu

the notorious resistance of successful intracellular pathogens to a number of other microbicidal effectors, autophagy can efficiently eliminate intracellular microorganisms [8]. These observations have been confirmed by several groups in different contexts, including a report showing that autolysosomes contain ubiquitin fragments that act as mycobactericidal peptides [33], a study linking TLR stimulation and autophagy [34], a screen for novel autophagy inducers [35] and a recent study [36] showing that the previously reported ATP stimulation of P2X7 receptor leading to an elimination of intracellular mycobacteria [37] does so through autophagy [36]. Furthermore, a paper has just been published in *Nature Medicine* showing that autophagy induction can improve the vaccine potency of bacillus Calmette-Guérin (BCG) [38]. Only recently did mechanistic studies of autophagy become possible. The first book [Deretic V. (ed): Autophagosome and Phagosome. Totowa, Humana Press, 2008] that compiles autophagy methods has just recently been published [39]. The present toolbox for autophagy studies is limited by having very few pharmacological agonists and antagonists, boiling down to 2: rapamycin, an inducer, and 3-methyladenine, an inhibitor. However, rapamycin has been used clinically in the treatment of chronic conditions and transplantation and thus holds promise for application in Crohn's disease.

Autophagy as a Mechanism for Cleaning up Cellular Interiors

Autophagy impacts every cell in the human body and plays a role in a broad range of health and disease states. Autophagy is a fundamental cytoplasmic homeostasis process enabling individual cells to clean up, in a highly regulated fashion, their own cytoplasm by sequestering portions of the cytoplasm and degrading the captured constituents [1–6]. This primordial function is evolutionarily preserved in all eukaryotes, from yeast to human. The main morphological feature of autophagy is a membrane that wraps around portions of the cytoplasm earmarked to be sequestered, forming a double-membrane organelle termed autophagosome. The formation of autophagosomes is heralded by the appearance of punctate structures in the cytoplasm representing newly formed phagophores and autophagosomes. The captured material, once corralled into an autophagosome, is degraded upon autophagosomal fusion with lysosomal organelles. Autophagy has many physiological roles and is often employed to remove damaged or surplus organelles. It is also used by cells to turn over long-lived proteins and other macromolecules, either to get rid of protein aggregates or to supply nutrients for essential anabolic needs under conditions of nutrient deprivation or growth factor withdrawal. The broad spectrum of autophagy functions is hard-wired into a wide range of health-related issues, including cancer, neurodegeneration, aging and infections [32, 40]. The most recent additions to the list of processes affected by autophagy are the control of intracellular pathogens [8, 10–12, 15–17, 40–42] and inflammatory conditions such as Crohn's disease [25–29].

Autophagy in Immunity

Autophagy plays a role in a wide spectrum of immunological processes [40, 43] with the list of immunological autophagy categories (dubbed 'immunophagy' [3, 4]) rapidly growing [44].

(1) *Autophagy in direct elimination of microbes:* Autophagy is an innate immunity mechanism for the cell-autonomous elimination of intracellular microbes [8, 10–12, 15–17, 40, 42]. In the context of infectious disease, autophagy – when induced by physiological (starvation), pharmacological (rapamycin) or immunological (IFN-γ) means – can eliminate a number of important intracellular pathogens, including prominently *M. tuberculosis* [8, 9, 33]. Attesting to the role of autophagy in eliminating microbes, many successful pathogens had to evolve ways to deal with or inhibit it [17, 45] as a part of their repertoire of anti-immune defenses.

(2) *Autophagy as an effector of PRR/TLR signaling:* Autophagy is an effector of TLR signaling [34, 46, 47], and can enhance or interfere with innate antiviral responses regulated by TLR7 [48] and RIG-I [49].

(3) *Autophagy as an effector of Th1/Th2 polarization:* Autophagy, in its role as an antimicrobial defense mechanism, is controlled by Th1/Th2 polarization [50]. The Th1 cytokines such as IFN-γ [8, 51], and TNF-α [52] also acting downstream of CD40 ligation [16], stimulate autophagy, whereas the Th2 cytokines IL-4 and IL-13 inhibit autophagy [50, 53–55].

(4) *Autophagy in immune cell homeostasis:* Autophagy controls T and B cell development, survival, and proliferation [23, 24, 56].

(5) *Autophagy, MHC II presentation and thymic selection:* Autophagy contributes to MHC-II-restricted endogenous (cytosolic) antigen presentation [18, 19, 57, 58] with a role in thymic selection, allergy and autoimmune diseases [59].

(6) *Autophagy and vaccines:* Recent studies have shown that this newly discovered power of autophagy (MHC II presentation of cytoplasmic antigens) can be used for vaccine betterment as in the case of the influenza virus antigens [19, 60] and the widely used tuberculosis vaccine BCG [38].

(7) *Autophagy in inflammation:* Autophagy has recently been implicated in predisposition to Crohn's disease, a prevalent inflammatory bowel disease [61–63]. This latest breakthrough, made possible by the powerful genome-wide association screenings, has uncovered the role of autophagy in Crohn's disease, clearly demonstrating the role of autophagy in innate immunity in human populations [25–27, 29, 64], and a need to target this process for the treatment of a broad range of infectious and inflammatory diseases.

Innate Immunity, Autophagy, ATG16L1 and IRGM in Crohn's Disease

Genetic predisposition to Crohn's disease has been linked to regulators of innate immunity, of which Nod proteins (specifically Nod2) [65, 66] and most recently autophagy factors, including ATG16L1 and IRGM [25, 27, 67], are now some of the most prominent examples [26]. The specific role of Nod2 in Crohn's disease pathophysiology provides an obvious link with innate immunity and inflammation. Nod2 has been extensively studied and a considerable body of literature exists on this topic, including a very recent review [68]. The latest breakthroughs made possible by the powerful genome-wide association screenings have uncovered its role in at least 2 additional immunity pathways [26]: (1) IL-12 and IL-23 (IL23R-Arg381Gln) driving the Th17 differentiation of Th1 cells, with the Th17 phenotype often associated with organ-specific autoimmunity and inflammation, and (2) autophagy, a fundamental cellular homeostatic process involved in innate immunity against intracellular pathogens [3, 4, 40] and in endogenous antigen presentation [19, 43].

In contrast to the extensively studied Nod2 pathway, almost nothing is known about the role of IRGM in Crohn's disease, due to the only very recent recognition of its linkage to Crohn's disease [25–27]. Interestingly, *IRGM* is the only human gene representative of an otherwise prolific class of innate immunity effectors in vertebrates, called immunity-related GTPases (IRG) [69], also known as p47 GTPases [70]. In the mouse, there are 24 IRG genes and many of them have been initially recognized by their role in the defense against a variety of in-

tracellular bacterial and protozoan pathogens. Intriguingly, humans and chimpanzees have only one IRG, *IRGM* [69], and now this gene has turned out to be a Crohn's disease predisposition locus [25–27].

Since the initial reports of an association of ATG16L1 and IRGM polymorphisms with Crohn's disease [25–29, 67], a growing number of replicating studies have confirmed this genetic link in general and in several specific populations [28, 71–79]. Although several risk loci are common to ulcerative colitis and Crohn's disease, the autophagy genes ATG16L1 and IRGM – along with NOD2 – appear to be specific to Crohn's disease [80] with some indications of the specificity of IRGM association with ileal disease in some populations [81]. A study including 2,731 Dutch and Belgian patients (1,656 with Crohn's disease and 1,075 with ulcerative colitis) and 1,086 controls showed association of ATG16L1 (rs2241880) and IRGM (rs4958847) specifically with Crohn's disease [79]. Single-nucleotide polymorphisms in the IRGM gene (rs1000113 and rs4958847) have confirmed that IRGM is a susceptibility locus specifically for Crohn's disease, either of adult or childhood onset, in Italian populations possibly being associated with fistulizing disease [79].

Function of ATG16L1 and IRGM

Functional information regarding the role of autophagy in humans in the context of Crohn's disease is still lacking. Some information has been gleaned from studies of ATG16L1 in vitro with cell lines or in vivo in mice, with the 3 published studies pointing to different, albeit potentially congruent, effects: (1) reduced capacity of the ATG16L1*300A allele to control intracellular enteric pathogens when examined in a human epithelial cell [82]; (2) susceptibility to dextran sulphate sodium-induced acute colitis in mice lacking *Atg16L1* in hematopoietic cells and increase in IL-1β signaling with possible proinflammatory action [83], and (3) direct or indirect effects on Paneth cells in the intestinal crypts of ATG16L1-hypomorphic mice [84]. The role of IRGM cannot be properly investigated in mice, as the mouse has 24 IRGM-like genes, while humans have only 1 (IRGM); albeit 1, *Irgm1*, of the 3 putative murine orthologs shows effects on hematopoietic stem cell proliferation and T cell survival [85, 86]. Some information on the direct function of the human IRGM in antibacterial defenses has been known even before autophagy loci have been linked with Crohn's disease [9]. Future work will be needed to establish the scope and extent of the role of autophagy in Crohn's disease.

Acknowledgement

This work was supported by a Senior Research Award (CCFA 2053) 'Autophagy in Crohn's Disease' from the Crohn's and Colitis Foundation of America to V.D.

Disclosure Statement

The author declares that no financial or other conflict of interest exists in relation to the content of the article.

References

1 Shintani T, Klionsky DJ: Autophagy in health and disease: a double-edged sword. Science 2004;306:990–995.

2 Lum JJ, DeBerardinis RJ, Thompson CB: Autophagy in metazoans: cell survival in the land of plenty. Nat Rev Mol Cell Biol 2005;6: 439–448.

3 Deretic V: Autophagy in innate and adaptive immunity. Trends Immunol 2005;26:523–528.

4 Deretic V, Levine B: Autophagy, immunity, and microbial adaptations. Cell Host Microbe 2009;5:527–549.

5 Levine B: Cell biology: autophagy and cancer. Nature 2007;446:745–747.

6 Rubinsztein DC, Gestwicki JE, Murphy LO, Klionsky DJ: Potential therapeutic applications of autophagy. Nat Rev Drug Discov 2007;6:304–312.

7 Klionsky DJ, Cregg JM, Dunn WA Jr, Emr SD, Sakai Y, Sandoval IV, Sibirny A, Subramani S, Thumm M, Veenhuis M, Ohsumi Y: A unified nomenclature for yeast autophagy-related genes. Dev Cell 2003;5:539–545.

8 Gutierrez MG, Master SS, Singh SB, Taylor GA, Colombo MI, Deretic V: Autophagy is a defense mechanism inhibiting BCG and *Mycobacterium tuberculosis* survival in infected macrophages. Cell 2004;119:753–766.

9 Singh SB, Davis AS, Taylor GA, Deretic V: Human IRGM induces autophagy to eliminate intracellular mycobacteria. Science 2006;313:1438–1441.

10 Ogawa M, Yoshimori T, Suzuki T, Sagara H, Mizushima N, Sasakawa C: Escape of intracellular Shigella from autophagy. Science 2005;307:727–731.

11 Nakagawa I, Amano A, Mizushima N, Yamamoto A, Yamaguchi H, Kamimoto T, Nara A, Funao J, Nakata M, Tsuda K, Hamada S, Yoshimori T: Autophagy defends cells against invading group A Streptococcus. Science 2004;306:1037–1040.

12 Birmingham CL, Smith AC, Bakowski MA, Yoshimori T, Brumell JH: Autophagy controls Salmonella infection in response to damage to the Salmonella-containing vacuole. J Biol Chem 2006;281:11374–11383.

13 Liu Y, Schiff M, Czymmek K, Tallóczy Z, Levine B, Dinesh-Kumar SP: Autophagy regulates programmed cell death during the plant innate immune response. Cell 2005; 121:567–577.

14 Checroun C, Wehrly TD, Fischer ER, Hayes SF, Celli J: Autophagy-mediated reentry of *Francisella tularensis* into the endocytic compartment after cytoplasmic replication. Proc Natl Acad Sci USA 2006;103:14578–14583.

15 Ling YM, Shaw MH, Ayala C, Coppens I, Taylor GA, Ferguson DJ, Yap GS: Vacuolar and plasma membrane stripping and autophagic elimination of *Toxoplasma gondii* in primed effector macrophages. J Exp Med 2006;203:2063–2071.

16 Andrade RM, Wessendarp M, Gubbels MJ, Striepen B, Subauste CS: CD40 induces macrophage anti-*Toxoplasma gondii* activity by triggering autophagy-dependent fusion of pathogen-containing vacuoles and lysosomes. J Clin Invest 2006;116:2366–2377.

17 Orvedahl A, Alexander D, Tallóczy Z, Sun Q, Wei Y, Zhang W, Burns D, Leib D, Levine B: HSV-1 ICP34.5 confers neurovirulence by targeting the Beclin 1 autophagy protein. Cell Host Microbe 2007;1:23–35.

18 Paludan C, Schmid D, Landthaler M, Vockerodt M, Kube D, Tuschl T, Münz C: Endogenous MHC class II processing of a viral nuclear antigen after autophagy. Science 2005; 307:593–596.

19 Schmid D, Pypaert M, Münz C: Antigen-loading compartments for major histocompatibility complex class II molecules continuously receive input from autophagosomes. Immunity 2007;26:79–92.

20 Dengjel J, Schoor O, Fischer R, Reich M, Kraus M, Müller M, Kreymborg K, Altenberend F, Brandenburg J, Kalbacher H, Brock R, Driessen C, Rammensee HG, Stevanovic S: Autophagy promotes MHC class II presentation of peptides from intracellular source proteins. Proc Natl Acad Sci USA 2005;102: 7922–7927.

21 Crotzer VL, Blum JS: Autophagy and intracellular surveillance: modulating MHC class II antigen presentation with stress. Proc Natl Acad Sci USA 2005;102:7779–7780.

22 Lum JJ, Bauer DE, Kong M, Harris MH, Li C, Lindsten T, Thompson CB: Growth factor regulation of autophagy and cell survival in the absence of apoptosis. Cell 2005;120:237–248.

23 Pua HH, Dzhagalov I, Chuck M, Mizushima N, He YW: A critical role for the autophagy gene *Atg5* in T cell survival and proliferation. J Exp Med 2007;204:25–31.

24 Li C, Capan E, Zhao Y, Zhao J, Stolz D, Watkins SC, Jin S, Lu B: Autophagy is induced in CD4+ T cells and important for the growth factor-withdrawal cell death. J Immunol 2006;177:5163–5168.

25 Wellcome Trust Case Control Consortium: Genome-wide association study of 14,000 cases of seven common diseases and 3,000 shared controls. Nature 2007;447:661–678.

26 Massey D, Parkes M: Common pathways in Crohn's disease and other inflammatory diseases revealed by genomics. Gut 2007;56: 1489–1492.

27 Parkes M, Barrett JC, Prescott NJ, Tremelling M, Anderson CA, Fisher SA, Roberts RG, Nimmo ER, Cummings FR, Soars D, Drummond H, Lees CW, Khawaja SA, Bagnall R, Burke DA, Todhunter CE, Ahmad T, Onnie CM, McArdle W, Strachan D, Bethel G, Bryan C, Lewis CM, Deloukas P, Forbes A, Sanderson J, Jewell DP, Satsangi J, Mansfield JC, Cardon L, Mathew CG: Sequence variants in the autophagy gene *IRGM* and multiple other replicating loci contribute to Crohn's disease susceptibility. Nat Genet 2007;39:830–832.

28 Prescott NJ, Fisher SA, Franke A, Hampe J, Onnie CM, Soars D, Bagnall R, Mirza MM, Sanderson J, Forbes A, Franke A, Lewis CM, Schreiber S, Mathew CG: A nonsynonymous SNP in ATG16L1 predisposes to ileal Crohn's disease and is independent of CARD15 and IBD5. Gastroenterology 2007; 132:1665–1671.

29 Rioux JD, Xavier RJ, Taylor KD, Silverberg MS, Goyette P, Huett A, Green T, Kuballa P, Barmada MM, Datta LW, Shugart YY, Griffiths AM, Targan SR, Ippoliti AF, Bernard EJ, Mei L, Nicolae DL, Regueiro M, Schumm LP, Steinhart AH, Rotter JI, Duerr RH, Cho JH, Daly MJ, Brant SR: Genome-wide association study identifies new susceptibility loci for Crohn disease and implicates autophagy in disease pathogenesis. Nat Genet 2007;39:596–604.

30 Deretic V, Klionsky DJ: How cells clean house. Sci Am 2008;298:74–81.

31 Klionsky DJ: Autophagy: from phenomenology to molecular understanding in less than a decade. Nat Rev Mol Cell Biol 2007;8:931–937.

32 Levine B, Kroemer G: Autophagy in the pathogenesis of disease. Cell 2008;132:27–42.

33 Alonso S, Pethe K, Russell DG, Purdy GE: Lysosomal killing of Mycobacterium mediated by ubiquitin-derived peptides is enhanced by autophagy. Proc Natl Acad Sci USA 2007;104:6031–6036.

34 Xu Y, Jagannath C, Liu XD, Sharafkhaneh A, Kolodziejska KE, Eissa NT: Toll-like receptor 4 is a sensor for autophagy associated with innate immunity. Immunity 2007;27:135–144.

35 Floto RA, Sarkar S, Perlstein EO, Kampmann B, Schreiber SL, Rubinsztein DC: Small molecule enhancers of rapamycin-induced TOR inhibition promote autophagy, reduce toxicity in Huntington's disease models and enhance killing of mycobacteria by macrophages. Autophagy 2007;3:620–622.

36 Biswas D, Qureshi OS, Lee WY, Croudace JE, Mura M, Lammas DA: ATP-induced autophagy is associated with rapid killing of intracellular mycobacteria within human monocytes/macrophages. BMC Immunol 2008;9:35.

37 Lammas DA, Stober C, Harvey CJ, Kendrick N, Panchalingam S, Kumararatne DS: ATP-induced killing of mycobacteria by human macrophages is mediated by purinergic P2Z (P2X7) receptors. Immunity 1997;7:433–444.

38 Jagannath C, Lindsey DR, Dhandayuthapani S, Xu Y, Hunter RL Jr, Eissa NT: Autophagy enhances the efficacy of BCG vaccine by increasing peptide presentation in mouse dendritic cells. Nat Med 2009;15:267–276.

39 Deretic V, Klionsky DJ: How cells clean house. Sci Am 2008;298:74–81.

40 Levine B, Deretic V: Unveiling the roles of autophagy in innate and adaptive immunity. Nat Rev Immunol 2007;7:767–777.

41 Py BF, Lipinski MM, Yuan J: Autophagy limits Listeria monocytogenes intracellular growth in the early phase of primary infection. Autophagy 2007;3:117–125.

42 Birmingham CL, Canadien V, Kaniuk NA, Steinberg BE, Higgins DE, Brumell JH: Listeriolysin O allows Listeria monocytogenes replication in macrophage vacuoles. Nature 2008;451:350–354.

43 Schmid D, Münz C: Innate and adaptive immunity through autophagy. Immunity 2007;27:11–21.

44 Deretic V, Master S, Singh S: Autophagy gives a nod and a wink to the inflammasome and Paneth cells in Crohn's disease. Dev Cell 2008;15:641–642.

45 Gutierrez MG, Vazquez CL, Munafo DB, Zoppino FC, Beron W, Rabinovitch M, Colombo MI: Autophagy induction favours the generation and maturation of the Coxiella-replicative vacuoles. Cell Microbiol 2005;7:981–993.

46 Sanjuan MA, Dillon CP, Tait SW, Moshiach S, Dorsey F, Connell S, Komatsu M, Tanaka K, Cleveland JL, Withoff S, Green DR: Toll-like receptor signalling in macrophages links the autophagy pathway to phagocytosis. Nature 2007;450:1253–1257.

47 Delgado MA, Elmaoued RA, Davis AS, Kyei G, Deretic V: Toll-like receptors control autophagy. EMBO J 2008;27:1110–1121.

48 Lee HK, Lund JM, Ramanathan B, Mizushima N, Iwasaki A: Autophagy-dependent viral recognition by plasmacytoid dendritic cells. Science 2007;315:1398–1401.

49 Jounai N, Takeshita F, Kobiyama K, Sawano A, Miyawaki A, Xin KQ, Ishii KJ, Kawai T, Akira S, Suzuki K, Okuda K: The Atg5 Atg12 conjugate associates with innate antiviral immune responses. Proc Natl Acad Sci USA 2007;104:14050–14055.

50 Harris J, de Haro SA, Master SS, Keane J, Roberts EA, Delgado M, Deretic V: T helper 2 cytokines inhibit autophagic control of intracellular Mycobacterium tuberculosis. Immunity 2007;27:505–517.

51 Inbal B, Bialik S, Sabanay I, Shani G, Kimchi A: DAP kinase and DRP-1 mediate membrane blebbing and the formation of autophagic vesicles during programmed cell death. J Cell Biol 2002;157:455–468.

52 Djavaheri-Mergny M, Amelotti M, Mathieu J, Besancon F, Bauvy C, Souquere S, Pierron G, Codogno P: NF-κB activation represses tumor necrosis factor-α-induced autophagy. J Biol Chem 2006;281:30373–30382.

53 Arico S, Petiot A, Bauvy C, Dubbelhuis PF, Meijer AJ, Codogno P, Ogier-Denis E: The tumor suppressor PTEN positively regulates macroautophagy by inhibiting the phosphatidylinositol 3-kinase/protein kinase B pathway. J Biol Chem 2001;276:35243–35246.

54 Petiot A, Ogier-Denis E, Blommaart EF, Meijer AJ, Codogno P: Distinct classes of phosphatidylinositol 3-kinases are involved in signaling pathways that control macroautophagy in HT-29 cells. J Biol Chem 2000;275:992–998.

55 Scarlatti F, Bauvy C, Ventruti A, Sala G, Cluzeaud F, Vandewalle A, Ghidoni R, Codogno P: Ceramide-mediated macroautophagy involves inhibition of protein kinase B and up-regulation of beclin 1. J Biol Chem 2004;279:18384–18391.

56 Miller BC, Zhao Z, Stephenson LM, Cadwell K, Pua HH, Lee HK, Mizushima NN, Iwasaki A, He YW, Swat W, Virgin HW 4th: The autophagy gene ATG5 plays an essential role in B lymphocyte development. Autophagy 2008;4:309–314.

57 Dörfel D, Appel S, Grünebach F, Weck MM, Müller MR, Heine A, Brossart P: Processing and presentation of HLA class I and II epitopes by dendritic cells after transfection with in vitro-transcribed MUC1 RNA. Blood 2005;105:3199–3205.

58 Dengjel J, Schoor O, Fischer R, Reich M, Kraus M, Müller M, Kreymborg K, Altenberend F, Brandenburg J, Kalbacher H, Brock R, Driessen C, Rammensee HG, Stevanovic S: Autophagy promotes MHC class II presentation of peptides from intracellular source proteins. Proc Natl Acad Sci USA 2005;102:7922–7927.

59 Nedjic J, Aichinger M, Emmerich J, Mizushima N, Klein L: Autophagy in thymic epithelium shapes the T-cell repertoire and is essential for tolerance. Nature 2008;455:396–400.

60 Münz C: Enhancing immunity through autophagy. Annu Rev Immunol 2009;27:423–449.

61 Crohn BB, Ginzburg L, Oppenheimer GD: Regional ileitis: a pathologic and clinical entity (1932). Mt Sinai J Med 2000;67:263–268.

62 Hanauer SB: Inflammatory bowel disease. N Engl J Med 1996;334:841–848.

63 Podolsky DK: Inflammatory bowel disease. N Engl J Med 2002;347:417–429.

64 Hampe J, Franke A, Rosenstiel P, Till A, Teuber M, Huse K, Albrecht M, Mayr G, de la Vega FM, Briggs J, Günther S, Prescott NJ, Onnie CM, Häsler R, Sipos B, Fölsch UR, Lengauer T, Platzer M, Mathew CG, Krawczak M, Schreiber S: A genome-wide association scan of nonsynonymous SNPs identifies a susceptibility variant for Crohn disease in ATG16L1. Nat Genet 2007;39:207–211.

65 Ogura Y, Bonen DK, Inohara N, Nicolae DL, Chen FF, Ramos R, Britton H, Moran T, Karaliuskas R, Duerr RH, Achkar JP, Brant SR, Bayless TM, Kirschner BS, Hanauer SB, Nunez G, Cho JH: A frameshift mutation in NOD2 associated with susceptibility to Crohn's disease. Nature 2001;411:603–606.

66 Hugot JP, Chamaillard M, Zouali H, Lesage S, Cezard JP, Belaiche J, Almer S, Tysk C, O'Morain CA, Gassull M, Binder V, Finkel Y, Cortot A, Modigliani R, Laurent-Puig P, Gower-Rousseau C, Macry J, Colombel JF, Sahbatou M, Thomas G: Association of NOD2 leucine-rich repeat variants with susceptibility to Crohn's disease. Nature 2001;411:599–603.

67 McCarroll SA, Huett A, Kuballa P, Chilewski SD, Landry A, Goyette P, Zody MC, Hall JL, Brant SR, Cho JH, Duerr RH, Silverberg MS, Taylor KD, Rioux JD, Altshuler D, Daly MJ, Xavier RJ: Deletion polymorphism upstream of IRGM associated with altered IRGM expression and Crohn's disease. Nat Genet 2008;40:1107–1112.

68 Kanneganti TD, Lamkanfi M, Nunez G: Intracellular NOD-like receptors in host defense and disease. Immunity 2007;27:549–559.

69 Bekpen C, Marques-Bonet T, Alkan C, Antonacci F, Leogrande MB, Ventura M, Kidd JM, Siswara P, Howard JC, Eichler EE: Death and resurrection of the human IRGM gene. PLoS Genet 2009;5:e1000403.

70 Taylor GA, Feng CG, Sher A: p47 GTPases: regulators of immunity to intracellular pathogens. Nat Rev Immunol 2004;4:100–109.

71 Baldassano RN, Bradfield JP, Monos DS, Kim CE, Glessner JT, Casalunovo T, Frackelton EC, Otieno FG, Kanterakis S, Shaner JL, Smith RM, Eckert AW, Robinson LJ, Onyiah CC, Abrams DJ, Chiavacci RM, Skraban R, Devoto M, Grant SF, Hakonarson H: Association of the T300A non-synonymous variant of the ATG16L1 gene with susceptibility to paediatric Crohn's disease. Gut 2007;56: 1171–1173.

72 Cummings JR, Cooney R, Pathan S, Anderson CA, Barrett JC, Beckly J, Geremia A, Hancock L, Guo C, Ahmad T, Cardon LR, Jewell DP: Confirmation of the role of ATG16L1 as a Crohn's disease susceptibility gene. Inflamm Bowel Dis 2007;13:941–946.

73 Roberts RL, Gearry RB, Hollis-Moffatt JE, Miller AL, Reid J, Abkevich V, Timms KM, Gutin A, Lanchbury JS, Merriman TR, Barclay ML, Kennedy MA: IL23R R381Q and ATG16L1 T300A are strongly associated with Crohn's disease in a study of New Zealand Caucasians with inflammatory bowel disease. Am J Gastroenterol 2007;102:2754–2761.

74 Fowler EV, Doecke J, Simms LA, Zhao ZZ, Webb PM, Hayward NK, Whiteman DC, Florin TH, Montgomery GW, Cavanaugh JA, Radford-Smith GL: ATG16L1 T300A shows strong associations with disease subgroups in a large Australian IBD population: further support for significant disease heterogeneity. Am J Gastroenterol 2008;103: 2519–2526.

75 Glas J, Konrad A, Schmechel S, Dambacher J, Seiderer J, Schroff F, Wetzke M, Roeske D, Török HP, Tonenchi L, Pfennig S, Haller D, Griga T, Klein W, Epplen JT, Folwaczny C, Lohse P, Göke B, Ochsenkühn T, Mussack T, Folwaczny M, Müller-Myhsok B, Brand S: The ATG16L1 gene variants rs2241879 and rs2241880 (T300A) are strongly associated with susceptibility to Crohn's disease in the German population. Am J Gastroenterol 2008;103:682–691.

76 Okazaki T, Wang MH, Rawsthorne P, Sargent M, Datta LW, Shugart YY, Bernstein CN, Brant SR: Contributions of IBD5, IL23R, ATG16L1, and NOD2 to Crohn's disease risk in a population-based case-control study: evidence of gene-gene interactions. Inflamm Bowel Dis 2008;14:1528–1541.

77 Weersma RK, Zhernakova A, Nolte IM, Lefebvre C, Rioux JD, Mulder F, van Dullemen HM, Kleibeuker JH, Wijmenga C, Dijkstra G: ATG16L1 and IL23R are associated with inflammatory bowel diseases but not with celiac disease in the Netherlands. Am J Gastroenterol 2008;103:621–627.

78 van Limbergen J, Russell RK, Nimmo ER, Drummond HE, Smith L, Anderson NH, Davies G, Gillett PM, McGrogan P, Weaver LT, Bisset LW, Mahdi G, Arnott ID, Wilson DC, Satsangi J: Autophagy gene ATG16L1 influences susceptibility and disease location but not childhood-onset in Crohn's disease in Northern Europe. Inflamm Bowel Dis 2008;14:338–346.

79 Latiano A, Palmieri O, Cucchiara S, Castro M, D'Inca R, Guariso G, Dallapiccola B, Valvano MR, Latiano T, Andriulli A, Annese V: Polymorphism of the IRGM gene might predispose to fistulizing behavior in Crohn's disease. Am J Gastroenterol 2009;104:110–116.

80 Fisher SA, Tremelling M, Anderson CA, Gwilliam R, Bumpstead S, Prescott NJ, Nimmo ER, Massey D, Berzuini C, Johnson C, Barrett JC, Cummings FR, Drummond H, Lees CW, Onnie CM, Hanson CE, Blaszczyk K, Inouye M, Ewels P, Ravindrarajah R, Keniry A, Hunt S, Carter M, Watkins N, Ouwehand W, Lewis CM, Cardon L, Lobo A, Forbes A, Sanderson J, Jewell DP, Mansfield JC, Deloukas P, Mathew CG, Parkes M, Satsangi J: Genetic determinants of ulcerative colitis include the ECM1 locus and five loci implicated in Crohn's disease. Nat Genet 2008;40:710–712.

81 Roberts RL, Hollis-Moffatt JE, Gearry RB, Kennedy MA, Barclay ML, Merriman TR: Confirmation of association of IRGM and NCF4 with ileal Crohn's disease in a population-based cohort. Genes Immun 2008;9: 561–565.

82 Kuballa P, Huett A, Rioux JD, Daly MJ, Xavier RJ: Impaired autophagy of an intracellular pathogen induced by a Crohn's disease associated ATG16L1 variant. PLoS One 2008;3:e3391.

83 Saitoh T, Fujita N, Jang MH, Uematsu S, Yang BG, Satoh T, Omori H, Noda T, Yamamoto N, Komatsu M, Tanaka K, Kawai T, Tsujimura T, Takeuchi O, Yoshimori T, Akira S: Loss of the autophagy protein Atg16L1 enhances endotoxin-induced IL-1β production. Nature 2008;456:264–268.

84 Cadwell K, Liu JY, Brown SL, Miyoshi H, Loh J, Lennerz JK, Kishi C, Kc W, Carrero JA, Hunt S, Stone CD, Brunt EM, Xavier RJ, Sleckman BP, Li E, Mizushima N, Stappenbeck TS, Virgin HW 4th: A key role for autophagy and the autophagy gene Atg16l1 in mouse and human intestinal Paneth cells. Nature 2008;456:259–263.

85 Feng CG, Weksberg DC, Taylor GA, Sher A, Goodell MA: The p47 GTPase Lrg-47 (Irgm1) links host defense and hematopoietic stem cell proliferation. Cell Stem Cell 2008;2:83–89.

86 Feng CG, Zheng L, Jankovic D, Bafica A, Cannons JL, Watford WT, Chaussabel D, Hieny S, Caspar P, Schwartzberg PL, Lenardo MJ, Sher A: The immunity-related GTPase Irgm1 promotes the expansion of activated CD4+ T cell populations by preventing interferon-γ-induced cell death. Nat Immunol 2008;9:1279–1287.

Dig Dis 2009;27:252–258
DOI: 10.1159/000228558

The Microbiota in Inflammatory Bowel Disease in Different Age Groups

Salvatore Cucchiara[a]   Valerio Iebba[b]   Maria Pia Conte[b]   Serena Schippa[b]

[a]Pediatric Gastroenterology and Liver Unit, Department of Pediatrics, and [b]Microbiology Unit, Department of Public Health Sciences, Sapienza University of Rome, Rome, Italy

Key Words
Microbiota · Inflammatory bowel disease · Biodiversity

Abstract
Background: Many efforts were made in the past decades to assess the role of gut microbiota in inflammatory bowel diseases (IBD), leading to the hypothesis that an altered microbial composition, other than the presence of a specific pathogen, could be involved in the pathogenesis of the disease. On the other hand, existing differences in gut microbial community between distinct classes of age make sense of an increasing research in microbial shifts in IBD. **Methods:** Cultural, molecular, metabolomic and metagenomic approaches are trying to define the human gut microbiota in different age groups. **Results and Conclusion:** An increase in anaerobic bacteria (Bacteroides vulgatus, Streptococcus faecalis) was observed in adult IBD, whereas an increase in aerobic and facultative-anaerobic (Escherichia coli) was found in pediatric IBD. Overall higher bacterial cell counts were observed in IBD, jointly with a general loss of biodiversity and a preponderance of Bacteroidetes and a parallel decrease of Firmicutes phylum: a predominance of potential harmful members of Proteobacteria (E. coli) and low abundance of beneficial species (Faecalibacterium prausnitzii) was also reported in pediatric and adult age groups, respectively. Microbial community of elderly subjects contains a wider range of different species than those of children and adults, both in healthy and IBD status.   Copyright © 2009 S. Karger AG, Basel

Introduction

The mucosal surface of the human gastrointestinal tract is approximately 200–300 m^2 in area and is colonized by 10^{14} bacteria of greater than 1,000 different species and subspecies as detected by ordinary culture methods. The number of bacterial cells within the gastrointestinal tract outnumbers the host cell populations by 10:1, highlighting the relative importance of microbiota composition and metabolic activity on host homeostasis. How Scheline said in the 1973, 'the gastrointestinal microbiota has the ability to act as an organ with a metabolic potential at least equal to the liver', pointing out a rising research interest in evaluating the gut bacterial community composition [1]. However, most of the bacterial species present within the gastrointestinal tract still remain to be characterized, as well as their role in healthy people and inflammatory bowel disease (IBD) patients. In a recent review, Frank and Pace [2] showed the presence of around 45,000 phylotypes in the human gut, with only 10 of >100 described phyla identified so far. Furthermore, phylum-level diversity is not evenly distributed, with the majority of bacteria identified in all human guts belonging to just two phyla: the Firmicutes and the Bacteroidetes [3]. Conversely, there is great diversity at lower taxonomic levels (genera and species), bringing out such a microbial 'fingerprint' an individual quality. The astounding potential of our gut microflora lies in its 'plasticity' due to the different composition in bacterial species and their relative abundances, both subjected to al-

Salvatore Cucchiara
Pediatric Gastroenterology Unit, Head Pediatric Inflammatory Bowel Disease Center
University of Rome La Sapienza, Viale Regina Elena 324
IT–00161 Rome (Italy)
Tel. +39 064 997 9326, Fax +39 064 997 9325, E-Mail salvatore.cucchiara@uniroma1.it

terations in the human host lifetime. The next generation metagenomic studies will be addressed towards a comprehensive knowledge of the existing cross-talk between microbiota and mucosa, taking in awareness the concept of human gut districts as various and changeable niches for bacterial colonization. Nonetheless, a so-called 'holistic' approach spanning from metagenomic to metabolomic, via an ecological background, will give further insights into the mechanisms underlying the multiple activities of human gut microflora in IBD.

Microbiotica in Healthy Gut

Bacterial populations are not distributed evenly throughout the gastrointestinal tract. Their spatial organization varies along cephalic-caudal and luminal-epithelial axes, as reported by Swidsinski et al. [4] in FISH experiments conducted on human and mice gut biopsies. Bacterial numbers in different parts of the gastrointestinal tract appear to be influenced by multiple factors, including pH, peristalsis, redox potential, bacterial adhesion sites, bacterial cooperation/quorum signaling, mucin secretion, nutrient availability, diet, and bacterial antagonism. In adults, because of the low pH of the stomach and the relatively swift peristalsis through the stomach and the small bowel, the stomach and the upper two-thirds of the small intestine (duodenum and jejunum) contain only low numbers of micro-organisms, which range from 10^3 to 10^4 bacteria per milliliter of the gastric or intestinal contents. These are primarily acid-tolerant lactobacilli and streptococci. In the distal small intestine (ileum), the microbiota begins to resemble those of the colon, with numbers approaching 10^7 to 10^8 bacteria per milliliter of the intestinal contents. With decreased peristalsis, acidity, and lower oxidation-reduction potentials, the ileum maintains a more diverse microbiota and a higher bacterial population. The colon is the primary site of microbial colonization in humans, probably because of slow intestinal motility and the low oxidation-reduction potential. The colon harbors tremendous numbers and species of bacteria, most of which are obligate anaerobes, with numbers approaching 10^{10} to 10^{12} bacteria per milliliter of the intestinal contents. Members of the anaerobic genera *Bacteroides*, *Eubacterium*, *Clostridium*, *Ruminococcus*, and *Faecalibacterium* have typically been found to comprise a large majority of this gut district. Such a huge bacterial diversity gives to the colon the properties of a 'bioreactor' capable to degrade many food and xenobiotic compounds, leading to the production of metabolites with positive (short-chain fatty acids, SCAFs) or negative (ammines) effects on mucosal homeostasis [5].

The gut microflora is acquired during the first 2 years of life. The ability of a species to establish itself durably in the colonic ecosystem depends on complex interactions between host and bacteria [6] as well as between the bacteria themselves. Relevant factors pertaining at birth, notably environmental conditions and hygiene, are currently a topic of great interest because of changes recently observed in intestinal colonization profiles in babies and possible links with the explosion of allergic disease in developed countries.

Continually exposed to novel bacteria, the baby's microbiota subsequently diversifies until a profile considered as more or less identical to that of an adult is established by the age of about two [7]. In normal conditions, the colonic redox potential is high at this stage of life, so strict anaerobes cannot grow and the first colonizing bacteria are aerobic species or facultative anaerobes (staphylococci, enterococci and enteric bacteria). These proliferate rapidly in the colon to reach a level of 10^{10} CFU per gram of contents. They consume oxygen thereby leading to a drop in the local redox potential: after about one week of life, strictly anaerobic species such as *Bifidobacterium*, *Bacteroides* and *Clostridium* colonize the colon. Conversely, oxygen level falls and density of aerobes decreases [7, 8]. All infants are initially colonized by large numbers of *E. coli* and streptococci. Within a few days, bacterial numbers reach 10^8 to 10^{10} per gram of feces [7, 9]. During the first week of life, these bacteria create a reducing environment favorable for the subsequent bacterial succession of strict anaerobic species mainly belonging to the genera *Bifidobacterium*, *Bacteroides*, *Clostridium* and *Ruminococcus* [10]. Breast-fed babies become dominated by bifidobacteria, possibly due to the contents of bifidobacterial growth factors in breast milk [11]. In contrast, the microbiota of formula-fed infants is more diverse with high numbers of Enterobacteriaceae, Enterococci, Bifidobacteria, Bacteroides, and Clostridia [12, 13]. After the introduction of solid food and weaning, the microflora of breast-fed infants becomes similar to that of formula-fed infants. By the second year of life the fecal microflora resembles that of adults.

We have to rule out the statement 'pediatric patients' as 'little people', because their developing gut microbial 'organ' has profound differences compared to that of adults, mainly in the intrinsic resistance and resilience properties. As described above, the infant GI microbiota is more variable in its composition and less stable over time. In the first year of life, the infant intestinal tract

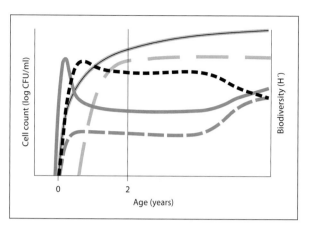

Fig. 1. Microbial community succession during life course. Relative bacterial abundances in fecal samples of newborn, pediatric, adult and elderly healthy patients. The vertical line shows the partition between pediatric and adult ages from an intestinal microbiota point of view. Bacterial species are depicted as follows: solid line = *Escherichia* spp., *Streptococcus* spp.; dotted line = *Bifidobacteria* spp.; dashed line = *Lactobacillus* spp.; long-dashed line = *Bacteroides* spp., *Peptococcus* spp. H'; solid bold line = Shannon-Weaver index of diversity, taking into account the number of species and their relative abundances.

progresses from sterility to extremely dense colonization, ending with a mixture of microbes that is broadly very similar to that found in the adult intestine [14], so the microbial succession is far more chaotic and driven by local changes due to perinatal exposures, genetic background and syntrophisms between colonizing bacterial species. In contrast, each adult's gut appears to have a unique microbial community, with a structure that remains stable on the time scale of years (fig. 1) [15, 16]. However, a recognizably climax (adult) community is not attained for several years after birth [17]. By then, the bifidobacterial population comprises just a few percent of the community. The remarkable population shifts that occur in the infant bowel during the first year of life coincide with the continuing development of immunological foci in the bowel mucosa. The stimuli evoked by bacterial antigens in early life might have long lasting, even lifelong, influences on the human immune system. Interestingly, differences in the species composition of bifidobacterial populations have been observed in children of different nationalities with different prevalence of atopic diseases, and between children of allergic and non-allergic status [18–21].

The composition of the microbiota varies from individual to individual and may also vary with changing

physiological and pathological conditions. Zoetendal et al. [15] estimate that a DGGE profile reveals between 90 and 99% of the bacteria present. In sixteen adults, they described highly variable profiles with differences in both the number and positions of bands. In contrast, the profile for any given individual remained very stable over time, suggesting that every healthy person has a distinct but fairly constant microbiota. A few bands were common to all subjects, and sequence analysis of these bands revealed strong homologies to *Ruminococcus obeum*, *Eubacterium hallii* and *Fusobacterium prausnitzii*, these species are often found in the human microbiota and probably play important functional roles [22, 23]. Franks et al. [24] used in situ hybridization combined with image analysis to study microfloral variability in 78 samples prepared at different times from a total of 9 subjects. There was more variability in the *Bacteroides* group than in the *Clostridium coccoides* group and in every single subject, it was the *Bifidobacterium* group which varied the most. Another study focused on temporal variations in *Bifidobacterium* in 5 adults: profiles proved to be host-specific and remained stable over the four weeks of the experiment [25]. DGGE has shown that *Lactobacillus* populations remain more constant in adults than they do in babies [26].

Finally, a few studies have focused on the intestinal microbiota in the elderly. Mitsuoka [27] showed rises in Clostridia, enteric bacteria and Enterococci. In the same vein, a more recent study combining a molecular dot-blot approach with fatty acid analysis showed that the number of anaerobes falls and the number of Enterobacteriaceae rises with age [28]. It has also been shown that microbiota diversity tends to increase with age, with routine probes only detecting about 50% of the microbiota of an elderly subject (compared with 80% in a normal adult) suggesting that species remain to be identified [29].

Microbiotica in IBD

As mammals have harbored their commensal partners for millennia, adaptive co-evolution has formed an inextricable bond between microbe and host [30]. Imbalances in the microbiota may contribute to some human diseases, and altered composition of the gut bacteria has been implicated in obesity [31]. Many studies point toward a pathogenic role of commensal gut microflora in IBD. Antibiotic treatment alleviates intestinal inflammation in humans and experimental animals. Germ-free rederivation of animals genetically susceptible to colitis

Table 1. Alterations of gut microbiota associated with IBD detected in fecal samples

Alteration in gut microbiota	Number of subjects	Method used	Reference
Enterobacteria observed more frequently in CD; more instability	17 CD, 16 controls	dot-blot TGGE	[48]
Firmicute phylotypes less diverse and less abundant	6 CD, 6 controls	metagenomic sequencing	[49]
Lower temporal stability of dominant bacteria in CD; lower diversity of lactic acid bacteria in CD	11 CD/remission, 5 CD/active, 18 controls	DGGE	[50]
Higher proportion of bacteria detected in control subjects with 6 probes; *Clostridium coccoides* group reduced in UC; *Clostridium leptum* group reduced in CD; *Bacteroides* group more abundant in IC	13 CD, 13 UC, 5 IC, 13 controls	FISH	[51]
Lower bacterial diversity in CD; healthy twins more similar than CD twins; alterations in abundances of *Bacteroides* species	10 CD monozygotic twin pairs, 8 control monozygotic twin pairs	TRFLP %G+C profiling	[52]

CD = Crohn's disease; DGGE = denaturing gradient gel electrophoresis; FISH = fluorescent in situ hybridization; %G+C = percent guanine plus cytosine profiling; IBD = irritable bowel disease; IC = infectious colitis; TGGE = temperature gradient gel electrophoresis; TRFLP = terminal restriction fragment length polymorphism; UC = ulcerative colitis.

prevents development of intestinal inflammation. Therefore, in animal models, the gut microflora is a crucial factor in the induction and maintenance of intestinal lesions [32]. This notion is highlighted by a recent study conducted on T-bet-deficient mice by Garrett and colleagues. This interesting research showed how in this immunodeficient mice the colonic environment facilitates the growth of colitogenic bacteria whose behavior is then modulated by cytokines, including TNF-α, leading to an increase in the growth rate of specific bacteria (anaerobic) and to enhance virulence attributes, including adherence and invasion. Once generated, this community of bacteria drives intestinal inflammation even in immunocompetent mice that express T-bet [33].

In humans and other animals, inflammatory responses are apparently directed towards specific subsets of commensal organisms that have pathogenic potential but are not typically infectious pathogenic agents. All mammals harbor these species, but it is unknown why inflammation arises only in those patients affected by IBD. Investigations aimed at detecting novel pathogens in Crohn's disease and ulcerative colitis patients achieved no such resounding results [34]. *Mycobacterium avium* ssp. *pseudotuberculosis* (MAP), the cause of Johne's disease in farm animals, has long been suspected to be the etiological agent of Crohn's disease, but convincing evidence of cause and effect has yet to be obtained [35]. *Escherichia coli* strains (Adherent Invasive *Escherichia Coli*, AIEC) that adhere to the mucosa of the terminal ileum have been de-

tected in some Crohn's disease patients and might be responsible for disease in a subset of patients [36].

Some investigators have predicted that, in addition to genetic factors, an imbalance in the normal microbiota without acquisition of an infectious organism is at least partially responsible for IBD [1, 37]. Metagenomic studies have shown that entire classes of bacteria are lost or over-represented as part of the IBD process [2, 3]. Perhaps in certain disorders where environmental factors are implicated, an imbalance between commensal bacteria with pathogenic potential (which we term pathobionts) and symbionts (commensal bacteria with beneficial potential) in the microbiota has a role in pathogenesis. Recently, it has been observed that the gut microbiotas of elderly subjects contain a wider range of different species than those of younger, healthy adults [38]. The same is true of the fecal microbiota of patients who suffer from Crohn's disease. Most light has been shed on the pathogenic role of the gut microflora in Crohn's disease by work on the model of endoscopic recurrence following surgery. After surgical resection of the terminal ileum followed by ileocolonic anastomosis, endoscopic recurrence occurred within one year in 73% of cases. It has been shown that the instillation of ileal contents into the excluded colon led to clinical recurrence within one week in 60% of patients with Crohn's disease in remission, suggesting that the gut microflora has a primordial role in the phenomenon.

Differences in bacterial species were observed between IBD children and adults. In adults, the intestinal mucosa

Table 2. Alterations of gut microbiota associated with IBD detected using mucosal biopsy samples

Alteration in gut microbiota	Number of subjects	Method used	Reference
Reduction in diversity due to loss of *Bacteroides*, *Eubacterium* and *Lactobacillus species*	57 IBD, 46 controls	SSCP rDNA sequencing Real-time PCR	[53]
Bacteria more abundant in IBD patients *Bacteroides* dominant in IBD *Eubacterium rectale-Clostridium coccoides* group dominant in IBS	50 CD, 60 non-CD controls	FISH	[54]
Distinctive clustering of DGGE fingerprints Greater variability among CD patients' microbiota *Clostridium* cluster XIVa more prevalent in CD *Ruminococcus torques*-like phylotype more prevalent in CD *Enterobacteriaceae* more prevalent in CD *Faecalibacterium prausnitzii*-like phylotype more prevalent in controls	19 CD, 15 controls, 1 UC, 1 IC	DGGE rDNA sequencing	[55]
Lower abundance of *Bacteroidetes* and higher abundance of *Firmicutes* associated with inflamed tissue of IBD patients Species richness highest in noninflamed tissue samples of IBD patients	10 CD, 15 UC, 16 controls	ARISA TRFLP	[56]
Faecalibacterium prausnitzii associated with lower risk of postoperative relapse in CD *Faecalibacterium prausnitzii* reduced severity of colitis and balanced dysbiosis induced in mice	9 UC, 9 controls	FISH real-time PCR	[57]
Clone libraries of CD, UC and non-IBD differ significantly *Lachnospiraceae* and *Bacteroidetes* less abundant in IBD	CD, UC non-IBD GI patients	rDNA sequencing real-time PCR	[58]
Low abundance of *F. prausnitzii* and high abundance of *Escherichia coli* associated with ileal CD	6 discordant monozygotic CD twin pairs 4 concordant monozygotic CD twin pairs	TRFLP rDNA sequencing real-time PCR	[59]

ARISA = Automated ribosomal intergenic spacer analysis; CD = Crohn's disease; DGGE = denaturing gradient gel electrophoresis; FISH = fluorescence in situ hybridization; IBD = inflammatory bowel disease; IBS = irritable bowel syndrome; IC = ischemic colitis; rDNA = ribosomal deoxyribonucleic acid; real-time PCR = real-time polymerase chain reaction; SSCP = single-strand conformation polymorphism; TRFLP = terminal restriction fragment length polymorphism; UC = ulcerative colitis.

of an IBD patient is colonized by an abundant gut microflora, especially in ulcers and fistulae. Cartun et al. [39] detected antigens of *Escherichia coli* and *Streptococcus* in 69 and 63%, respectively, of resected tissues from patients with Crohn's disease. In a number of studies, high levels of antibodies directed against various bacteria of the saprophytic microflora (notably *Bacteroides*, *Streptococcus faecalis* and *E. coli*) have been measured in the blood of patients with Crohn's disease. Most studies so far of the gut microflora of patients suffering from Crohn's disease and ulcerative colitis have been based on fecal and mucosal samples (tables 1, 2). Such studies have shown increased densities of anaerobic bacteria, notably of *Bacteroides vulgatus* and certain Gram-positive cocci (*Eubacterium*, *Peptostreptococcus* and *Coprococcus*). This pattern could be

genetically determined since, in a prospective study, Van de Merwe et al. [40] showed that one-third of the children (who were symptom-free) of patients with Crohn's disease had higher fecal densities of anaerobic bacteria than control subjects, although this observation has not yet been confirmed. Keighley et al. [41] detected significant increases in the numbers of *Escherichia coli* and *Bacteroides fragilis* in the ileum and colon of patients with Crohn's disease. In three distinct cohorts of adult UC patients, Hartley et al. [42] observed reduced numbers of *Bifidobacterium* and increased colonization by *E. coli* in the involved segments. In another study on the microflora associated with the ileal mucosa, Enterobacteria were isolated more often from biopsies from patients with Crohn's disease than from control subjects [43].

About 15% of IBD patients are diagnosed before the age of 18 years with an incidence of 12 new cases every 100,000 each year [44], and few studies were addressed in understanding the microbiota involvement. A pilot study [45] in pediatric IBD conducted on 12 CD, 7 UC, 6 CI and 10 control patients found a higher number of mucosa-associated aerobic and facultative-anaerobic bacteria with high cell count of *E. coli*, a potentially harmful commensal, and a parallel decrease in *Bacteroides vulgatus* levels. This increase in members of *Enterobacteriaceae* family, in which Gram-negative bacteria predominate, could promote an enhanced mucosal inflammation due to the enormous amounts of bacterial antigens and micrometabolites. Recently, a second study [46] conducted on *E. coli* strains isolated from the aforementioned patients showed a well-defined clustering of pulsed field gel electrophoresis (PFGE) profiles according to CD, UC and control groups. This result supports the idea about a disease-associated gut microenvironment that selects similar *E. coli* clones: nonetheless, the existence of subgroups in the same cluster may be the consequence of actual subtypes of CD and UC.

An interesting study reported that the bacterial profiles associated with biopsies are not different between inflamed and noninflamed mucosa [47]. In this proposition, the genetic predisposition of patients to abnormal permeability of the bowel mucosa enables entry of commensal antigens into subepithelial tissues. It might be more useful to identify bacterial antigens and metabolites against which the immune cells of Crohn's disease and ulcerative colitis patients react, and to determine simultaneous shifts in community composition. Future studies (most of which are running) will be focused on this latter approach to get a 'holistic' knowledge of the intimate cross-talk existing between the gut microbiota community and the mucosal surface.

Disclosure Statement

The authors declare that no financial or other conflict of interest exists in relation to the content of the article.

References

1 O'Hara AM, Shanahan F: The gut flora as a forgotten organ. EMBO Rep 2006;7:688–693.
2 Frank DN, Pace NR: Gastrointestinal microbiology enters the metagenomics era. Curr Opin Gastroenterol 2008;24:4–10.
3 Peterson DA, Frank DN, Pace RN, Gordon JI: Metagenomic approaches for defining the pathogenesis of inflammatory bowel diseases. Cell Host Microbe 2008;3:417–427.
4 Swidsinski A, Loening-Baucke V, Lochs H, Hale LP: Spatial organization of bacterial flora in normal and inflamed intestine: a fluorescence in situ hybridization study in mice. World J Gastroenterol 2005;11:1131–1140.
5 Neish AS: Microbes in gastrointestinal health and disease. Gastroenterology 2009; 136:65–80.
6 Khachatryan ZA, Ktsoyan ZA, Manukyan GP, et al: Predominant role of host genetics in controlling the composition of gut microbiota. PLoS One 2008;3:e3064.
7 Mackie R, Sghir A, Gaskins HR: Developmental microbial ecology of the neonatal gastrointestinal tract. Am J Clin Nutr 1999; 69:1035S–1045S.
8 Heavey PM, Rowland IR: The gut microflora of the developing infant: microbiology and metabolism. Microbial Ecol Health Dis 1999; 11:75–83.

9 Schwiertz A, Gruhl B, Lobnitz M, Michel P, Radke M, Blaut M: Development of the intestinal bacterial composition in hospitalized preterm infants in comparison with breast-fed, full-term infants. Pediatr Res 2003;54: 393–399.
10 Favier CF, Vaughan EE, De Vos WM, Akkermans AD: Molecular monitoring of succession of bacterial communities in human neonates. Appl Envir Microbiol 2002;68: 219–226.
11 Coppa GV, Bruni S, Morelli L, Soldi S, Gabrielli O: The first prebiotics in humans: human milk oligosaccharides. J Clin Gastroenterol 2004;38:S80–S83.
12 Harmsen HJ, Wildeboer-Veloo AC, Raangs GC, Wagendorp AA, Klijn N, Bindels JG, Welling GW: Analysis of intestinal flora development in breast-fed and formula-fed infants by using molecular identification and detection methods. J Pediatr Gastroenterol Nutr 2000;30:61–67.
13 Fanaro S, Chierici R, Guerrini P, Vigi V: Intestinal microflora in early infancy: composition and development. Acta Paediatr 2003; 91:48–55.
14 Palmer C, Bik EM, DiGiulio DB, Relman DA, Brown PO: Development of the human infant intestinal microbiota. PLoS Biol 2007;5:e177.

15 Zoetendal EG, Akkermans ADL, De Vos WM: Temperature gradient gel electrophoresis analysis of 16S rRNA from human fecal samples reveals stable and host-specific communities of active bacteria. Appl Environ Microbiol 1998;64:3854–3859.
16 Eckburg PB, Bik EM, Bernstein CN, et al: Diversity of the human intestinal microbial flora. Science 2005;308:1635–1638.
17 Tannock GW, Cook G: Enterococci as members of the intestinal microflora of humans; in Gilmore MS (ed): The Enterococci: Pathogenesis, Molecular Biology, and Antibiotic Resistance. Washinghton, ASM Press, 2002, pp 101–132.
18 Gore C, et al: *Bifidobacterium pseudocatenulatum* is associated with atopic eczema: a nested case-control study investigating the fecal microbiota of infants. J Allergy Clin Immunol 2008;121:135–140.
19 Young SL, et al: Bifidobacterial species differentially affect expression of cell surface markers and cytokines of dendritic cells harvested from cord blood. Clin Diagn Lab Immunol 2004;11:686–690.
20 Ouwehand AC, et al: Differences in Bifidobacterium flora composition in allergic and healthy infants. J Allergy Clin Immunol 2001;108:144–145.

21 Sepp E, et al: Intestinal microflora of Estonian and Swedish infants. Acta Paediatr 1997;86:956–961.

22 Suau A, Bonnet R, Sutren M, et al: Direct analysis of genes encoding 16S rRNA from complex communities reveals many novel molecular species within the human gut. Appl Environ Microbiol 1999;65:4799–4807.

23 Zoetendal EG, Ben-Amor K, Harmsen HJM, Schut F, Akkermans ADL, De Vos WM: Quantification of uncultured *Ruminococcus obeum*-like bacteria in human fecal samples by fluorescent in situ hybridization and flow cytometry using 16S rRNA-targeted probes. Appl Environ Microbiol 2002;68:4225–4232.

24 Franks AH, Harmsen HJM, Raangs GC, Jansen GJ, Schut F, Welling GW: Variations of bacterial populations in human feces measured by fluorescent in situ hybridization with group-specific 16S rRNA-targeted oligonucleotide probes. Appl Environ Microbiol 1998;64:3336–3345.

25 Satokari RM, Vaughan EE, Akkermans ADL, Saarela M, De Vos WM: Bifidobacterial diversity in human feces detected by genus-specific PCR and denaturing gradient gel electrophoresis. Appl Environ Microbiol 2001;67:504–513.

26 Heilig HG, Zoetendal EG, Vaughan EE, Marteau P, Akkermans ADL, De Vos WM: Molecular diversity of *Lactobacillus* spp. and other lactic acid bacteria in the human intestine as determined by specific amplification of 16S ribosomal DNA. Appl Environ Microbiol 2002;68:114–123.

27 Mitsuoka T: Intestinal flora and aging. Nutr Rev 1992;50:438–446.

28 Hopkins MJ, Sharp R, Macfarlane GT: Age and disease related changes in intestinal bacterial populations assessed by cell culture. 16S rRNA abundance and community cellular fatty acid profiles. Gut 2001;48:198–205.

29 Saunier K, Dore J: Gastrointestinal tract and the elderly: functional foods, gut microflora and healthy ageing. Dig Liver Dis 2002;34:S19–S24.

30 Liu CH, Lee SM, Vanlare JM, Kasper DL, Mazmanian SK: Regulation of surface architecture by symbiotic bacteria mediates host colonization. Proc Natl Acad Sci USA 2008;105:3951–3956.

31 Turnbaugh PJ, et al: An obesity-associated gut microbiome with increased capacity for energy harvest. Nature 2006;444:1027–1031.

32 Sartor RB: Microbial influences in inflammatory bowel diseases. Gastroenterology 2008;134:577–594.

33 Garrett WS, Lord GM, Punit S, et al: Communicable ulcerative colitis induced by T-bet deficiency in the innate immune system. Cell 2007;131:33–45.

34 Strober W, et al: The fundamental basis of inflammatory bowel disease. J Clin Invest 2007;117:514–521.

35 Peyrin-Biroulet L, et al: Antimycobacterial therapy in Crohn's disease: game over? Gastroenterology 2007;132:2594–2598.

36 Darfeuille-Michaud A, et al: High prevalence of adherent-invasive *Escherichia coli* associated with ileal mucosa in Crohn's disease. Gastroenterology 2004;127:412–421.

37 Tannock GW: The search for disease-associated compositional shifts in bowel bacterial communities of humans. Trends Microbiol 2008;16:488–495.

38 Guigoza Y, Doré JI, Schiffrina EJ: The inflammatory status of old age can be nurtured from the intestinal environment. Curr Opin Clin Nutr Metab Care 2008;11:13–20.

39 Cartun RW, Van Kruiningen HJ, Pedersen CA, et al: An immunocytochemical search for infectious agents in Crohn's disease. Mod Pathol 1993;6:212–219.

40 Van de Merwe JP, Schroder AM, Wensinck F, Hazenberg MP: The obligate anaerobic faecal flora of patients with Crohn's disease and their first-degree relatives. Scand J Gastroenterol 1988;23:1125–1131.

41 Keighley MR, Arabi Y, Dimock F, Burdon DW, Allan RN, Alexander-Williams J: Influence of inflammatory bowel disease on intestinal microflora. Gut 1978;19:1099–1104.

42 Hartley MG, Hudson MJ, Swarbrick ET, et al: The rectal mucosa-associated microflora in patients with ulcerative colitis. J Med Microbiol 1992;36:96–103.

43 Peach S, Lock MR, Katz D, Todd IP, Tabaqchali S: Mucosal-associated bacterial flora of the intestine in patients with Crohn's disease and in a control group. Gut 1978;19:1034–1042.

44 Nieuwenhuis EES, Escher JC: Early onset IBD: what's the difference? Dig Liver Dis 2008;40:12–15.

45 Conte MP, Schippa S, et al: Gut-associated bacterial microbiota in paediatric patients with inflammatory bowel disease. Gut 2006;55:1760–1767.

46 Schippa S, Conte MP, et al: Dominant genotypes in mucosa-associated *Escherichia coli* strains from pediatric patients with inflammatory bowel disease. Inflamm Bowel Dis 2009;15:661–672.

47 Vasquez N, Mangin I, et al: Patchy distribution of mucosal lesions in ileal Crohn's disease is not linked to differences in the dominant mucosa-associated bacteria: a study using fluorescence in situ hybridization and temporal temperature gradient gel electrophoresis. Inflamm Bowel Dis 2007;13:684–692.

48 Seksik P, Rigottier-Gois L, Gramet G, Sutren M, Pochart P, Marteau P, Jian R, Doré J: Alterations of the dominant faecal bacterial groups in patients with Crohn's disease of the colon. Gut 2003;52:237–242.

49 Manichanh C, Rigottier-Gois L, Bonnaud E, Gloux K, Pelletier E, Frangeul L, Nalin R, Jarrin C, Chardon P, Marteau P, Roca J, Doré J: Reduced diversity of faecal microbiota in Crohn's disease revealed by a metagenomic approach. Gut 2006;55:205–211.

50 Scanlan PD, Shanahan F, O'Mahony C, Marchesi JR: Culture-independent analyses of temporal variation of the dominant fecal microbiota and targeted bacterial subgroups in Crohn's disease. J Clin Microbiol 2006;44:3980–3988.

51 Sokol H, Seksik P, Rigottier-Gois L, Lay C, Lepage P, Podglajen I, Marteau P, Doré J: Specificities of the fecal microbiota in inflammatory bowel disease. Inflamm Bowel Dis 2006;12:106–111.

52 Dicksved J, Halfvarson J, Rosenquist M, Jarnerot G, Tysk C, Apajalahti J, Engstrand L, Jansson JK: Molecular analysis of the gut microbiota of identical twins with Crohn's disease. ISME J 2008;2:716–727.

53 Ott SJ, Musfeldt M, Wenderoth DF, Hampe J, Brant O, Folsch UR, Timmis KN, Schreiber S: Reduction in diversity of the colonic mucosa associated bacterial microflora in patients with active inflammatory bowel disease. Gut 2004;53:685–693.

54 Weber AJ, Loening-Baucke V, Hale LP, Lochs H: Spatial organization and composition of the mucosal flora in patients with inflammatory bowel disease. J Clin Microbiol 2005;43:3380–3389.

55 Martinez-Medina M, Aldeguer X, Gonzalez-Huix F, Acero D, Garcia-Gil LJ: Abnormal microbiota composition in the ileocolonic mucosa of Crohn's disease patients as revealed by polymerase chain reaction-denaturing gradient gel electrophoresis. Inflamm Bowel Dis 2006;12:1136–1145.

56 Sepehri S, Kotlowski R, Bernstein CN, Krause DO: Microbial diversity of inflamed and noninflamed gut biopsy tissues in inflammatory bowel disease. Inflamm Bowel Dis 2007;13:675–683.

57 Sokol H, Pigneur B, Watterlot L, Lakhdari O, Bermúdez-Humarán LG, Gratadoux JJ, Blugeon S, Bridonneau C, Furet JP, Corthier G, Grangette C, Vasquez N, Pochart P, Trugnan G, Thomas G, Blottière HM, Doré J, Marteau P, Seksik P, Langella P: *Faecalibacterium prausnitzii* is an anti-inflammatory commensal bacterium identified by gut microbiota analysis of Crohn disease patients. Proc Natl Acad Sci USA 2008;105:16731–16736.

58 Frank DN, St Amand AL, Feldman RA, Boedeker EC, Harpaz N, Pace NR: Molecular phylogenetic characterization of microbial community imbalances in human inflammatory bowel diseases. Proc Natl Acad Sci USA 2007;104:13780–13785.

59 Willing B, Halfvarson J, Dicksved J, Rosenquist M, Järnerot G, Engstrand L, Tysk C, Jansson JK: Twin studies reveal specific imbalances in the mucosa-associated microbiota of patients with ileal Crohn's disease. Inflamm Bowel Dis 2009;15:653–660.

Dig Dis 2009;27:259–268
DOI: 10.1159/000228559

What Is the Role of Serological Markers in IBD? Pediatric and Adult Data

Marla Dubinsky

Pediatric IBD Center, Cedars-Sinai Medical Center, David Geffen School of Medicine, Los Angeles, Calif., USA

Key Words
Crohn's disease · Ulcerative colitis · Perinuclear
anti-neutrophil antibody · Anti-*Saccharomyces cerevisiae*
antibody · Natural history

Abstract
Physicians rely heavily on the presence of disease markers to support or even at times modify their clinical impression for certain diseases that can only be diagnosed clinically. Typically these markers play an important role in helping to establish a diagnosis and to evaluate the activity of a chronic disease over time. The diagnosis of inflammatory bowel disease (IBD), however, is not based solely on clinical grounds. Invasive endoscopic and radiological as well as histopathological criteria need to be met in order to make a correct diagnosis and differentiate disease subtypes. The search for novel diagnostic approaches that accurately distinguishes a group of patients with IBD from those unaffected by the disease has become a focus in IBD research. This search, however, has taken a very exciting turn in the direction of finding biologic and genetic markers that can assess the natural history and predict the course of individual's disease including response to treatments over time.

Copyright © 2009 S. Karger AG, Basel

Introduction

The search for the underlying trigger of the abnormal intestinal inflammatory reaction characteristic of inflammatory bowel disease (IBD) has led to the discovery of antibodies present specifically in the blood of patients with Crohn's disease (CD) and/or ulcerative colitis (UC). Immune responses to resident intestinal flora in humans have been reported. Duchmann et al. [1] demonstrated that CD patients boast reactivity to hundreds of bacterial antigens created from sonification of multiple bacterial specifies including enterobacteria, bacteroides and bifidobacterium.

Perinuclear anti-neutrophil antibody (pANCA) is noted for its association with UC or a UC-like phenotype. This IBD-specific ANCA displays a unique perinuclear highlighting (pANCA) on immunofluorescence staining and is DNAse sensitive [2]. Although it remains undefined, it has been suggested that the antigen to which pANCA is directed is a nuclear histone (H1) [3]. This antigen is clearly distinct from the proteinase 3 or the myeloperoxidase reactivity observed in those pANCA and cANCA patients with vasculitic disorders. pANCA is likely an autoantibody that is representative of a cross-reactivity with a luminal bacterial antigen [4–6]. pANCA has been shown repeatedly to be prevalent in the sera of approximately 60 and 20% of UC and CD patients, re-

Marla Dubinsky, MD
Director, Pediatric IBD Center, Cedars-Sinai Medical Center
David Geffen School of Medicine
Los Angeles, CA 90048 (USA)
E-Mail dubinskym@csmc.edu

spectively [7–13]. ASCA (anti-*Saccharomyces cerevisiae* antibody) is another important antibody marker that is present in the blood of individuals with IBD. Studies in both the adult and pediatric IBD population have demonstrated that ASCA is found in the blood of approximately 60% of CD, 10% of UC and <5% of non-IBD patients [7–9]. Antibodies to *S. cerevisiae* (ASCA) was the first CD-specific immune response thought to be targeted towards microbial antigens. IgA and IgG antibodies are directed against a specific oligomannosidic epitope present on the cell wall of the yeast saccharomyces that shares homology with intestinal bacteria [14]. To date, it remains unclear as to the specific bacterial drive behind ASCA production. One interesting study published in *World Journal of Gastroenterology* looked at whether or not ASCA in the serum was correlated with *S. cerevisiae* present in the mucosa [15]. The investigators found that the presence of *S. cerevisiae* in the colonic mucosal biopsy was very rare. This attempted to examine whether there was some cross-reactivity with yeast in the mucosa, but there did not appear to be an association. ASCA is part of the family of anti-glycan (carbohydrate) antibodies. Other anti-glycan antibodies, antibodies against laminaribioside (ALCA) and chitobioside (ACCA) have been studied in IBD [16].

In addition to the anti-glycan antibodies, 3 additional markers representative of microbial driven immune responses have been identified; antibodies to the *Escherichia coli* outer-membrane porin C (OmpC), the *Pseudomonas fluorescens* CD-related protein (anti-CD-related bacterial sequence I2) and the CBir1 flagellin. Antibodies to OmpC, whose antigen is purified from commensal *E. coli* [6, 17], have been reported in 37–55% of patients with CD and 2–11% of patients with UC, while no more than 5% of non-IBD individuals express anti-OmpC [18–20]. I2 was isolated from affected colonic mucosa in CD patients yet not in the unaffected segments [17]. Immune responses to this antigen are present in up to 55% of CD patients; it has also been detected in the serum of UC patients (10%) and in up to 20% of non-IBD patients rendering this marker less specific for CD [17, data on file Prometheus Labs]. Serologic expression cloning was used to identify an immunodominant antigen, CBir1 flagellin, to which strong immune responses (B cell and CD4T cell) occurred in colitic mice [21]. Subsequent human studies reported 50% prevalence of seroreactivity to CBir1 in CD patients whereas UC, inflammatory and healthy controls exhibited little to no reactivity to this flagellin [22]. As seen with the genetic and clinical heterogeneity of CD, studies have shown immune response (immune pheno-

type) heterogeneity exists among CD patients. Landers et al. [17] analyzed immune response heterogeneity in 330 patients and found that ASCA was detected in 56% of patients; 55% were seroreactive to OmpC C, 50% were seroreactive to I2, and 23% were pANCA. Eighty-five percent responded to at least 1 antigen; only 4% responded to all 4. Among microbial antigens (ASCA, OmpC, I2), 78% responded to at least 1, and 57% were double positive, but only 26% responded to all 3. The level of response was stable over time and with change in disease activity. Among patients with the same qualitative antigen-response profiles, quantitative response differed. Moreover, this study demonstrated that CD patients could be clustered into 4 distinct groups depending on their immune response patterns to microbial or autoantigens. One cluster was ASCA, a second was antibodies to OmpC and I2, the third pANCA and the fourth was low or no immune response to any tested antigens. Subsequent analyses incorporating CBir1 demonstrated that antibodies to CBir1 are present in approximately 40% of CD patients negative for antibodies to specific microbial antigens (ASCA, OmpC and I2) which suggests a unique immune phenotype [21]. Immune reactivity to CBir1 may further define CD phenotypes in that anti-CBir1 expression is present in 40–44% of pANCA-positive CD patients versus only 4% in pANCA-positive UC patients. This difference may denote a unique etiopathogenic mechanism of disease that helps to further stratify patients based on immunogenetic phenotypes.

Given the CD- and UC-specific characteristics of ASCA and pANCA, these markers were initially introduced as markers used to differentiate CD from UC in indeterminate cases. However, as the number of identified antibody markers increased as well as improved test sensitivity, consideration has been given to these tests as adjunctive diagnostic tools and as possible prognostic indicators, given their association with disease phenotype.

Differentiating IBD from Non-IBD

The recognition of IBD and subsequent diagnostic evaluation, in most cases, can be straightforward when the clinical presentation is unambiguous. However, a diagnostic challenge arises in patients who present with overlapping, nonspecific and indolent symptoms that are characteristic of both organic and nonorganic disorders. In the face of diagnostic uncertainty clinicians are often obligated to exclude IBD using invasive diagnostic testing, in particular contrast radiography and colonoscopy with biopsies. Suspicion of IBD commonly results in extensive diagnostic investigations of patients who are ultimately found to have a functional bowel disorder. In contrast, the diagnosis of IBD, particularly CD, can be missed or delayed due to the nonspecific nature of both the intestinal and extraintestinal symptoms at presentation. Given these clinical challenges, the search has intensified for an accurate noninvasive diagnostic marker to aid clinicians in the prompt recognition of IBD and the differentiation of these disorders from mimickers.

The ideal noninvasive diagnostic test is both highly sensitive and specific. Moreover, it should be as good as the gold standard. To date, no such test has been developed; however, advances in testing strategies and the addition of novel markers have helped the characteristics of available tests. Numerous studies have examined the diagnostic value of these markers, ASCA and pANCA in particular, in IBD and non-IBD patients. Peeters et al. [23] found that positivity for both markers was significantly lower in healthy and non-IBD controls. The sensitivity, specificity, PPV, and NPV for differentiating IBD from controls were: ASCA+: 60% (243/407), 91% (345/378), 88% (243/276), and 68% (345/509); pANCA+: 50% (73/147), 95% (605/638), 69% (73/106), and 89% (605/679); ASCA+/pANCA−: 56% (229/407), 94% (355/378), 91% (229/252), and 67% (355/533); and pANCA+/ASCA−: 44% (65/147), 97% (620/638), 78% (65/83), and 88% (620/702). This study concluded that the specificity of serological markers for IBD is high, but low sensitivity making them less useful as diagnostic tests. The combination, however, of these tests is probably more powerful as a tool to differentiate IBD from non IBD. A similar study was performed in the pediatric age group [24]. Serum was collected from 120 children with new or established diagnoses of UC (n = 25) or CD (n = 20) and non-IBD patients (n = 74). This group also confirmed that the highest sensitivity for detecting inflammatory bowel disease, 71%, was achieved by using ANCA and ASCA together. A prospective study was then performed in children with non-alarm-type symptoms undergoing a complete diagnostic evaluation to rule in or out IBD (small bowel follow through and EGD and colonoscopy), at the same time they underwent serologic testing [25]. Diagnosis of IBD versus non-IBD was made based on gold standard and blinded to serological analyses. The test characteristics of these markers were then examined using a sequential diagnostic testing strategy. In this study the modified serodiagnostic assay was more sensitive (81 vs.

69%), whereas the traditional assay had a higher specificity (96 vs. 72%) for IBD (p < 0.05). The results of this study suggested that by sequencing from a sensitive test to a more specific test the false-positive diagnoses would have been reduced by 81%, yielding an overall sequential testing strategy accuracy of 84%. A decision analysis followed which reported that the sequential serodiagnostic strategies resulted in the largest cost savings (USD 550 per average patient) with an average cost per correct diagnosis of USD 1,640 compared to USD 2,188 for standard invasive testing. Cost savings were attributable to a 39% reduction in the use of invasive tests [26]. This sequential testing strategy is no longer commercially available, and results from a similar study design using more updated diagnostic algorithms are needed to truly evaluate the accuracy of noninvasive serodiagnostic markers in children with symptoms suggestive of, but not diagnostic of, IBD. Subsequent pediatric studies confirmed the specificity of these markers for IBD but continued to question the sensitivity of these tests as a screening tool to differentiate IBD from non-IBD [27]. The addition of CD-specific CBir1 and OmpC to serodiagnostic panels has the potential to improve the sensitivity of these markers for CD versus UC and versus IBD. The same can be said perhaps for the anti-glycan antibodies. Dotan et al. [16] found that in addition to ASCA, antibodies to laminaribioside (ALCA) and chitobioside (ACCA) had the highest discriminative capability between CD and UC (p < 0.001 and p < 0.05, respectively). Importantly, 44% (12/27) of ASCA-negative CD patients were positive for ALCA or ACCA. In patients with inflammatory bowel disease positive for antibodies against either ALCA, ACCA, or ASCA, the diagnosis of CD was suggested with a sensitivity of 77.4% and specificity of 90.6%. Having at least 2 of these antibodies increased the specificity to 99.1%. In CD, higher levels of antibodies against ALCA or ASCA were significantly associated with small intestinal disease (p = 0.03 and p < 0.0001, respectively). Although conflicting, studies do support the use of these markers, particularly in children, to guide clinicians in cases of diagnostic uncertainty [9, 23, 25]. The addition of new markers and the use of algorithmic testing based on pattern recognition rather than ROC determined cut offs should lead to increased accuracy of these tests in both children and adults. Further studies are needed in prospective cohorts where these tests are compared to gold standard diagnostic criteria in cases of diagnostic uncertainty.

Differentiating CD from UC: Indeterminate Colitis

Although UC and CD may share epidemiologic, immunologic, therapeutic and clinical features, they are currently considered to be two distinct subtypes of IBD. Clinical, endoscopic, histopathologic and radiographic criteria have been put forth to help clinicians differentiate between these two diseases. However, despite published criteria, this discrimination may still prove to be difficult in patients with disease limited to the large bowel. This entity referred to as indeterminate colitis (IC) occurs in approximately 10–15% of IBD patients. Classically this term had applied to those patients whose diagnosis remained unknown even after careful examination of resected surgical specimens. There still remains, however, a lot of inconsistency in the literature when defining IC since it is generally based on imprecise clinical definitions and very small retrospective studies. It must be emphasized that both surgical options and perhaps medical treatment rely on a correct diagnosis. There is always a hesitation when offering IC patients pouch surgery because of concern of pouch failure, refractory pouchitis, and a postoperative diagnosis of CD. Yu et al. [28] compared the 10-year outcome of IC and chronic UC patients undergoing ileal-pouch anal anastomosis (IPAA). Those patients going into surgery with a diagnosis of IC had significantly more episodes of pelvic sepsis (17% indeterminate colitis vs. 7% chronic UC; p < 0.001), pouch fistula (31 vs. 9%; p < 0.001), and pouch failure (27 vs. 11%; p < 0.001). Moreover, 15% of patients with IC, but only 2% of patients with chronic UC, had their original diagnosis changed to CD (p < 0.001).

Given the CD specificity of ASCA and the UC specificity of pANCA, these antibodies have been widely studied and have become with the addition of novel markers more widely accepted as useful discriminatory markers that help clinicians differentiate UC from Crohn's colitis. However, the discriminatory strength of these markers is amplified when they are evaluated in combination. A pANCA+/ASCA– serological profile was shown to be 19 times more likely to be present in the serum of a patient with UC than CD. Conversely, pANCA–/ASCA+ is 16 times more likely in CD than UC [29]. Quinton et al. obtained serum samples from 100 patients with CD, 101 patients with UC, 27 patients with other miscellaneous diarrheal illnesses, and 163 healthy controls [30]. The combination of a positive pANCA test and a negative ASCA test yielded a sensitivity, specificity, and positive predictive value of 57, 97, and 92.5% respectively for UC. The combination of a positive ASCA test and a negative

pANCA test yielded a sensitivity, specificity, and positive predictive value of 49, 97, and 96% respectively for CD. It should be noted that in patients with pure colonic CD, the prevalence of ASCA positivity is relatively low. Ruemmele et al. [7] also studied ASCA and pANCA in cases of colitis among children with IBD. IgA and IgG ASCA titers were significantly greater and highly specific for CD (95% for either, 100% if both positive). pANCA was 92% specific for UC and absent in all non-IBD controls. The majority of patients with CD positive for pANCA had a UC-like presentation. A meta-analysis was performed to examine the test characteristics of ASCA and pANCA [31]. Sensitivity, specificity, and likelihood ratios (LR+, LR–) were calculated for different test combinations for CD, UC, and for IBD compared with controls. A total of 60 studies comprising 3,841 UC and 4,019 CD patients were included. The ASCA+ with pANCA– test offered the best sensitivity for CD (54.6%) with 92.8% specificity and an area under the receiver operating characteristic (ROC) curve (AUC) of 0.85 (LR+ = 6.5, LR– = 0.5). Sensitivity and specificity of pANCA+ tests for UC were 55.3 and 88.5%, respectively (AUC of 0.82; LR+ = 4.5, LR– = 0.5). Sensitivity and specificity were improved to 70.3% and 93.4% in a pediatric subgroup when combined with an ASCA-negative test. Meta-regression analysis showed decreased diagnostic precision of ASCA for isolated colonic CD (RDOR = 0.3). This study concluded that ASCA and pANCA testing are specific but not sensitive for CD and UC. It may be particularly useful for differentiating between CD and UC in the pediatric population. The first prospective study was conducted in IC patients and reported by Joossens et al. [32] in 2001. They enrolled 97 predefined IC patients and followed them prospectively over time blinded to their ASCA and pANCA status. Over 6 years, 17 of 97 patients were diagnosed with CD, 66 of the 97 patients remained indeterminate, and 14 patients of the 97 declared as UC. Thus, a definitive diagnosis was reached for 31 of 97 patients (32%). Their initial serum antibody characterization demonstrated that 48% of the population was ASCA–/pANCA–, 27% were ASCA+/pANCA–, 21% were ASCA–/pANCA+, and 4% were ASCA+/pANCA+. ASCA+/pANCA– correlated with CD in 8 of 10 (80%) patients, whereas ASCA–/pANCA+ correlated with UC in 7 of 11 (63.6%) patients. The remaining 4 cases became CD, clinically behaving as UC-like CD. Thus 100% of UC or UC-like CD were pANCA-positive. At the time of last follow-up, almost half of the patients (47 of 97, 48.5%) were negative for ASCA and pANCA. Only 7 seronegative cases (14.9%) became CD or UC compared with 48% (24 of 50) of seropositive patients (p < 0.001). The conclusions of this study are that IC may represent a distinct form of IBD based on the lack of IBD-associated antibodies.

Four years later, the same group investigated if anti-OmpC and anti-I2 were additive to ASCA and pANCA in their IC cohort and if patients who remained unclassified over time also lacked response to these microbial antigens in addition to ASCA and pANCA [33]. The results of this study indicated that by adding anti-OmpC and anti-I2, the predictive capacity of serological tests only increases marginally and specificity drops significantly. Despite another 1.5 years of follow-up, there still remained a large group of IC patients who remained negative for serological markers and may represent a separate phenotype. The entity of a UC-like Crohn's phenotype was first introduced by Vasiliauskas et al. [34] in 1996. pANCA-positive patients with CD were reported to have endoscopically and/or histopathologically documented left-sided colitis and symptoms of left-sided colonic inflammation, clinically reflected by rectal bleeding and mucus discharge, urgency, and treatment with topical agents. One hundred percent of patients with CD expressing pANCA had 'UC-like' features. The presence of pANCA in up to 25% of CD patients however limits its ability to distinguish UC form CD on its own. Novel antibodies like anti-CBir1 may help to dissect the pANCA-positive IBD group. Targan et al. found CBir1 reactivity in 44% of pANCA-positive CD patients versus only 4% of pANCA-positive UC patients [21]. This suggests that pANCA-positive/antiCBir1-positive colonic CD patients may represent a unique UC-like phenotype. It is unclear as to whether the natural history of UC-like CD is different from chronic UC, especially when it comes to therapeutic responses and postoperative outcomes.

Phenotypic Stratification

If indeed these immune responses represent the sum of a genetic and environmental predisposition to IBD, quantitative and qualitative expression of these immune responses may serve as an immunologic risk marker for IBD phenotypes. Vasiliauskas et al. [35] introduced the notion of immune response stratification when they first reported that high ASCA levels were found to be associated with fibrostenosing (FS) and internal penetrating (IP) disease as well as the need for small bowel surgery. Similar associations were then reported between NOD2/CARD15 and small bowel fibrostenosing CD [36–39]. These studies, however, did not take into account the im-

mune responses as a confounding variable to all reported associations. Another cross-sectional study demonstrated that patients who were ASCA IgA- or IgG-positive were 8.5 and 5.5 times more likely to undergo early surgery (within 3 years of diagnosis) than ASCA IgA- or IgG-negative patients [40]. Mow et al. [41] examined the association of multiple immune responses and disease phenotype. Reactivity to OmpC was independently associated with IP disease, while reactivity to anti-I2 was independently associated with FS disease and the need for surgery. Both the presence and magnitude of the immune response was associated with more aggressive disease behaviors. A similar study in a Scottish CD cohort reported that the cumulative reactivity to ASCA, I2 and OmpC was associated with small bowel complications [42]. Antibodies to CBir1 were examined in a later study and were found to be independently associated with small bowel disease, IP and FS disease [21]. Xue et al. [43] demonstrated that reactivity to ASCA, OmpC and CBir1 was associated with early disease onset, FS and IP disease and the need for surgery. Cross-sectional studies confirm that there is a significant association between the presence of microbial-driven immune responses and more aggressive disease phenotypes. More recent pediatric cohort studies suggest that these markers are present in patients before a complication occurs and thus predictive of disease progression from uncomplicated to complicated state. This could address the suggestion that a complication leads to an alteration in mucosal permeability and hence seroreactivity to microbial antigens. Desir et al. [44] demonstrated that baseline ASCA reactivity was associated with a more relapsing course in a pediatric CD cohort (IgA: OR 2.9; 95% CI 1.33–6.35). Serial antibody measurements did not predict the occurrence of clinical outcomes and that there was a limited variability in the antibodies over time. A multicenter study examined the association of ASCA, anti-I2, anti-OmpC, and anti-CBir1 reactivity with disease course in 196 pediatric CD patients [45]. The qualitative and quantitative reactivity to I2, and OmpC were each independently associated with the development of IP and FS disease behavior and the frequency of development of disease complication increased in parallel with reactivity to increasing numbers of antigens. The OR for the development of IP/FS disease was 5.3 and 11.0 for children with reactivity to 3, and 4 antigens, respectively. Furthermore, survival analysis demonstrated that reactivity to at least one microbial antigen was associated with the development of IP/FS disease faster as compared to patients negative for all markers, suggesting that these markers may predict more ag-

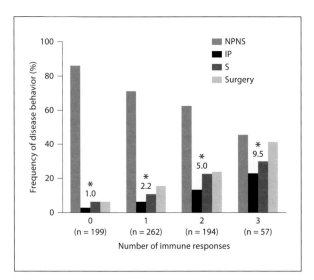

Fig. 1. The frequency of disease behavior (nonpenetrating, nonstricturing disease (NPNS), internal penetrating (IP) stricturing (S) and surgery) based on number of immune responses. The test for trend demonstrated a positive linear trend in the frequency of patients with IP disease as the number of positive immune responses toward, OmpC, ASCA and CBir1 increased (p < 0.0001). The ORs reflect the odds of having internal penetrating when positive for any 1, combination of 2, or all 3 immune responses, as compared to those patients negative for all immune responses (baseline group).

gressive disease behaviors. This cohort has now been expanded to include close to 800 pediatric patients. The data confirms that increasing number of immune responses as well as the magnitude of the immune response is predictive of a more rapid disease progression [46] (fig. 1). Amre et al. [47] also studied a cohort of pediatric CD patients who had sera drawn at diagnosis and were studied for the subsequent development of complications of their disease. Survival analysis revealed that the time to first complication was more rapid for ASCA-positive patients than those who were ASCA negative. Moreover, the relative risk of a recurrent complication (RR = 3.68) and needs for an additional surgery (RR = 1.95) was significantly higher in ASCA-positive patients. Data now exists that links seroreactivity to microbial antigens to underlying genetically determined innate immune defects *(NOD2)* [39, 48–50]. Devlin et al. [48] demonstrated that a significant proportion of the cumulative seroreactivity to microbial antigens was determined by the presence of variants in the *NOD2* gene in CD patients. Ippoliti et al. [51] also demonstrated an association between

NOD2/CARD15 and magnitude of immune response in patients with fibrostenosing CD. Those patients homozygote for NOD2/CARD15 had higher levels of immune reactivity as compared to those heterozygote and homozygote wild type, respectively. Thus, it is hypothesized that the more defective the innate immunity is (NOD2–/NOD2– vs. NOD2+/NOD2+), the more intolerant/maladaptive the adaptive immune response is as expressed by higher immune responses. This in turn translates to a more aggressive clinical phenotype [48]. Papp similarly observed a serological dosage effect between gASCA and AMCA antibodies and NOD2/CARD15, in addition to a gene-dosage effect [52].

As compared to the positive association between ASCA, antibodies to OmpC, I2 and CBir1 and disease complication, pANCA has been shown to be associated with a more benign, UC-like disease course and negatively associated with small bowel complicating disease [34, 35]. High pre-colectomy levels of pANCA (>100 EU/ml) have been prospectively shown to be associated with the development of chronic pouchitis in IBD patients undergoing IPAA [53]. More recently, the same group reported that anti-CBir1 may accelerate the development of chronic pouchitis in the face of high pANCA levels [54]. Melmed et al. [55] demonstrated that ASCA positivity and a family history of CD was most predictive of CD of the pouch after IPAA. This information may not change the need for colectomy, but the surgical procedure chosen and the postoperative management would certainly be impacted by this prognostic information.

Predictor of Response to Therapy

If indeed these B cell responses are a surrogate marker for antigen-driven specific T cell pathways, it is conceivable that individuals with certain immune response profiles will respond better to specific therapeutic targets. To date, most of the interest has been on the immune responses and infliximab. It is clear from both the clinical trials and clinical experience that not all patients respond to infliximab therapy. Taylor et al. [56] were the first to report on the negative association between pANCA and infliximab response. A subsequent study could not confirm that either ASCA or pANCA could predict response to treatment. However, lower response rates were observed for patients with refractory intestinal disease carrying the pANCA+/ASCA– combination (p = 0.67) [57].

The use of infliximab in UC has added another level of treatment for patients in whom colectomy may have

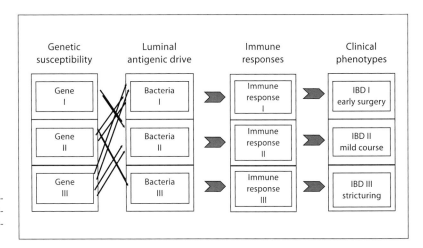

Fig. 2. The classification of IBD: Phenotype stratification based on immune response categories reflective of the genetic-bacterial interaction.

been the only alternative. That being said, however, not all patients respond to infliximab and the a priori knowledge of which patients are unlikely to respond to therapy may help clinicians and patients make the appropriate decision regarding medical versus surgical therapy. One hundred UC patients followed at a single center were enrolled to examine predictors of early clinical response to infliximab [58]. Of the 100 patients, 60 (60%) had pancolitis, 63% were on concomitant immunosuppressive therapy, 9% were active smokers, 64% had C-reactive protein > or = 5 mg/dl, and 44% were pANCA+/ASCA–. Only 5 patients in this study received IFX because of severe acute colitis refractory to intravenous corticosteroids. Early complete and partial clinical responses were observed in 41 and 24% of patients. Patients who were pANCA+/ASCA– had a significantly lower early clinical response (55 vs. 76%; OR = 0.40 (0.16–0.99), p = 0.049). Concomitant immunosuppressive therapy and the use of an IFX induction scheme did not influence early clinical response.

Predictor of Disease Susceptibility

The results from a very thought provoking study from Israel suggested that immune reactivity to microbial antigens could occur in advance of clinical presentation in CD [59]. Sera were collected from members of the Israeli Defense Force (IDF), at the time of recruitment. Thirty-two individuals subsequently developed CD at a mean of 38 months postrecruitment. Over 30% of patients who subsequently developed CD were ASCA positive at the

time of recruitment into the IDF. There has been interest in evaluating whether immune responses are familial traits due to genetic factors. Sutton et al. demonstrated that the quantitative and qualitative expression of ASCA may be familial [60]. Studies in a twin population demonstrated an agreement in ASCA titers within concordant monozygotic twin pairs with CD and suggested that the level of increase (magnitude) is genetically determined [61]. A very recent study has shown that antibodies to OmpC have a strong familial aggregation pattern [62]. Preliminary studies in a pediatric cohort suggest that the quantitative but more so the qualitative expression of immune responses to microbial antigens is increased in the parents of pediatric CD patients, suggesting that the immune dysregulation observed in such patients is a familial trait [63]. Further research in a larger number of parents will increase our understanding of the role of familial expression of serological immune response. It will be important to further evaluate the subclinical or even preclinical nature of these markers of disease.

Conclusion

This chapter highlighted the recent advances in the area of diagnostic and prognostic immune markers, focusing on serologic immune markers as well as discussing the spectrum of utility and their feasibility. Research and technological advancements have fostered a novel approach to understanding the intricate relationship between genetic and clinical expression of disease. Serum immune markers, as well as genetic markers, hold the most promise in helping researchers better comprehend disease heterogeneity and natural history. Although our current gold standard diagnostic tests do not possess this capability, prospective research studies now suggest that IBD-specific genetic and antibody markers may serve as predictors of an individual's disease course (fig. 2). Thus, the foundation has been laid upon which the discovery of novel IBD-specific and IBD-sensitive markers will enable researchers to identify at-risk individuals, as well as diagnose IBD and stratify patients into homogeneous subtypes with certainty. Clinicians can then create and implement individual treatment plans designed to improve the long-term prognosis of this chronic disease.

Disclosure Statement

Consultant Prometheus Labs, San Diego, Calif., USA.

References

1 Duchmann R, May E, Heike M, Knolle P, Neurath M, Meyer zum Buschenfelde KH: T cell specificity and cross reactivity towards enterobacteria, bacteroides, bifidobacterium, and antigens from resident luminal flora in humans. Gut 1999;44:812–818.

2 Vidrich A, Lee J, James E, Cobb L, Targan S: Segregation of pANCA antigenic recognition by DNase treatment of neutrophils: ulcerative colitis, type 1 autoimmune hepatitis, and primary sclerosing cholangitis. J Clin Immunol 1995;15:293–299.

3 Eggena M, Cohavy O, Parseghian MH, Hamkalo BA, Clemens D, Targan SR, Gordon LK, Braun J: Identification of histone H1 as a cognate antigen of the ulcerative colitis-associated marker antibody pANCA. J Autoimmun 2000;14:83–97.

4 Cohavy O, Harth G, Horwitz M, Eggena M, Landers C, Sutton C, Targan SR, Braun J: Identification of a novel mycobacterial histone H1 homologue (HupB) as an antigenic target of pANCA monoclonal antibody and serum immunoglobulin A from patients with Crohn's disease. Infect Immunol 1999; 67:6510–6517.

5 Seibold F, Brandwein S, Simpson S, Terhorst C, Elson CO: pANCA represents a cross-reactivity to enteric bacterial antigens. J Clin Immunol 1998;18:153–160.

6 Cohavy O, Bruckner D, Gordon LK, Misra R, Wei B, Eggena ME, Targan SR, Braun J: Colonic bacteria express an ulcerative colitis pANCA-related protein epitope. Infect Immunol 2000;68:1542–1548.

7 Ruemmele FM, Targan SR, Levy G, Dubinsky M, Braun J, Seidman EG: Diagnostic accuracy of serological assays in pediatric inflammatory bowel disease. Gastroenterology 1998;115:822–829.

8 Quinton JF, Sendid B, Reumaux D, Duthilleul P, Cortot A, Grandbastien B, Charrier G, Targan SR, Colombel JF, Poulain D: Anti-Saccharomyces cerevisiae mannan antibodies combined with antineutrophil cytoplasmic autoantibodies in inflammatory bowel disease: prevalence and diagnostic role. Gut 1998;42:788–791.

9 Hoffenberg EJ, Fidanza S, Sauaia A: Serologic testing for inflammatory bowel disease. J Pediatr 1999;134:447–452.

10 Duerr RH, Targan SR, Landers CJ, Sutherland LR, Shanahan F: Anti-neutrophil cytoplasmic antibodies in ulcerative colitis: comparison with other colitides/diarrheal illnesses. Gastroenterology 1991;100:1590–1596.

11 Proujansky R, Fawcett PT, Gibney KM, Treem WR, Hyams JS: Examination of antineutrophil cytoplasmic antibodies in childhood inflammatory bowel disease. J Pediatr Gastroenterol Nutr 1993;17:193–197.

12 Winter HS, Landers CJ, Winkelstein A, Vidrich A, Targan SR: Anti-neutrophil cytoplasmic antibodies in children with ulcerative colitis. J Pediatr 1994;125:707–711.

13 Oberstadt K, Schaedel W, Weber M, Classen M, Deusch K: P-ANCA as a differential diagnostic marker in inflammatory bowel disease. Adv Exp Med Biol 1995;371B:1313–1316.

14 Sendid B, Colombel JF, Jacquinot PM, Faille C, Fruit J, Cortot A, Lucidarme D, Camus D, Poulain D: Specific antibody response to oligomannosidic epitopes in Crohn's disease. Clin Diagn Lab Immunol 1996;3:219–226.

15 Mallant-Hent RC, Mooij M, von Blomberg BM, Linskens RK, van Bodegraven AA, Savelkoul PH: Correlation between Saccharomyces cerevisiae DNA in intestinal mucosal samples and anti-Saccharomyces cerevisiae antibodies in serum of patients with IBD. World J Gastroenterol 2006;12:292–297.

16 Dotan I, Fishman S, Dgani Y, Schwartz M, Karban A, Lerner A, Weishauss O, Spector L, Shtevi A, Altstock RT, Dotan N, Halpern Z: Antibodies against laminaribioside and chitobioside are novel serologic markers in Crohn's disease. Gastroenterology 2006;131:366–378.

17 Landers CJ, Cohavy O, Misra R, Yang H, Lin YC, Braun J, Targan SR: Selected loss of tolerance evidenced by Crohn's disease-associated immune responses to auto- and microbial antigens. Gastroenterology 2002;123:689–699.

18 Beaven SW, Abreu MT: Biomarkers in inflammatory bowel disease. Curr Opin Gastroenterol 2004;20:318–327.

19 Mow WS, Vasiliauskas EA, Lin YC, Fleshner PR, Papadakis KA, Taylor KD, Landers CJ, Abreu-Martin MT, Rotter JI, Yang H, Targan SR: Association of antibody responses to microbial antigens and complications of small bowel Crohn's disease. Gastroenterology 2004;126:414–424.

20 Arnott ID, Landers CJ, Nimmo EJ, Drummond HE, Smith BK, Targan SR, Satsangi J: Sero-reactivity to microbial components in Crohn's disease is associated with disease severity and progression, but not NOD2/CARD15 genotype. Am J Gastroenterol 2004;99:2376–2384.

21 Targan SR, Landers CJ, Yang H, Lodes MJ, Cong Y, Papadakis KA, Vasiliauskas E, Elson CO, Hershberg RM: Antibodies to CBir1 flagellin define a unique response that is associated independently with complicated Crohn's disease. Gastroenterology 2005;128:2020–2028.

22 Lodes MJ, Cong Y, Elson CO, Mohamath R, Landers CJ, Targan SR, Fort M, Hershberg RM: Bacterial flagellin is a dominant antigen in Crohn disease. J Clin Invest 2004;113:1296–1306.

23 Peeters M, Joossens S, Vermeire S, et al: Diagnostic value of anti-Saccharomyces cerevisiae and antineutrophil cytoplasmic autoantibodies in inflammatory bowel disease. Am J Gastroenterol 2001;96:730–734.

24 Hoffenberg EJ, Fidanza S, Sauaia A: Serologic testing for inflammatory bowel disease. J Pediatr 1999;134:447–452.

25 Dubinsky MC, Ofman JJ, Urman M, Targan SR, Seidman EG: Clinical utility of serodiagnostic testing in suspected pediatric inflammatory bowel disease. Am J Gastroenterol 2001;96:758–765.

26 Dubinsky MC, Johanson JF, Seidman EG, Ofman JJ: Suspected inflammatory bowel disease: the clinical and economic impact of competing diagnostic strategies. Am J Gastroenterol 2002;97:2333–2342.

27 Zholudev A, Zurakowski D, Young W, Leichtner A, Bousvaros A: Serologic testing with ANCA, ASCA, and anti-OmpC in children and young adults with Crohn's disease and ulcerative colitis: diagnostic value and correlation with disease phenotype. Am J Gastroenterol 2004;99:2235–2241.

28 Yu CS, Pemberton JH, Larson D: Ileal pouch-anal anastomosis in patients with indeterminate colitis: long-term results. Dis Colon Rectum 2000;43:1487–1496.

29 Panaccione R, Sandborn WJ: Is antibody testing for inflammatory bowel disease clinically useful? Gastroenterology 1999;116:1001–1002; discussion 1002–1003.

30 Quinton JF, Sendid B, Reumaux D, Duthilleul P, Cortot A, Grandbastien B, Charrier G, Targan SR, Colombel JF, Poulain D: Anti-Saccharomyces cerevisiae mannan antibodies combined with antineutrophil cytoplasmic autoantibodies in inflammatory bowel disease: prevalence and diagnostic role. Gut 1998;42:788–791.

31 Reese GE, Constantinides VA, Simillis C, Darzi AW, Orchard TR, Fazio VW, Tekkis PP: Diagnostic precision of anti-Saccharomyces cerevisiae antibodies and perinuclear antineutrophil cytoplasmic antibodies in inflammatory bowel disease. Am J Gastroenterol 2006;101:2410–2422.

32 Joossens S, Reinisch W, Vermeire S, et al: The value of serologic markers in indeterminate colitis: a prospective follow-up study. Gastroenterology 2002;122:1242–1247.

33 Joossens S, Colombel JF, Landers C, Poulain D, Geboes K, Bossuyt X, Targan S, Rutgeerts P, Reinisch W: Anti-outer membrane of porin C and anti-I2 antibodies in indeterminate colitis. Gut 2006;55:1667–1669.

34 Vasiliauskas EA, Plevy SE, Landers CJ, Binder SW, Ferguson DM, Yang H, Rotter JI, Vidrich A, Targan SR: Perinuclear antineutrophil cytoplasmic antibodies in patients with Crohn's disease define a clinical subgroup. Gastroenterology 1996;110:1810–1819.

35 Vasiliauskas EA, Kam LY, Karp LC, Gaiennie J, Yang H, Targan SR: Marker antibody expression stratifies Crohn's disease into immunologically homogeneous subgroups with distinct clinical characteristics. Gut 2000;47:487–496.

36 Lesage S, Zouali H, Cezard JP, Colombel JF, Belaiche J, Almer S, Tysk C, O'Morain C, Gassull M, Binder V, Finkel Y, Modigliani R, Gower-Rousseau C, Macry J, Merlin F, Chamaillard M, Jannot AS, Thomas G, Hugot JP: CARD15/NOD2 mutational analysis and genotype-phenotype correlation in 612 patients with inflammatory bowel disease. Am J Hum Genet 2002;70:845–857.

37 Ahmad T, Armuzzi A, Bunce M, Mulcahy-Hawes K, Marshall SE, Orchard TR, Crawshaw J, Large O, de Silva A, Cook JT, Barnardo M, Cullen S, Welsh KI, Jewell DP: The molecular classification of the clinical manifestations of Crohn's disease. Gastroenterology 2002;122:854–866.

38 Cuthbert AP, Fisher SA, Mirza MM, King K, Hampe J, Croucher PJ, Mascheretti S, Sanderson J, Forbes A, Mansfield J, Schreiber S, Lewis CM, Mathew CG: The contribution of NOD2 gene mutations to the risk and site of disease in inflammatory bowel disease. Gastroenterology 2002;122:867–874.

39 Abreu MT, Taylor KD, Lin YC, Hang T, Gaiennie J, Landers CJ, Vasiliauskas EA, Kam LY, Rojany M, Papadakis KA, Rotter JI, Targan SR, Yang H: Mutations in NOD2 are associated with fibrostenosing disease in patients with Crohn's disease. Gastroenterology 2002;123:679–688.

40 Forcione DG, Rosen MJ, Kisiel JB, Sands BE: Anti-Saccharomyces cerevisiae antibody (ASCA) positivity is associated with increased risk for early surgery in Crohn's disease. Gut 2004;53:1117–1122.

41 Mow WS, Vasiliauskas EA, Lin YC, Fleshner PR, Papadakis KA, Taylor KD, Landers CJ, Abreu-Martin MT, Rotter JI, Yang H, Targan SR: Association of antibody responses to microbial antigens and complications of small bowel Crohn's disease. Gastroenterology 2004;126:414–424.

42 Arnott ID, Landers CJ, Nimmo EJ, Drummond HE, Smith BK, Targan SR, Satsangi J: Sero-reactivity to microbial components in Crohn's disease is associated with disease severity and progression, but not NOD2/CARD15 genotype. Am J Gastroenterol 2004;99:2376–2384.

43 Xue S, Stempak JM, Elkadri AA, Greenberg GR, Walters TD, Griffiths AM, Steinhart H, Silverberg MS: Serological markers are associated with severity of disease and need for surgery in IBD patients. Gastroenterology 2006;130:S1303.

44 Desir B, Amre DK, Lu SE, Ohman-Strickland P, Dubinsky M, Fisher R, Seidman EG: Utility of serum antibodies in determining clinical course in pediatric Crohn's disease. Clin Gastroenterol Hepatol 2004;2:139–146.

45 Dubinsky MC, Lin YC, Dutridge D, Picornell Y, Landers CJ, Farrior S, Wrobel I, Quiros A, Vasiliauskas EA, Grill B, Israel D, Bahar R, Christie D, Wahbeh G, Silber G, Dallazadeh S, Shah P, Thomas D, Kelts D, Hershberg RM, Elson CO, Targan SR, Taylor KD, Rotter JI, Yang H: Serum immune responses predict rapid disease progression among children with Crohn's disease: immune responses predict disease progression. Am J Gastroenterol 2006;101:360–367.

46 Dubinsky MC, Kugathasan S, Mei L, Picornell Y, Nebel J, Wrobel I, Quiros JA, Silber G, Wahbeh G, Vasiliauskas EA, Bahar RJ, Otley A, Mack DR, Evans J, Rosh JR, Oliva Hemker M, Leleiko NS, Crandall WV, Langton C, Taylor KD, Targan SR, Rotter JI, Markowitz JF, Hyams JS: Increased immune reactivity predicts aggressive complicating Crohn's disease in children. Gastroenterology 2007;132:A17.

47 Amre DK, Lu SE, Costea F, Seidman EG: Utility of serological markers in predicting the early occurrence of complications and surgery in pediatric Crohn's disease patients. Am J Gastroenterol 2006;101:645–652.

48 Devlin SM, Yang H, Ippoliti A, Taylor KD, Landers CJ, Su X, Abreu MT, Papadakis KA, Vasiliauskas EA, Melmed GY, Fleshner PR, Mei L, Rotter JI, Targan SR: NOD2 variants and antibody response to microbial antigens in Crohn's disease patients and their unaffected relatives. Gastroenterology 2007;132:576–586.

49 Cruyssen BV, Peeters H, Hoffman IE, Laukens D, Coucke P, Marichal D, Cuvelier C, Remaut E, Veys EM, Mielants H, De Vos M, De Keyser F: CARD15 polymorphisms are associated with anti-Saccharomyces cerevisiae antibodies in Caucasian Crohn's disease patients. Clin Exp Immunol 2005;140:354–359.

50 Annese V, Lombardi G, Perri F, D'Inca R, Ardizzone S, Riegler G, Giaccari S, Vecchi M, Castiglione F, Gionchetti P, Cocchiara E, Vigneri S, Latiano A, Palmieri O, Andriulli A: Variants of CARD15 are associated with an aggressive clinical course of Crohn's disease: an IG-IBD study. Am J Gastroenterol 2005;100:84–92.

51 Ippoliti AF, Devlin S, Yang H, Mei L, Papadakis K, Vasiliauskas E, Melmed G, Shaye O, Enyati G, Chen J, Nataskin I, Patel Y, Mehdikhani E, Taylor KD, Landers C, Rotter JI, Targan S: The relationship between abnormal innate and adaptive immune function and fibrostenosis in Crohn's disease patients. Gastroenterology 2006;130:A127.

52 Papp M, Altorjay I, Dotan N, Palatka K, Foldi I, Tumpek J, Sipka S, Udvardy M, Dinya T, Lakatos L, Kovacs A, Molnar T, Tulassay Z, Miheller P, Norman G, Szamosi T, Papp J, Lakatos P: New serological markers for inflammatory bowel disease are associated with earlier age at onset, complicated disease behavior, risk for surgery, and NOD2/CARD15 genotype in a Hungarian IBD cohort. Am J Gastroenterol 2008;103:665–681.

53 Fleshner PR, Vasiliauskas EA, Kam LY, Fleshner NE, Gaiennie J, Abreu-Martin MT, Targan SR: High level perinuclear antineutrophil cytoplasmic antibody (pANCA) in ulcerative colitis patients before colectomy predicts the development of chronic pouchitis after ileal pouch-anal anastomosis. Gut 2001;49:671–677.

54 Fleshner P, Vasiliauskas E, Dubinsky M, Mei L, Landers C, Ippoliti A, Papadakis K, Targan S: Both preoperative pANCA and CBir1 flagellin expression in ulcerative colitis (UC) patients influence pouchitis development after ileal pouch-anal anastamosis (IPAA). Gastroenterology 2006;130:A130.

55 Melmed GY, Fleshner PR, Bardakcioglu O, Ippoliti A, Vasiliauskas EA, Papadakis KA, Dubinsky M, Landers C, Rotter JI, Targan SR: Family history and serology predict Crohn's disease after ileal pouch-anal anastomosis for ulcerative colitis. Dis Colon Rectum 2008;51:100–108.

56 Taylor KD, Plevy SE, Yang H, Landers CJ, Barry MJ, Rotter JI, Targan SR: ANCA pattern and LTA haplotype relationship to clinical responses to anti-TNF antibody treatment in Crohn's disease. Gastroenterology 2001;120:1347–1355.

57 Esters N, Vermeire S, Joossens S, Noman M, Louis E, Belaiche J, De Vos M, Van Gossum A, Pescatore P, Fiasse R, Pelckmans P, Reynaert H, Poulain D, Bossuyt X, Rutgeerts P, Belgian Group of Infliximab Expanded Access Program in Crohn's Disease: Serological markers for prediction of response to anti-tumor necrosis factor treatment in Crohn's disease. Am J Gastroenterol 2002;97:1458–1462.

58 Ferrante M, Vermeire S, Katsanos KH, Noman M, Van Assche G, Schnitzler F, Arijs I, De Hertogh G, Hoffman I, Geboes JK, Rutgeerts P: Predictors of early response to infliximab in patients with ulcerative colitis. Inflamm Bowel Dis 2007;13:123–128.

59 Israeli E, Grotto I, Gilburd B, Balicer RD, Goldin E, Wiik A, Shoenfeld Y: Anti-*Saccharomyces cerevisiae* and antineutrophil cytoplasmic antibodies as predictors of inflammatory bowel disease. Gut 2005;54:1232–1236.

60 Sutton CL, H Yang, Li Z, Rotter JI, Targan SR, Braun J: Familial expression of anti-*Saccharomyces cerevisiae* mannan antibodies in affected and unaffected relatives of patients with Crohn's disease. Gut 2000;46:58–63.

61 Halfvarson J, Standaert-Vitse A, Järnerot G, Sendid B, Jouault T, Bodin L, Duhamel A, Colombel JF, Tysk C, Poulain D: Anti-*Saccharomyces cerevisiae* antibodies in twins with inflammatory bowel disease. Gut 2005; 54:1237–1243.

62 Mei L, Targan SR, Landers CJ, Dutridge D, Ippoliti A, Vasiliauskas EA, Papadakis K, Fleshner PR, Rotter JI, Yang HY: Familial expression of anti-*Escherichia coli* outer membrane porin (OmpC) in relatives of patients with Crohn's disease. Gastroenterology 2006;130:1078–1085.

63 Dubinsky M, Mei L, Landers C, Katzir L, Farrior S, Wrobel I, Quiros A, Bahar R, Wahbeh G, Grill B, Silber G, Pietzak M, Vasiliauskas E, Dallazadeh S, Kelts D, Elson C, Hershberg R, Huiying Y, Targan S, Rotter J, Western Regional Pediatric IBD Research Alliance, Los Angeles, CA; Cedars-Sinai Medical Center, Los Angeles, CA; University of Alabama, Birmingham, AL; Dendreon Corporation, Seattle, WA: Familial expression of serological immune responses in pediatric IBD. J Pediatr Gastroenterol Nutr 2005;41:A150.

Dig Dis 2009;27:269–277
DOI: 10.1159/000228560

Inflammatory Bowel Diseases: Controversies in the Use of Diagnostic Procedures

Boris Vucelic

Division of Gastroenterology and Hepatology, Department of Medicine, University Hospital Rebro, Zagreb, Croatia

Key Words

Inflammatory bowel disease · Ulcerative colitis · Crohn's disease · Diagnostic procedure · Endoscopy · Imaging methods

Abstract

The term inflammatory bowel disease (IBD) denotes a genetically, immunologically and histopathologically heterogeneous group of inflammatory bowel disorders classified at present time as ulcerative colitis (UC), Crohn's disease (CD) and indeterminate colitis (IC). Diagnosis of IBD is based on a non-strictly defined combination of clinical and diagnostic parameters. In order to guide the treatment, patients must be assessed by determining IBD phenotype, disease extension and distribution, extraintestinal manifestations, disease behavior, disease severity and drug responsiveness. Each element of the diagnostic process cannot be looked at alone, but has to be incorporated into general clinical assessment, bearing in mind that different phenotypes and age groups require specific diagnostic solutions. Advances in technology provided the possibility for the assessment of the entire digestive system with endoscopy leading the way. Sophisticated imaging methods made the analysis of the bowel wall with its vascularity and adjacent mesentery possible. The challenge is still the small bowel, where a combination of endoscopy and imaging methods is used. The use of imaging methods should be, among other things, guided by level of irradiation which is especially important in young patients and in patients requiring repeated investigations. Using abdominal ultrasound as a low-cost, noninvasive procedure, one has to take into account that it is very operator-dependent method. In UC, endoscopy is used for the evaluation of the extent and activity of the disease and to assess complications like stricture, dysplasia and cancer. UC is classified by the disease extent into proctitis, left-sided colitis and extensive colitis beyond the splenic flexure. Pediatric patients with UC have more extensive disease than adults with rectal sparing in up to 30% of patients. The severity of mucosal changes are reported as Baron endoscopic score. Endoscopic findings correlate well with clinical activity and are commonly incorporated into Mayo index, combination of clinical Truelove Witts index and Baron score. Complications like strictures require imaging methods as supplement to endoscopy. The incidence of CD, particularly in children and adolescents, has risen during the past decade, with children often having extensive and severe disease The nature of CD requires the use of wide array of endoscopic and imaging methods, placed properly in the diagnostic algorithms for specific disease phenotypes and complications and adapted for specific age groups. Endoscopic features of CD are very variable and can be quantified as Crohn's Disease Endoscopic Index of Severity (CDEIS) or Simple Endoscopic Score for CD (SES-CD). Disease activity is most commonly assessed by CDAI. Perianal disease activity should be measured by PDAI due to low CDAI scores in these patients. The activity of CD in children should be assessed by the Pediatric Activity Index. IC is part of the IBD spectrum where chronic colitis cannot be defined as either UC or CD after sequential colonoscopies and colonic biopsies or at colectomy.

Copyright © 2009 S. Karger AG, Basel

Prof. Boris Vucelic, MD
Division of Gastroenterology and Hepatology, Department of Medicine
University Hospital Rebro, Kispaticeva 12
HR–10000 Zagreb (Croatia)
Tel./Fax +385 1 2421 844, E-Mail boris.vucelic@zg.t-com.hr

Introduction

The term inflammatory bowel disease (IBD) denotes a genetically, immunologically and histopathologically heterogeneous group of inflammatory bowel disorders. At present, it is classified as either ulcerative colitis (UC) or Crohn's disease (CD). However, IBD in some individuals escapes the usual criteria for either UC or CD and is referred to as indeterminate colitis (IC). Further, CD itself represents a heterogeneous entity comprising a variety of complex phenotypes.

The therapeutic goals in IBD are rapid control of symptoms and induction of remission, maintenance of remission as long as possible, reduction of number of surgeries and hospitalizations and improvement in quality of life. In order to achieve these goals, each patient must be assessed in an appropriate way, guiding the often complex treatment.

The assessment includes the determination of IBD phenotype which often requires prolonged observation of the clinical course (disease behavior), extension and severity of the disease, detection of extraintestinal manifestations and analysis of drug responsiveness, all in most objective and reliable manner possible. Embarking on the difficult road to proper diagnosis in a widest sense of the word, we must take into account the age of our IBD patients with particular care for extremes, pediatric age group and older patients. The current view is that the diagnosis is established by a non-strictly defined combination of clinical presentation, endoscopic appearance, radiology, histology, serology and surgical findings.

Indeterminate Colitis (IC)

The term IC is originally referred to 10–15% of IBD cases in which there was difficulty distinguishing between UC and CD in the colectomy specimens. These were patients with fulminant colitis without antecedent definition of the underlying disease. Fulminant colitis caused such intense destruction and hemorrhage with comparatively little inflammatory changes that the diagnostic features of CD or UC were absent or obscured. The term IC evolved with time and is increasingly used in chronic colitis when a definitive diagnosis of UC or CD cannot be made at sequential colonoscopies and colonic biopsies or at colectomy, making it a clinicopathological entity [1]. Whether IC is really a separate entity is currently unknown. Most patients with IC evolve to a definitive diagnosis of CD or UC at the long-term follow-up,

but some remain IC, particularly those with both negative pANCA and ASCA. The present view is that a diagnosis of IC could be made, apart from fulminant colitis, in all cases with endoscopic, radiographic and histologic evidence of IBD confined to the colon, but without fulfilment of diagnostic criteria for UC or CD and only after exhaustive clinical, radiographic and anatomic pathologic assessment, has guaranteed that no new information will be forthcoming and no decisive distinction between CD and UC can be made [2, 3]. The view that IC is a distinct category of IBD is supported by several clinical features. Fulminant colitis is more common in patients with IC. These patients require more surgery and have a higher incidence of complications and a greater risk of pouch failure [4].

The diagnosis of IC is based on macroscopic evaluation of the colon performed by the endoscopist and adequate pathohistological analysis of the endoscopic biopsy samples that have to be multiple and obtained in all segments of the colon and terminal ileum [5]. The problem is that there are no generally accepted microscopic criteria for the diagnosis of IC [4, 6, 7]. The latest proposal is to make a diagnosis of IC when endoscopy is equivocal and microscopy shows features of IBD but absence of diagnostic features for either CD or UC in mucosal biopsies from different segments of the colon, obtained at least at two sequential determinations, in a patient with a history of chronic or relapsing colitis. The pathologist analyzing the samples with the diagnosis of IC is faced with several scenarios [1, 7]. The first is fulminant colitis or refractory phase of chronic colitis. The histologic distinction of UC and CD is more difficult in the fulminant setting because the histologic features overlap. Some gross and microscopic features that are useful in distinguishing two diseases in the chronic state are common to both in this phase. Relative rectal sparing, intermittent ulceration, regular glandular pattern and lack of mucin depletion favor the diagnosis of CD. Some argue that intensive steroid treatment for fulminant disease may lead to the histologic appearance of IC. The second scenario is a chronic phase of colitis. There is sometimes development of non-diffuse distribution, normal rectal mucosa and variation in extent of involvement over time. It has to be remembered that medical treatment can have a profound effect on mucosal histology.

The third scenario is the early stage of disease. The microscopic features used for the diagnosis of IBD are often not present in the very early stage of the disease, especially in children who may show relative or complete sparing or even patchiness of disease at initial presentation. The final problem is the interobserver bias in the diagnosis and classification of colonic IBD, which can result in a change of diagnosis. One study showed that 43% of the cases initially diagnosed as UC were changed to CD or IC, whereas 17% initially diagnosed CD were changed to UC or IC. No diagnosis of IC was made by general pathologist, whereas the gastroenterological pathologist reclassified the IBD as IC in 24% of cases [6].

Serologic evaluation of pANCA and ASCA could be of help in patients with IC. Combined testing for pANCA and ASCA was performed in a prospective study of 97 patients with IC. It was found that 47 patients (48.5%) were negative for both pANCA and ASCA. Forty-two of these 47 patients remained IC patients after a mean follow-up of 8.8 years. Only 5 (10.6%) of the seronegative patients could eventually be classified as having either CD or UC compared with 40% (20/50) who had positive serology (p < 0.001) [8]. Patients with IC and negative serology may, therefore, present an undefined subgroup of IBD, which needs to be confirmed [9].

The natural history of patients with IC is unclear making therapeutic recommendations difficult. IC is basically treated like UC. Acute IC is managed like acute UC. Patients with chronic IC have not been evaluated in randomized clinical trials, result being the lack of evidence-based recommendations. Based on available data, IC is not a contraindication for ileal pouch-anal anastomosis following proctocolectomy.

Ulcerative Colitis (UC)

The discussion on diagnostic approach to UC should start with comments about the disease itself. The inflammation of the colon commences in the rectum and extends proximally in a continuous, confluent and concentric manner to affect variable extent of the colon or its entire mucosal surface. The proximal extent of inflammation may progress or regress over time, but after the disease regression the distribution of inflammation tends to match the extent of previous episodes in case of relapse. There are several situations that require our understanding. Macroscopic and microscopic rectal sparing has been described in children with UC prior to treatment [10]. In adults, normal rectum or patchy rectal inflammation is likely to be due to topical or systemic therapy [11]. Patchy inflammation in the cecum is called cecal patch and is usually seen in patients with left-sided colitis. The natural history of these patients is similar to those with isolated left-sided UC [12]. Involvement of the appendix

as a skip lesion is reported in up to 75% of patients with UC. Appendiceal inflammation has been associated with a more responsive course of disease and with a higher risk of pouchitis after proctocolectomy with IPAA. Backwash ileitis represents continuous extension of macroscopic or histological inflammation from the cecum into the distal ileum and is observed in 20% of patients with pancolitis. This form of UC seems to have more refractory course. Sometimes, these macroscopic changes of the terminal ileum require differentiation from CD [13].

Symptoms of UC are visible blood in the stools, loose stools, chronic diarrhea with rectal bleeding, rectal urgency, tenesmus, passage of mucopurulent exudates, nocturnal defecation and crampy abdominal pain. Proctitis may cause severe constipation. Simple fistule may occur, but recurrent or complex fistulae always raise suspicion of Crohn's colitis. Symptoms depend on the extent and severity of disease, presence of extraintestinal manifestations and concurrent therapy. There is no gold standard for diagnosis of UC and the diagnosis is made on the basis of combination of medical history, clinical evaluation and endoscopic and histologic findings, with infectious causes being excluded. In case that there is a doubt about the diagnosis, diagnostic work-up should be repeated after an interval. In 10% of patients initially diagnosed as UC, the diagnosis will be changed during the 5-year period after the initial onset of symptoms.

Initial evaluation includes a full medical history, careful description of symptoms, history of recent travels, food intolerances, nocturnal diarrhea, extraintestinal manifestations, recent medications (particularly antibiotics and NSAIDs), smoking habit, sexual practice, family history and previous appendectomy. Physical examination may be unremarkable in mild or even moderate disease.

Initial laboratory evaluation should give information on inflammatory activity and severity and help in differential diagnosis of acute colitis. Complete blood count gives a lot of information: thrombocytosis indicates chronic inflammatory response, anemia is reflection of severity and chronicity, leukocytosis indicates infectious complications. Inflammatory marker CRP is less good marker for assessing disease activity in UC than in CD, but correlates well with disease activity in acute severe UC, both in adults and children. For example, CRP >45 mg/l at day 3 following hospital admission for severe colitis together with more than 8 stools a day is highly predictive for need for colectomy. CRP, however, does not correlate with severity of disease in proctitis. Stool microbiology testing on *Clostridium difficile* toxins A and B,

Campylobacter spp., enteropathogenic *Escherichia coli* and *Cytomegalovirus* is very important in differential diagnosis of acute colitis, particularly recognition of the reactivation of CMV infection. Multiple intranuclear inclusions are usually significant, whereas occasional intranuclear inclusion bodies consistent with CMV on histopathology do not necessarily indicate clinically significant infection [14, 15]. Other initial important tests are urea, creatinine, electrolytes, liver enzymes and iron studies.

Endoscopy is used in UC to confirm the diagnosis, to evaluate the extent of disease, to assess the activity of disease, to evaluate disease unresponsive to therapy and to assess complications like stricture, dysplasia and cancer. No endoscopic feature is specific for UC. Most useful finding is rectal involvement and continuous and confluent colonic involvement with clear demarcation of inflammation. Mild inflammation is characterized with erythema, vascular congestion of the mucosa and loss of visible vascular pattern. Moderate inflammation appears as coarse granular appearance with mucosal erosions and friability. Spontaneous bleeding and ulcerations mark severe inflammation, where deep ulcers represent bad prognostic sign. The described degrees of severity are frequently reported as Baron endoscopic score [16]. Chronic inflammation is characterized by mucosal atrophy, loss of haustral folds, luminal narrowing and pseudopolyps. Since endoscopic findings correlate reasonably well with clinical activity, they tend to be incorporated into indices like Mayo score [17], which is a combination of clinical Truelove Witts index and endoscopic Baron scale. Patients with UC should be classified not only according to severity but also by disease extent. The extent of inflammation influences the management and choice of delivery system for a given therapy, for example topical therapy as suppositories for proctitis, enemas for left-sided colitis and oral plus topical treatment for extensive disease beyond splenic flexure. The extent of disease determines the start and frequency of surveillance program for CRC, since pancolitis carries greater risk for CRC than more limited disease.

Endoscopic classification therefore recognizes proctitis, left-sided colitis and extensive colitis beyond splenic flexure [18].

The endoscopic procedure of choice is colonoscopy with ileoscopy and segmental biopsies. However, one should avoid colonoscopy in severe UC and use flexible sigmoidoscopy to confirm diagnosis and exclude infection, particularly CMV infection. Bowel preparation itself, both safer phosphate preparations and more dangerous purgative preparations, can provoke colonic dilatation and carries risk of colonic perforation.

Plain abdominal radiograph is very useful in severe UC, not as a diagnostic test but as a valuable test in initial assessment of patients with severe UC. It is used to exclude colonic dilatation (≥ 6 cm), to estimate the extent of disease and to look for features that predict poor response to treatment (mucosal islands, more than two gas-filled loops of small bowel).

Abdominal ultrasound is a low-cost, non-invasive procedure, but very operator-dependent with low specificity for UC comparing with other causes of colonic inflammation. Hydrocolonic US has apparently high sensitivity for active colitis, but it is too cumbersome for daily practice [19]. Doppler US of superior and inferior mesenteric artery has been used to evaluate activity and risk of relapse, but it is not a standard procedure [20].

Small bowel radiology is not routinely recommended in UC. It should be done only in cases with diagnostic difficulties like rectal sparing, atypical symptoms and macroscopic backwash ileitis.

Leukocyte scintigrafy is a safe, noninvasive procedure used for the assessment of presence, extent and activity of disease. Unfortunately, it lacks specificity and is unreliable in patients on corticosteroids [21].

Virtual colonoscopy is an evolving technology with conflicting results. Subtle changes of the mucosa such as erosions or flat polyps are insufficiently visualized. It is not an alternative for colonoscopy.

Histopathology is a very important part of diagnostic process. It is important for diagnosis since normal mucosal biopsies exclude active UC as a cause of symptoms. Other important tasks are the assessment of disease activity and identification of intraepithelial neoplasia (dysplasia). Microscopic features can be classified into three categories: architectural changes (crypt branching and distorsion, crypt atrophy and surface irregularity), epithelial abnormalities (mucin depletion, Paneth cell metaplasia), and inflammatory features (increased lamina propria cellularity, basal plasmacytosis, basal lymphoid aggregates, lamina propria eosinophils). Diagnosis of UC is based on the combination of basal plasmacytosis (presence of plasma cells around or below the crypts), diffuse transmucosal lamina propria cell increase and widespread mucosal and crypt architectural distorsion [22]. Villous surface is an important feature of UC, since it is present in 17–63% of cases compared with 0–24% cases in CD and 0–7% cases in infective colitis. It is also present in one third of the initial biopsies of children with UC [23]. In adults, villous surface is present in 23% patients presenting 16–30 days after initial symptoms, but not in earlier biopsies [24]. Reliable histologic diagnosis of UC can be made with multiple biopsies (minimum of two samples) from five sites around colon (including rectum) and the ileum. Repeated biopsies after an interval may help solve differential diagnostic problems and establish definitive diagnosis in adults. In young children or patients with aberrant presentation of colitis, UC should always be considered in differential diagnosis even if pathology is not typical. Colonic stenosis always raises the suspicion of colorectal carcinoma. Multiple biopsies should be taken from the stenotic area. If the stenosis cannot be reached by endoscopy, imaging procedures like double contrast barium enema, CT and or MRI/colonography should be done.

Finally, all assembled data should be combined in order to assess disease activity and severity, guiding patient's management. Indices of UC severity have not been adequately validated. Indices used in daily practice are modifications of the original Truelove and Witts' criteria [25] and modified Mayo score that incorporates both clinical and endoscopic information [17]. A distinction should be made between disease activity at a point in time (remission, mild, moderate, severe) and the response of disease to treatment (steroid-refractory, biologic-dependent, etc.). The two should not be confused by terminology such as describing mildly active steroid-dependent disease as severe disease.

Pediatric UC

10–15% of patients with IBD are diagnosed before the age of 18 years. During puberty, the incidence is 7 per 100,000 per year and increases further during adolescence. In children, most cohort studies show lower incidence of UC compared with CD. In contrast to adults, clinical presentation of UC is more often severe in children, which may be explained by the predominance of pancolitis (70–80% of children) at the time of diagnosis [26, 27]. The leading clinical manifestation of UC is bloody diarrhea accompanied by tenesmus. Infective etiology should be excluded, although its presence does not exclude a diagnosis of IBD of either phenotype. A shorter interval from symptoms to diagnosis of UC explains why growth failure is half as common compared with CD. Growth failure is a unique complication of pediatric IBD, caused by inadequate calorie intake, increased losses and active inflammation. When catch-up growth does not occur after growth failure at diagnosis, or when height velocity decreases during maintenance treatment, it is highly likely that there is persistent disease activity, so

therapy should be more aggressive and an adequate calorie intake ensured.

Ileocolonoscopy and biopsies should be performed in all children or adolescents with a suspicion of UC. Pediatric patients with UC have more extensive disease than adults with rectal sparing in up to 30% of patients, warranting complete diagnostic work-up in children with bloody diarrhea [28]. Upper GI endoscopy is recommended when ileocolonoscopy does not confirm a diagnosis of UC. In children and adolescents (up to 16–18 years of age), endoscopy should be performed by a specialist with experience in pediatric gastroenterology in a setting that is suitable for diagnosing and treating children with IBD (pediatric hospital, access to general anesthesia).

Crohn's Disease (CD)

CD represents a heterogeneous entity comprising a variety of complex phenotypes. It is most commonly diagnosed in late adolescence or early adulthood, but there is significant increase in number of pediatric cases. Symptoms at presentation vary depending on the location, behavior and severity of disease, as well as extraintestinal manifestations and medication.

The evaluation should start with a full history that includes detailed questioning about the onset of symptoms, recent travel, food intolerances, contact with enteric illnesses, medications (including antibiotics and NSAIDs), smoking, family history and past history of appendectomy. Careful questioning about nocturnal symptoms, features of extraintestinal manifestations involving the mouth, skin, eye, joints, episodes of perianal abscess or anal fissure are mandatory.

Detailed physical examination should include, besides the usual parameters, careful evaluation of the nutritional status.

Laboratory tests should detect signs of acute and chronic inflammatory response, anemia, fluid depletion and signs of malnutrition/malabsorption. Initially, CRP, ESR and CBC should be looked at. CRP correlates well with disease activity assessed by standard indices and indicates serial changes in inflammatory activities owing to its short half-life of 19 h. CBC may reveal anemia, leukocytosis or thrombocytosis. ESR measures intestinal inflammation in CD less accurately, reflecting changes of plasma protein concentration and hematocrit. It increases with disease activity, but correlates better with colonic rather than ileal disease. Neither of these parameters is specific enough to allow differentiation from UC or enteric infections. Careful microbiology testing should be done to exclude infectious diarrhea.

The first-line endoscopic procedure is ileocolonoscopy with biopsies from the terminal ileum and each colonic segment to look for microscopic evidence of CD. The most useful endoscopic features of CD are partially or not involved rectum, asymmetric affection, discontinuous involvement ('skip' lesions), aphthous lesions, linear and serpiginous lesions, ulcerations within normal appearing mucosa, 'cobblestone' appearance, anal lesions and presence of fistulae and stenoses. Colonoscopy predicts the anatomical severity of CD colitis with a high probability [29]. In view of effects of biologic therapy, assessment of mucosal healing becomes important but remains difficult and prognostic value has to be shown in prospective studies. The value of colonoscopy is limited in case of severe active disease by a higher risk of bowel perforation. It is safer in those circumstances to do flexible proctosigmoidoscopy and postpone ileocolonoscopy until the clinical condition improves. Esophagogastroduodenoscopy is recommended in patients with upper gastrointestinal symptoms, where CD involving the upper GI tract is almost always accompanied by small or large bowel involvement. Endoscopy with biopsy by a push endoscope is safe and useful procedure in selected patients with suggestive symptoms and failure of conventional radiology. Ileoscopy is superior for the diagnosis of CD of the terminal ileum when compared to small bowel radiology, whether performed as SBFT, enteroclysis or meal with pneumocolon [30].

Biopsies obtained by endoscopy are helpful for the diagnosis of CD but are often to superficial and nonrepresentative. Characteristic histological features are granulomas, focal (segmental or discontinuous) crypt architectural abnormalities, focal or patchy chronic inflammation and mucin preservation at active sites. Presence of granuloma and at least one other feature is needed for the diagnosis. More accurate is histologic analysis of full-thickness bowel wall obtained as surgical specimen.

The scoring of endoscopic disease activity in CD is usually preserved for clinical studies. Endoscopic indices used in clinical practice are Crohn's Disease Endoscopic Index of Severity (CDEIS) [31] and Simple Endoscopic Score for CD (SES-CD) [32]. CDEIS is reliable, reproducible and validated and is presently gold standard for evaluation of endoscopic activity. However, it has poor correlation with clinical activity, it is time-consuming, elaboration of the score requires analogue scale transformation, and therefore is unsuitable for everyday clinical practice. SES-CD is easier and faster to score and calculate than CDEIS and the results are reproducible and reliably correlate with clinical activity.

In patients with evidence of CD determined by ileocolonoscopy, further investigations are recommended to examine the location and extent of CD in the small bowel. CD may affect the ileum out of reach of an endoscope or involve more proximal small bowel. Several techniques are used. Radiographic techniques for imaging the small intestine are divided into non-intubation and intubation studies. Non-intubation studies (small bowel follow through – SBFT, small bowel enema – SBE, oral MR or CT enterography) cannot ensure even distension of the small bowel for accurate assessment of strictures. Intubation studies (enteroclysis, CT and MRI enteroclysis) provide additional information on bowel wall thickening-associated changes in vascularity and in the adjacent mesentery. MRI has the ability to detect extramural complications (abscess, fistula, sacroiliitis, gall stones and renal calculi). The current standards for assessing the small intestine are SBFT and SBE. In routine practice, SBFT is simpler and superior to SBE for detecting mucosal disease, fistulae or gastroduodenal involvement, but it is operator dependent and not as good for strictures. Intestinal imaging with CT enteroclysis or CT enterography has improved and it is claimed to be complementary or even superior to barium studies for detection of involved segments. The radiation burden from fluoroscopy and CT is appreciable, so alternatives as US and MRI should be used where possible.

Wireless endoscopy capsule is advancement for small bowel imaging. It is considered in symptomatic patients with suspected small bowel disease in whom stricture/stenosis has been excluded, endoscopy of terminal ileum is normal or not possible, and in whom fluoroscopic or cross-sectional imaging have not revealed lesions. The accuracy of capsule endoscopy remains to be defined.

US is because of its nonionizing character suitable for the initial examination of a young population, especially for ileal CD [33]. Its sensitivity is 87–95% when performed by a specialist, but is even more operator dependent. The role of color, power Doppler and contrast-enhanced power Doppler investigation of the bowel wall for defining disease activity remains to be determined.

Leukocyte scintigraphy is safe, non-invasive and allows assessment of the presence, extent and activity of inflammation in patients not taking steroids but lacks specificity. Abdominal plain radiography is valuable in the initial assessment of patients with severe CD by providing evidence of small bowel or colonic dilatation, calcified calculi, sacroiliitis or impression of the mass in the right iliac fossa.

Stricturing CD often represents diagnostic challenge. The most reliable criterion for defining stricture is localized, relatively short persistent narrowing, whose functional effects may be judged from pre-stenotic dilatation. Suspected small bowel stenosis is best assessed by enteroclysis because it distends the bowel and reveals the extent and number of strictures. Enteroclysis most reliably differentiates irreversible stenosis from functional spasm. MRI enteroclysis is comparable to classical enteroclysis [34]. Plain film radiography and CT have similar accuracy in identifying small bowel obstruction. US is helpful in detecting prestenotic dilatation in small bowel strictures in severe cases that are candidates for surgery. If colonoscopy cannot reach the stricture or is incomplete due to stricture, barium enema is usually used. CT colonography can reveal mucosal pattern and show colitis proximal to a stricture, but may not identify all strictures seen on colonoscopy [35]. Differentiation between inflammatory and fibrostenotic strictures is crucial to the choice of therapy. Disease activity at a stricture is inferred from the presence or absence of ulceration that indicates active inflammation. Contrast-enhanced Doppler US may be valuable in determining disease activity within strictures. Both CT and MRI can illustrate mural changes with disease activity, MRI being more sensitive [36, 37].

Extramural complications of CD are clinically very important. US is an operator-dependent but readily available diagnostic tool for the diagnosis of fistulae and abscesses. CT and MRI are highly accurate in complicated CD, especially for the detection of fistulae, abscesses and phlegmons. MRI is superior to CT in that regard because it has higher sensitivity, provides capability of selecting cross-sectional planes (transverse, coronal, sagittal) and absence of radiation exposure.

Activity assessment of CD is based on noninvasive indices (clinical parameters), invasive indices (include endoscopy), biochemical markers of activity and quality of life measures. The main problem with assessment of activity using indices is the fact that they are combination of subjective and objective measurements. The most commonly used activity indices in CD are Crohn Disease Activity Index (CDAI) [38], Harvey-Bradshaw Index [39] and Van Hees Index [40]. CDAI is a complex index, difficult to calculate in daily clinical practice, with predominance of subjective symptoms and sizable interobserver variation (up to 100 points), with poor correlation with endoscopic and laboratory data and with inadequate rep-

resentation of EIMs, perianal disease and postoperative recurrence. In addition, it is not suitable for measuring perianal disease activity because these patients have low CDAI scores. Therefore, we have to use the Perianal Disease Activity Index [41] for perianal disease. Perianal disease should be assessed by MRI, proctosigmoidoscopy (to assess inflammatory activity), EUA (examination under anesthesia) which is a gold standard in hands of experienced surgeons and anorectal US which is sometimes difficult or impossible to perform due to local complications. Fistulography is not recommended.

Pediatric CD
The incidence of CD in children and adolescents has risen during the past decade. The disease presents before the age of 18 years in about 25% of all patients, and CD is becoming more common even in very young children aged <2 years. Certain features are unique to pediatric CD, like growth failure (10–40% of affected children) and abdominal pain due to stricturing disease. Family history of IBD is often present in children (up to 40%).

The IBD working party of the European Society of Pediatric Gastroenterology Hepatology and Nutrition (ESPGHAN) has reached a consensus on the diagnosis of IBD in children, which have been summarized as the 'Porto Criteria' [42]. This group feels that it is essential to establish a diagnosis of the type of disease, as well as to determine severity, localization and extent of the disease before treatment is started. The ECCO Consensus also agrees that all children suspected of CD should have a complete examination at the time of diagnosis.

The endoscopic procedure of choice is colonoscopy with ileal intubation and not rectosigmoidoscopy [43, 44]. In children, upper GI endoscopy is very important because both retrospective and prospective studies show that histology of the upper GI tract may confirm a diagnosis of CD that would otherwise have been missed in 11–29% of cases [45]. Endoscopy in children is best carried out under general anesthesia: it is safe and preferred for ethical reasons [46].

Small bowel radiology should be a part of the initial investigation because the small bowel may be abnormal even though the terminal ileum is normal. In addition, SBFT or enteroclysis will give information on the extent and possible complications of small bowel CD including strictures or internal fistulas. Transabdominal ultrasound is not a substitute, but may be used for initial assessment of symptoms or to look for complications.

The activity of CD in children can be assessed by the specific Pediatric Activity Index [47].

Conclusions

IBD denotes a very heterogeneous group of inflammatory bowel disorders. The diagnosis of IBD is, due to the nature of these diseases, frequently established by a non-strictly defined combination of clinical and diagnostic parameters.

Indeterminate colitis represents the type of chronic colitis where a definitive diagnosis of UC or CD cannot be made in spite of numerous colonoscopies and colonic biopsies or at colectomy. Diagnosis of IC is based on endoscopic and pathohistological analysis, problem being nonspecific endoscopic colonic changes and lack of generally accepted microscopic criteria for the diagnosis of IC. The microscopic evaluation is further burdened with lack of IBD features in the early stage of the disease, especially in children, and with the interobserver bias in the classification of colonic IBD. Negative pANCA and ASCA are features of a subgroup of IC patients.

UC, characterised by the continuous inflammation of the rectum and colon, can present with rectal sparing in children prior to treatment. The features of UC like cecal patch, appendiceal inflammation as a skip lesion and backwash ileitis have to be understood. There is no gold standard for the diagnosis of UC and the diagnosis is made on the basis of combination of medical history, clinical evaluation and endoscopic and histologic findings. In 10% of patients initially diagnosed as UC, the diagnosis will be changed during the 5-year period after the initial onset of symptoms.

There is no endoscopic feature specific for UC. Endoscopic changes usually correlate well with clinical activity. UC is classified by the disease extent into proctitis, left-sided colitis and extensive colitis beyond the splenic flexure. Colonoscopy, otherwise diagnostic procedure of choice, should be avoided in severe colitis. Virtual colonoscopy is not an alternative for colonoscopy.

Reliable histologic diagnosis of UC requires multiple biopsies from five sites around the colon including the rectum and ileum. Normal mucosal biopsies exclude active UC as a cause of symptoms. Villous surface is a feature more specific for UC in IBD spectrum, particularly in children. Repeated biopsies after an interval may help solve many diagnostic problems.

Pediatric patients with UC have more extensive disease than adults with rectal sparing in up to 30% of patients. Ileocolonoscopy is the endoscopic procedure of choice in children and should be performed, like all other endoscopic procedures, by an endoscopist with experience in pediatric gastroenterology in a setting suitable for diagnosing children with IBD. Growth failure is half as common compared with CD due to a shorter interval from symptoms to diagnosis of UC. Failure of catch-up growth indicates persistent disease activity.

CD is a heterogeneous entity with recent significant increase in number of pediatric cases. Symptoms are very variable depending on the location, behavior and severity of disease. Advances in technology provided the possibility for the assessment of the entire digestive system with endoscopy leading the way. The challenge is still the small bowel, where combination of endoscopy and imaging methods is used. Sophisticated imaging methods made the analysis of the bowel wall with its vascularity and adjacent mesentery possible. The problem of the assessment of inflammatory activity in a stricture is solvable by using combination of endoscopy, contrast-enhanced Doppler US and CT and MRI, MRI being more sensitive for mural changes with disease activity. Perianal disease should be assessed by MRI, proctosigmoidoscopy and examination under anesthesia which is a gold standard in the hands of an experienced surgeon. CDAI is the most commonly used activity index in CD but is not suitable for measuring perianal disease activity due to low CDAI scores in these patients. Instead, the Perianal Disease Activity Index (PDAI) should be used.

The incidence of CD in children and adolescents has risen significantly during the past decade. A high number of children with CD have extensive and severe disease resulting clinically in growth failure. Children require extensive endoscopic evaluation which is best carried out under general anesthesia. The activity of CD in children should be assessed by the Pediatric Activity Index.

Disclosure Statement

The author declares that no financial or other conflict of interest exists in relation to the content of the article.

References

1 Guindi M, Riddell RH: Indeterminate colitis. J Clin Pathol 2004;57:1233–1244.
2 Ekbom A: Indeterminate IBD: the magnitude of the problem. Inflamm Bowel Dis 2000;6:S14–S15.
3 Domizio P: Pathology of chronic inflammatory bowel disease in children. Baillieres Clin Gastroenterol 1994;8:35–63.
4 Rudolph WG, Uthoff SMS, McAuliffe TL, et al: Indeterminate colitis: the real story. Dis Colon Rectum 2002;45:1528–1534.

5 Bentley E, Jenkins D, Campbell F, et al: How could pathologists improve the initial diagnosis of colitis? Evidence from an international workshop. J Clin Pathol 2002;55:955–960.

6 Farmer M, Petras R, Hunet LE, et al: The importance of diagnostic accuracy in colonic inflammatory disease. Am J Gastroenterol 2000;95:3184–3188.

7 Yantiss RK, Odze RD: Diagnostic difficulties in inflammatory bowel disease pathology. Histopathology 2006;48:116–132.

8 Joosens S, Reinisch W, Vermeire S, et al: The value of anti-*Saccharomyces cerevisiae* antibodies and perinuclear antineutrophil cytoplasmic antibodies in indeterminate colitis: a prospective follow-up study. Gastroenterology 2002;122:1242–1247.

9 Geboes K, De Hertogh G: Indeterminate colitis. Inflamm Bowel Dis 2003;9:324–331.

10 Rajwal SR, Puntis JW, McClean P, et al: Endoscopic rectal sparing in children with untreated ulcerative colitis. J Pediatr Gastroenterol Nutr 2004;38:66–69.

11 Kim B, Barnett JL, Kleer CG, Appelman HD: Endoscopic and histologic patchiness in treated ulcerative colitis. Am J Gastroenterol 1999;94:3258–3262.

12 Ladefoged K, Munck LK, Jorgensen F, Engel P: Skip inflammation of the appendiceal orifice: a prospective endoscopic study. Scand J Gastroenterol 2005;40:1192–1196.

13 Abdelrazeq AS, Wilson TR, Leitch DL, et al: Ileitis in ulcerative colitis: is it backwash? Dis Colon Rectum 2005;48:2038–2046.

14 Hommes DW, Sterringa G, Van Deventer SJH, Tytgat GNJ: The pathogenicity of *Cytomegalovirus* in inflammatory bowel disease. Inflamm Bowel Diseas 2004;10:245–250.

15 Kojima T, Watanabe T, Hata K, et al: *Cytomegalovirus* infection in ulcerative colitis. Scand J Gastroenterol 2006;41:706–711.

16 Baron JH, Connell AM, Lennard-Jones JE: Variation between observers in describing mucosal appearances in proctocolitis. Br Med J 1964;i:89–92.

17 Schroeder KW, Tremaine WJ, Ilstrup DM: Coated oral 5-ASA therapy for mildly to moderately active ulcerative colitis. A randomized study. N Engl J Med 1987;317:1625–1629.

18 Satsangi J: Silverberg MS, Vermeire S, Colombel JF: The Montreal classification of inflammatory bowel disease: controversies, consensus and implications. Gut 2006;55:749–753.

19 Dixit R, Chowdary V, Kumar N: Hydrocolonic sonography in the evaluation of colonic lesions. Abdom Imaging 1999;34:1103–1107.

20 Ludwig D, Wiener S, Bruning A, et al: Mesenteric blood flow is related to disease activity and risk of relapse in ulcerative colitis: a prospective follow-up study. Gut 1999;45:546–552.

21 Koutroubakis IE, Koukouraki SI, Dimoulios PD, et al: Active inflammatory bowel disease: evaluation with 99mTc (V) DMSA scintigraphy. Radiology 2003;229:70–74.

22 Bentley E, Jenkins D, Campbell F, Warren BF: How could pathologists improve the initial diagnosis of colitis? Evidence from an international workshop. J Clin Pathol 2002;55:955–960.

23 Washington K, Greenson JK, Montgomery E, et al: Histopathology of ulcerative colitis in initial rectal biopsy in children. Am J Surg Pathol 2002;26:1441–1449.

24 Schumacher G, Kollberg B, Sandstedt B: A prospective study of first attacks of inflammatory bowel disease and infectious colitis: histologic course during the first year after presentation. Scand J Gastroenterol 1994;29:318–332.

25 Truelove CS, Witts LJ: Cortisone in ulcerative colitis: final report on a therapeutic trial. Br Med J 1955;ii:1041–1048.

26 Sawczenko A, Sandhu BK: Presenting features of inflammatory bowel disease in Great Britain and Ireland. Arch Dis Child 2003;88:995–1000.

27 Griffiths AM: Specificities of inflammatory bowel disease in childhood. Best Pract Res Clin Gastroenterol 2004;18:509–523.

28 Glickman JN, Bousvaros A, Farraye FA, et al: Pediatric patients with untreated ulcerative colitis may present initially with unusual morphologic findings. Am J Surg Pathol 2004;28:190–197.

29 Nahon S, Bouhnik Y, Lavergne-Slove A, et al: Colonoscopy accurately predicts the anatomical severity of colonic Crohn's disease attacks: correlation with findings from colectomy specimens. Am J Gastroenterol 2002;97:102–107.

30 Marschall LK, Cawdron R, Zealley I, et al: Prospective comparison of small bowel meal with pneumocolon versus ileocolonoscopy for the diagnosis of ileal Crohn's disease. Am J Gastroenterol 2004;99:1321–1329.

31 Groupe D'Etudes Therapeutiques Des Affections Inflammatories Du Tube Digestif (GETAID), presented by Mary JY, Modigliani R: Development and validation of an endoscopic index of the severity of Crohn's disease: a prospective multicentre study. Gut 1989;30:983–989.

32 Daperno M, D'Haens G, Van Assche G, et al: Development and validation of a new, simplified endoscopic activity score for Crohn's disease: the SES-CD. Gastrointest Endosc 2004;60:505–512.

33 Bremner AR, Pridgeon J, Fairhurst J, Beattie RM: Ultrasound scanning may reduce the need for barium radiology in the assessment of small bowel Crohn's disease. Acta Pediatr 2004;93:479–481.

34 Rohr A, Rohr D, Kuhbacher T, et al: Radiologic assessment of small bowel obstructions: value of conventional enteroclysis and dynamic MR-enteroclysis. Rofo 2002;174:1158–1164.

35 Biancone L, Fiori R, Tosti C, et al: Virtual colonoscopy compared with conventional colonoscopy for stricturing postoperative recurrence in Crohn's disease. Inflamm Bowel Dis 2003;9:343–350.

36 Maccioni F, Viscido A, Broglia L, et al: Evaluation of Crohn disease activity with magnetic resonance imaging. Abdom Imaging 2000;25:219–228.

37 Koh DM, Miao Y, Chinn RJ, et al: MR imaging evaluation of the activity of Crohn's disease. AJR Am J Roentgenol 2001;177:1325–1332.

38 Best WR, Becktel JM, Singleton JW: Rederived values of eight coefficients of the Crohn's Disease Activity Index (CDAI). Gastroenterology 1979;77:843–846.

39 Harvey RF, Bradshaw JM: A simple index of Crohn's disease activity. Lancet 1980;1:514.

40 Van Hees PAM, van Elteren PH, van Lier HJJ, van Tongeren JHM: An index of inflammatory activity in patients with Crohn's disease. Gut 1980;21:279–286.

41 Irvine EJ: Usual therapy improves perianal Crohn's disease as measured by a new disease activity index. McMaster IBD Study Group. J Clin Gastroenterol 1995;20:27–32.

42 Escher JC, Amil Dias J, Bochenek K, et al: Inflammatory Bowel Disease in children and adolescents. Recommendations for Diagnosis: The Porto criteria. Medical Position Paper: IBD working group of the European Society of Pediatric Gastroenterology Hepatology and Nutrition (ESPGHAN). J Pediatr Gastroenterol Nutr 2005;41:1–7.

43 Escher JC, Ten KF, Lichtenbelt K, et al: Value of rectosigmoidoscopy with biopsies for diagnosis of inflammatory bowel disease in children. Inflamm Bowel Dis 2002;8:16–22.

44 Batres LA, Maller ES, Ruchelli E, et al: Terminal ileum intubation in pediatric colonoscopy and diagnostic value of conventional small bowel contrast radiography in pediatric inflammatory bowel disease. J Pediatr Gastroenterol Nutr 2002;35:320–323.

45 Castellaneta SP, Afzal NA, Greenberg M, et al: Diagnostic role of upper gastrointestinal endoscopy in pediatric inflammatory bowel disease. J Pediatr Gastroenterol Nutr 2004;39:257–261.

46 Wengrower D, Gozal D, Gozal Y, et al: Complicated endoscopic pediatric procedures using deep sedation and general anesthesia are safe in the endoscopy suite. Scand J Gastroenterol 2004;39:283–286.

47 Hyams JS, Ferry GD, Mandel FS, et al: Development and validation of a pediatric Crohn's disease activity index. J Pediatr Gastroenterol Nutr 1991;12:439–447.

Dig Dis 2009;27:278–284
DOI: 10.1159/000228561

Risk of Radiation and Choice of Imaging

Hans Herfarth   Lena Palmer

Department of Medicine, Division of Gastroenterology and Hepatology, University of North Carolina,
Chapel Hill, N.C., USA

Key Words
Inflammatory bowel diseases · Diagnostic medical
radiation · Magnetic resonance imaging · Computed
tomography · Fluoroscopy

Abstract
Radiological imaging plays an important role in the diagnosis and management of patients with inflammatory bowel
diseases (IBD). The barium or contrast techniques enteroclysis (SBE) and small bowel follow through (SBFT) are still the
mainstays in small bowel imaging. However, abdominal CT
and MRI, including enteroclysis, have comparable sensitivity
and specificity in detecting intestinal pathologies and have
gained in popularity over conventional techniques. The cancer risk associated with diagnostic procedures employing radiation has been receiving increasing attention over the last
few years. The cumulative exposure to ionizing radiation
may be a specific concern in young patients with IBD, who
are more susceptible than adults to the risks of ionizing radiation. Substantial exposure to radiation seems to be mainly caused by CT examinations of the abdomen. For that reason, imaging methods such as MRI or ultrasound should be
considered first when debating between alternative imaging strategies, particularly in young IBD patients. The major
drawbacks of MRI are its limited availability and greater costs
compared to CT. Moreover, the diagnostic accuracy of abdominal ultrasound is clearly operator dependent, which
limits the range of its applications. In light of these concerns,
diagnostic imaging studies using radiation will continue to
play an important role in the evaluation of patients with IBD.

Therefore, we need to develop low-radiation imaging protocols or improve access to MRI imaging procedures. We also
need to identify subsets of IBD patients who are at greater
risk of a significant lifetime exposure to radiation and develop methods to monitor their radiation exposure rate.

Copyright © 2009 S. Karger AG, Basel

Imaging Modalities in Inflammatory Bowel Diseases

The upper and lower gastrointestinal tract is generally
accessible with endoscopy, but only recently has the small
bowel, with its length of 3–4 m, become accessible by different imaging procedures. Capsule endoscopy and single or double balloon or spiral enteroscopy have allowed
direct visualization of nearly the entire small bowel.
These techniques are promising but not yet used as first-
line diagnostic tools. The first line of small bowel imaging remains radiological modalities (table 1). These are
employed in the following settings: (a) initial evaluation
of the patient for the purpose of establishing a diagnosis,
(b) in the preoperative situation to determine the full extent of the disease, (c) during clinical exacerbations to
determine if complications are present, or (d) to evaluate
extraintestinal manifestations of IBD.

Abdominal Ultrasound
Abdominal ultrasound offers the possibility to visu-
alize not only the gastrointestinal tract but also to evaluate the patient for extraintestinal complications such
as cholecystolithiasis or nephrolithiasis in the same ses-

Hans Herfarth, MD
Division of Gastroenterology and Hepatology, Department of Medicine
University of North Carolina, Bioinformatics Bldg., CB#7080
Chapel Hill, NC 27599 (USA)
Tel. +1 919 966 6806, Fax +1 919 966 7592, E-Mail hherf@med.unc.edu

Table 1. Comparison of the advantages and disadvantages of different imaging procedures for the evaluation of the small bowel in patients with IBD

	Small bowel follow through	Enteroclysis with nasojejunal intubation[1]	MRI/CT with nasojejunal intubation	MRI	CT	Ultra-sound
Peristaltic assessment	+	+	–	–	–	+
Lumen distension	+	++	++	+/–	+/–	+[2]
Functional stenosis	++	++	++	+	+	+
Detailed mucosal surface	+/–	+	–	–	–	+/–
Extraluminal pathology	–	–	+	+	+	+/–
Ionizing radiation	+	+	– (MRI)/+ (CT)	–	+	–
Pleasant procedure	+/–	–	–	+	+	+

[1] Nasojejunal intubation according to the technique of Herlinger [51].
[2] Employing oral contrast-enhanced bowel sonography as described by Parente et al. [5].

Table 2. Meta-analysis of studies investigating the per-patient sensitivity of abdominal ultrasound, scintigraphy, CT and MRI in patients with suspected or proven IBD [2]

	Number of studies	Pa-tients	Sensitivity, % (range)	Specificity, % (range)
Ultrasound	9	1,000	90 (78–96)	96 (67–100)
Scintigraphy	3	152	88 (76–95)	85 (78–93)
CT	4	113	84 (77–87)	95 (67–100)
MRI	7	292	93 (82–100)	93 (71–100)

The gold standard for the evaluation in all the studies was SBFT or SBE and/or surgery.

Table 3. Meta-analysis of studies investigating the per-intestinal segment sensitivity of abdominal ultrasound, scintigraphy, CT and MRI in patients with suspected or proven IBD [2]

	Number of studies	Pa-tients	Sensitivity, % (range)	Specificity, % (range)
Ultrasound	2	52	73 (70–78)	93 (92–93)
Scintigraphy	6	139	77 (73–87)	90 (76–96)
CT	3	86	67 (60–74)	90 (84–95)
MRI	5	131	70 (44–93)	94 (91–100)

The gold standard for the evaluation in all the studies was SBFT or SBE and/or surgery.

sion [1]. The sensitivity of high resolution abdominal ultrasound to detect small or large bowel inflammation in patients with suspected or proven IBD is in the range of 78–96% and 89–100%, respectively [2] (tables 2, 3). However, the sensitivity appears to be dependent on the localization of inflammation in the gastrointestinal tract. The method demonstrates good and reliable sensitivity if inflammation is present in the colon or terminal ileum, but is less likely to detect inflammatory lesions in the duodenum, proximal jejunum or rectum [3]. The use of oral and/or intravenous contrast media may be advantageous in detecting more subtle changes; however, multi-center studies examining such advanced ultrasound techniques are still missing [4, 5]. Several studies have also evaluated the clinical value of abdominal ultrasound in the detection of typical complications of Crohn's disease such as strictures, abscesses or intesti-

nal fistulizing disease. The sensitivity and specificity was described between 78–100% and 93–100%, respectively [4, 6, 7].

The advantages of abdominal ultrasound include its broad availability, ease of the examination, and lack of radiation exposure. The disadvantages, however, are the lack of standardized documentation, the variability of diagnostic accuracy by operator, and the limited diagnostic value in obese patients.

Small Bowel Follow Through (SBFT) and Small Bowel Enteroclysis (SBE)
SBFT after the application of oral barium is commonly performed to assess the presence or absence of inflammatory or strictured lesions in patients with IBD. This technique is considered to be reliable and reproducible in the daily clinical setting, provided it is a dedicated study

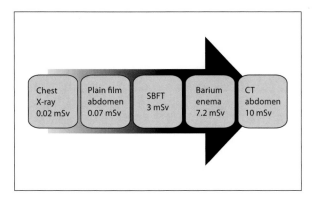

Fig. 1. Dose of diagnostic radiation for commonly used imaging studies in patients with IBD (according to Brenner and Hall [41]). The average exposure to environmental radiation of an individual person each year is 3 mSV.

incorporating fluoroscopy with manual palpation to compress individual loops properly [8, 9]. Whereas in North America SBFT is the preferred technique, in Europe SBE is favored. For SBE, a naso-gastric tube is placed behind the ligament of Treitz [10, 11]. With this technique, early mucosal pathologies of Crohn's disease in the small bowel can be visualized, including mucosal granularity, small aphthoid ulcerations, or diffuse fold thickening. However, given the need for placing and positioning the naso-gastric tube for contrast application, this type of examination is often considered extremely unpleasant by the patients.

Computed Tomography (CT) and Magnetic Resonance Imaging (MRI)
CT- or MRI-based imaging provides cross-sectional imaging in multiple planes. Both are able to demonstrate segmental thickening of the bowel wall, strictures or prestenotic dilatations and fistulas. CT or MR enteroclysis, with or without naso-jejunal intubation, is equal in sensitivity to conventional small bowel examinations in the assessment of severe and advanced Crohn's lesions [12–28].

The advantages of MRI and CT as compared to conventional radiological methods are the acquisition of additional information of extraluminal pathologies. Several studies comparing CT or MRI and conventional enteroclysis revealed further pathological extra-enteric abnormalities in 11–58% of the cases [20, 28–33]. Whereas the majority of the extraintestinal findings need no further clinical work-up or therapy, 12% of the findings

are of major clinical relevance [34], necessitating often a change in the medical or surgical management of IBD patients [35].

Which Technique Should Be Used?

In a recent meta-analysis, similar sensitivities and specificities for the various radiologic methods including abdominal ultrasound were reported [2] (tables 2, 3). Therefore, the choice of imaging probably is mostly dependent on local expertise, costs and availability of specific techniques. Only a few studies have compared the value of more than two different imaging techniques and including capsule endoscopy for the diagnostic approach of small bowel lesions in patients with suspected or proven IBD [36, 37]. The consensus of these studies seems to be that a combination of endoscopic and radiologic techniques are more reliable than a single imaging modality in the diagnosis of suspected IBD. Furthermore, capsule endoscopy demonstrates a superior sensitivity compared to radiological approaches. However, imaging studies such as SBFT, CT or MRI are generally performed anyway prior to capsule endoscopy in patients with suspected or proven IBD in order to identify potential strictures in the small bowel, as the risk of capsule retention is high in this patient group [38].

Diagnostic Medical Radiation and Cancer Risk

The technological improvements in the field of CT technology in the last 10–15 years lead to faster and more accurate imaging possibilities but have also significantly increased the risk of exposure to substantial cumulative diagnostic radiation doses over time compared to other imaging modalities (fig. 1). Currently, CT is the major source of diagnostic ionizing radiation [39]. In 2006 alone, over 63 million CT scans were performed in the United States. Radiation exposure imparts physiologic damage through various mechanisms, including DNA single or double strand breaks or base damage. Faulty DNA repair results in point mutations, chromosomal translocations, or gene fusions, all of which are implicated in the pathogenesis of cancer [40].

The cancer risks associated with the exposure to diagnostic radiation (X-ray or gamma-ray exposure) have been widely discussed in the medical literature in recent years, and it has been suggested that in the US the radiation exposure from CT examinations alone may be responsible for 0.5–2% of all cancers [41, 42]. Other studies have demonstrated a cumulative cancer risk of 0.6% in the United Kingdom, 1.5% in Germany and 3.2% in Japan [43]. These estimates were derived suggesting a linear dose effect ('linear no-threshold dose-effect model'), which postulates the possibility of carcinogenesis even with an exposure to low-dose radiation. Opponents to this model argue that extrapolating the cancer risk from high-dose exposure (>100 mSv) to lower doses may result in overestimation of the overall cancer risk.

Originally, risk estimates were derived from studies of survivors of the atomic bombs dropped on Japan in 1945, who were exposed to a range of doses of 0–4 Gy (table 4), and other risk groups such as the Colorado uranium miners' cohort or a cohort of Chinese tin miners [44]. More recently, several studies analyzed the risk of protracted low-dose radiation exposure (50–75 mSv) in nuclear industry workers and demonstrated an increased cancer-related mortality especially for lung cancer and multiple myeloma [45, 46]. Therefore, the postulation of an existing cancer risk associated with recurrent exposure to low-dose radiation seems to be reasonable; however, it is difficult to give an exact estimate of the magnitude of this risk.

Radiation and IBD

In recent years, the diagnostic approach for the evaluation of the small bowel in IBD patients in North America changed dramatically. This change is illustrated by the data of the Mayo Clinic demonstrating a decrease of 65% from 2,800 SBFT exams in 2003–2004 to 975 studies in 2007, while CT enterography increased by 840% from 375 studies in 2003 to 3,166 studies in 2007 [47]. Given the higher radiation exposure of patients undergoing CT examinations compared to SBFT exams, this shift in examination techniques already suggests that patients with IBD probably are at significantly higher risk for exposure to high amounts of diagnostic radiation compared to 10–15 years ago. So far only a few studies have evaluated radiation exposure in patients with IBD. In a retrospective analysis of 215 patients with either Crohn's disease or ulcerative colitis and a mean follow-up of approximately 9 years, Peloquin et al. at the Mayo Clinic found a median cumulative effective dose of diagnostic ionizing radiation of 26.6 mSv (range 0–279) in 103 patients with Crohn's disease and 10.5 mSv in 112 patients with UC [47]. The annual median effective dose of diagnostic ionizing radiation was 3.1 mSv/year in Crohn's disease patients and 1.2 mSv/year in patients with ulcerative colitis. The dif-

Table 4. Definitions used to quantify radiation exposure

Gray (Gy)	Energy (Joule) absorbed per unit of mass Used for calculations of organ doses Can be measured in anthropomorphic phantoms
Sievert (Sv)	Used for dose distributions, which are not homogenous (such as CT radiation) Provides an approximate estimate of the biological effects of radiation

ference of the effective radiation dose was primarily due to twice the number of abdomino-pelvic CT scans performed in Crohn's disease patients. Newnham et al. [48] from the Box Hill Hospital in Australia analyzed radiation exposure of 100 consecutive IBD patients at a tertiary referral center and found that 23% of the patients received an effective dose of diagnostic radiation >25 mSv and 11% received >50 mSv. The radiation exposure of 409 patients with Crohn's disease in a tertiary referral center in Ireland was analyzed between 1992 and 2007 by Desmond et al. [49]. They found results similar to those described above by the Mayo Clinic showing an increase of CT exams of nearly 400% over the 15-year study period. In the last 5-year period of their study (2002–2007), CT scans accounted for 84.7% of the overall diagnostic radiation. The mean cumulative dose of diagnostic radiation received by the patients was 36.1 mSv and exceeded 75 mSv in 15.5% of patients. The authors also analyzed risk factors for higher radiation exposure and found that certain medications and surgery were associated with cumulative effective doses >75 mSv, but not age at diagnosis, gender or smoking history (table 5). The largest study so far analyzed an insurance claims database for the radiation exposure in children [50]. 965 children with Crohn's disease and 628 with ulcerative colitis were identified and the radiation exposure was analyzed over a 24-month period. 34% of Crohn's disease patients and 23% of ulcerative colitis patients were exposed to moderate diagnostic radiation (OR 1.71, 95% CI 1.36–2.14) as defined by at least one CT examination or three fluoroscopic procedures during the observation period. For Crohn's disease patients, moderate radiation exposure was associated with hospitalization (OR 4.89, 95% CI 3.37–7.09), surgery (OR 2.93, 95% CI 1.59–5.39), emergency department encounter (OR 2.65, 95% CI 1.93–3.64), use of oral steroids (OR 2.25, 95% CI 1.50–3.38), and use of budesonide (OR 1.80, 95% CI 1.10–3.06). Interestingly, an inverse association was seen with immunomodulator

Table 5. Association between patient factors and total cumulative effective dose >75 mSv in patients with Crohn's disease (adapted from Desmond et al. [49])

Disease course and behavior	OR	95% CI	p value
Disease distribution			
Colonic	0.9	0.4–2.1	<0.71
Ileocolonic	2.1	1.0–4.2	<0.06
Upper gastrointestinal disease	2.4	1.2–4.9	<0.02
Perianal disease	1.3	0.6–2.3	<0.48
Disease behavior			
Stricturing	0.6	0.3–1.5	<0.3
Penetrating	2.0	1.0–3.9	<0.05
Medications			
Oral steroids	3.8	1.1–12.7	<0.01
Intravenous steroids	3.7	2.0–6.6	<0.0001
Immunosuppression	1.6	0.9–2.9	<0.12
Infliximab	2.3	1.2–4.4	<0.01
Surgical history			
One surgery only	1.8	0.7–4.4	<0.23
Multiple surgeries (>1)	2.7	1.4–5.4	<0.001
First surgery during study period	3.6	1.7–7.5	<0.001

use (OR 0.67, 95% CI 0.47–0.97). Similar relationships were seen in ulcerative colitis patients. These data are clearly provocative, since children are at greater risk than adults from the negative long-term effects of radiation. Children are inherently more radiosensitive and they have more remaining years of life during which a radiation-induced cancer could develop.

Providers at all levels of care are recognizing the risks of radiation-based imaging, and efforts are underway to minimize the potential for future harm from diagnostic testing. National coalitions have undertaken large-scale educational initiatives, such as the Image Gently™ campaign (http://www.pedrad.org/associations/5364/ig/), that inform both patients and providers of the risks of diagnostic testing. The National Quality Forum has made pediatric dose-reduction a patient-safety priority by including it as one of the consensus measure the *2009 Safe Practices for Better Healthcare* [http://www.qualityforum. org/publications/reports/safe_practices_2009.asp]. Providers can also involve patients in the risk-reduction effort through the use of a personal 'radiation diary' that tracks the cumulative radiation exposure they receive. An accurate and easily accessible account of radiation exposure may influence the choice of diagnostic imaging in patients who are likely to have higher risks of radiation exposure, such as those with perforating disease or a history of multiple surgeries.

Conclusions

Compared to 20 years ago, a broad range of imaging modalities are available as diagnostic procedures for patients with IBD. However, at least in North America and parts of Europe, CT-based imaging has evolved as the primary imaging tool in the diagnosis of suspected IBD or evaluation of complications in the course of disease. This is likely due to increased availability and more efficient performance of CT in terms of speed and diagnostic accuracy as compared to MRI. The cost of MRI is also a barrier to more widespread use of this modality. Use of CT, though, may add a significant risk of future neoplasia from radiation exposure to a group of patients who are already at increased risk of malignancy from other causes. Therefore, in future studies, risk factors for excessive radiation exposure must be identified, and patients and providers must be aware of the risk of diagnostic radiation when choosing between diagnostic approaches in the evaluation and management of inflammatory bowel disease.

Disclosure Statement

The authors declare that no financial or other conflict of interest exists in relation to the content of the article.

References

1 Hirche TO, Russler J, Schroder O, Schuessler G, Kappeser P, Caspary WF, Dietrich CF: The value of routinely performed ultrasonography in patients with Crohn disease. Scand J Gastroenterol 2002;37:1178–1183.

2 Horsthuis K, Bipat S, Bennink RJ, Stoker J: Inflammatory bowel disease diagnosed with US, MR, scintigraphy, and CT: meta-analysis of prospective studies. Radiology 2008;247:64–79.

3 Parente F, Greco S, Molteni M, Cucino C, Maconi G, Sampietro GM, Danelli PG, Cristaldi M, Bianco R, Gallus S, Bianchi Porro G: Role of early ultrasound in detecting inflammatory intestinal disorders and identifying their anatomical location within the bowel. Aliment Pharmacol Ther 2003;18:1009–1016.

4 Parente F, Greco S, Molteni M, Anderloni A, Bianchi Porro G: Imaging inflammatory bowel disease using bowel ultrasound. Eur J Gastroenterol Hepatol 2005;17:283–291.

5 Parente F, Greco S, Molteni M, Anderloni A, Sampietro GM, Danelli PG, Bianco R, Gallus S, Bianchi Porro G: Oral contrast enhanced bowel ultrasonography in the assessment of small intestine Crohn's disease. A prospective comparison with conventional ultrasound, X-ray studies, and ileocolonoscopy. Gut 2004;53:1652–1657.

6 Gasche C, Moser G, Turetschek K, Schober E, Moeschl P, Oberhuber G: Transabdominal bowel sonography for the detection of intestinal complications in Crohn's disease. Gut 1999;44:112–117.

7 Parente F, Maconi G, Bollani S, Anderloni A, Sampietro G, Cristaldi M, Franceschelli N, Bianco R, Taschieri AM, Bianchi Porro G: Bowel ultrasound in assessment of Crohn's disease and detection of related small bowel strictures: a prospective comparative study versus X-ray and intraoperative findings. Gut 2002;50:490–495.

8 Bernstein CN, Boult IF, Greenberg HM, van der Putten W, Duffy G, Grahame GR: A prospective randomized comparison between small bowel enteroclysis and small bowel follow-through in Crohn's disease. Gastroenterology 1997;113:390–398.

9 Marshall JK, Cawdron R, Zealley I, Riddell RH, Somers S, Irvine EJ: Prospective comparison of small bowel meal with pneumocolon versus ileo-colonoscopy for the diagnosis of ileal Crohn's disease. Am J Gastroenterol 2004;99:1321–1329.

10 Herlinger H: A modified technique for the double-contrast small bowel enema. Gastrointest Radiol 1978;3:201–207.

11 Herlinger H: The small bowel enema and the diagnosis of Crohn's disease. Radiol Clin North Am 1982;20:721–742.

12 Schunk K, Kern A, Oberholzer K, Kalden P, Mayer I, Orth T, Wanitschke R: Hydro-MRI in Crohn's disease: appraisal of disease activity. Invest Radiol 2000;35:431–437.

13 Rieber A, Wruk D, Potthast S, Nussle K, Reinshagen M, Adler G, Brambs HJ: Diagnostic imaging in Crohn's disease: comparison of magnetic resonance imaging and conventional imaging methods. Int J Colorectal Dis 2000;15:176–181.

14 Madsen SM, Thomsen HS, Munkholm P, Schlichting P, Davidsen B: Magnetic resonance imaging of Crohn's disease: early recognition of treatment response and relapse. Abdom Imaging 1997;22:164–166.

15 Madsen SM, Thomsen HS, Schlichting P, Dorph S, Munkholm P: Evaluation of treatment response in active Crohn's disease by low-field magnetic resonance imaging. Abdom Imaging 1999;24:232–239.

16 Umschaden HW, Szolar D, Gasser J, Umschaden M, Haselbach H: Small-bowel disease: comparison of MR enteroclysis images with conventional enteroclysis and surgical findings. Radiology 2000;215:717–725.

17 Maccioni F, Viscido A, Marini M, Caprilli R: MRI evaluation of Crohn's disease of the small and large bowel with the use of negative superparamagnetic oral contrast agents. Abdom Imaging 2002;27:384–393.

18 Maccioni F, Viscido A, Broglia L, Marrollo M, Masciangelo R, Caprilli R, Rossi P: Evaluation of Crohn disease activity with magnetic resonance imaging. Abdom Imaging 2000; 25:219–228.

19 Shoenut JP, Semelka RC, Magro CM, Silverman R, Yaffe CS, Micflikier AB: Comparison of magnetic resonance imaging and endoscopy in distinguishing the type and severity of inflammatory bowel disease. J Clin Gastroenterol 1994;19:31–35.

20 Holzknecht N, Helmberger T, von Ritter C, Gauger J, Faber S, Reiser M: MRI of the small intestine with rapid MRI sequences in Crohn disease after enteroclysis with oral iron particles. Radiologe 1998;38:29–36.

21 Koh DM, Miao Y, Chinn RJ, Amin Z, Zeegen R, Westaby D, Healy JC: MR imaging evaluation of the activity of Crohn's disease. AJR Am J Roentgenol 2001;177:1325–1332.

22 Small WC, DeSimone-Macchi D, Parker JR, et al: A multisite phase III study of the safety and efficacy of a new manganese chloride-based gastrointestinal contrast agent for MRI of the abdomen and pelvis. J Magn Reson Imaging 1999;10:15–24.

23 Kettritz U, Isaacs K, Warshauer DM, Semelka RC: Crohn's disease. Pilot study comparing MRI of the abdomen with clinical evaluation. J Clin Gastroenterol 1995;21: 249–253.

24 Low RN, Sebrechts CP, Politoske DA, Bennett MT, Flores S, Snyder RJ, Pressman JH: Crohn disease with endoscopic correlation: single-shot fast spin-echo and gadolinium-enhanced fat-suppressed spoiled gradient-echo MR imaging. Radiology 2002;222:652–660.

25 Low RN, Francis IR, Politoske D, Bennett M: Crohn's disease evaluation: comparison of contrast-enhanced MR imaging and single-phase helical CT scanning. J Magn Reson Imaging 2000;11:127–135.

26 Marcos HB, Semelka RC: Evaluation of Crohn's disease using half-fourier RARE and gadolinium-enhanced SGE sequences: initial results. Magn Reson Imaging 2000;18: 263–268.

27 Frokjaer JB, Larsen E, Steffensen E, Nielsen AH, Drewes AM: Magnetic resonance imaging of the small bowel in Crohn's disease. Scand J Gastroenterol 2005;40:832–842.

28 Bernstein CN, Greenberg H, Boult I, Chubey S, Leblanc C, Ryner L: A prospective comparison study of MRI versus small bowel follow-through in recurrent Crohn's disease. Am J Gastroenterol 2005;100:2493–2502.

29 Aschoff AJ, Zeitler H, Merkle EM, Reinshagen M, Brambs HJ, Rieber A: MR enteroclysis for nuclear spin tomographic diagnosis of inflammatory bowel diseases with contrast enhancement. Rofo 1997;167:387–391.

30 Rieber A, Wruk D, Nussle K, Aschoff AJ, Reinshagen M, Adler G, Brambs HJ, Tomczak R: MRI of the abdomen combined with enteroclysis in Crohn disease using oral and intravenous Gd-DTPA. Radiologe 1998; 38:23–28.

31 Jamieson DH, Shipman PJ, Israel DM, Jacobson K: Comparison of multidetector CT and barium studies of the small bowel: inflammatory bowel disease in children. AJR Am J Roentgenol 2003;180:1211–1216.

32 Mako EK, Mester AR, Tarjan Z, Karlinger K, Toth G: Enteroclysis and spiral CT examination in diagnosis and evaluation of small bowel Crohn's disease. Eur J Radiol 2000;35: 168–175.

33 Fishman EK, Wolf EJ, Jones B, Bayless TM, Siegelman SS: CT evaluation of Crohn's disease: effect on patient management. AJR Am J Roentgenol 1987;148:537–540.

34 Herfarth H, Grunert M, Klebl F, Strauch U, Feuerbach S, Scholmerich J, Rogler G, Schreyer AG: Frequency and nature of incidental extra-enteric lesions found on magnetic resonance enterography (MR-E) in patients with inflammatory bowel diseases (IBD). PLoS One 2009;4:e4863.

35 Booya F, Akram S, Fletcher JG, Huprich JE, Johnson CD, Fidler JL, Barlow JM, Solem CA, Sandborn WJ, Loftus EV Jr: CT enterography and fistulizing Crohn's disease: clinical benefit and radiographic findings. Abdom Imaging 2009;34:467–475.

36 Albert JG, Martiny F, Krummenerl A, Stock K, Lesske J, Gobel CM, Lotterer E, Nietsch HH, Behrmann C, Fleig WE: Diagnosis of small bowel Crohn's disease: a prospective comparison of capsule endoscopy with magnetic resonance imaging and fluoroscopic enteroclysis. Gut 2005;54:1721–1727.

37 Solem CA, Loftus EV Jr, Fletcher JG, et al: Small-bowel imaging in Crohn's disease: a prospective, blinded, 4-way comparison trial. Gastrointest Endosc 2008;68:255–266.

38 Triester SL, Leighton JA, Leontiadis GI, Gurudu SR, Fleischer DE, Hara AK, Heigh RI, Shiff AD, Sharma VK: A meta-analysis of the yield of capsule endoscopy compared to other diagnostic modalities in patients with non-structuring small bowel Crohn's disease. AJR Am J Gastroenterol 2006;101:954–964.

39 Martin DR, Semelka RC: Health effects of ionising radiation from diagnostic CT. Lancet 2006;367:1712–1714.

40 Barcellos-Hoff MH: Cancer as an emergent phenomenon in systems radiation biology. Radiat Environ Biophys 2008;47:33–38.

41 Brenner DJ, Hall EJ: Computed tomography: an increasing source of radiation exposure. N Engl J Med 2007;357:2277–2284.

42 Doll R, Peto R: The causes of cancer: quantitative estimates of avoidable risks of cancer in the United States today. J Natl Cancer Inst 1981;66:1191–1308.

43 Berrington de Gonzalez A, Darby S: Risk of cancer from diagnostic X-rays: estimates for the UK and 14 other countries. Lancet 2004; 363:345–351.

44 Krewski D, Zielinski JM, Hazelton WD, Garner MJ, Moolgavkar SH: The use of biologically based cancer risk models in radiation epidemiology. Radiat Prot Dosimetry 2003; 104:367–376.

45 Cardis E, Vrijheid M, Blettner M, et al: The 15-Country Collaborative Study of Cancer Risk among Radiation Workers in the Nuclear Industry: estimates of radiation-related cancer risks. Radiat Res 2007;167:396–416.

46 Vrijheid M, Cardis E, Blettner M, et al: The 15-Country Collaborative Study of Cancer Risk Among Radiation Workers in the Nuclear Industry: design, epidemiological methods and descriptive results. Radiat Res 2007;167:361–379.

47 Peloquin JM, Pardi DS, Sandborn WJ, Fletcher JG, McCollough CH, Schueler BA, Kofler JA, Enders FT, Achenbach SJ, Loftus EV Jr: Diagnostic ionizing radiation exposure in a population-based cohort of patients with inflammatory bowel disease. Am J Gastroenterol 2008;103:2015–2022.

48 Newnham E, Hawkes E, Surender A, James SL, Gearry R, Gibson PR: Quantifying exposure to diagnostic medical radiation in patients with inflammatory bowel disease: are we contributing to malignancy? Aliment Pharmacol Ther 2007;26:1019–1024.

49 Desmond AN, O'Regan K, Curran C, McWilliams S, Fitzgerald T, Maher MM, Shanahan F: Crohn's disease: factors associated with exposure to high levels of diagnostic radiation. Gut 2008;57:1524–1529.

50 Palmer L, Porter C, Kappelman M: Diagnostic ionizing radiation exposure in a population-based cohort of children with inflammatory bowel disease. Inflamm Bowel Dis 2008;12(suppl 3):S4–S5.

51 Herlinger H: Guide to imaging of the small bowel. Gastroenterol Clin North Am 1995; 24:309–329.

Dig Dis 2009;27:285–290
DOI: 10.1159/000228562

Bowel Ultrasound and Mucosal Healing in Ulcerative Colitis

F. Parente[a] M. Molteni[a] B. Marino[a] A. Colli[b] S. Ardizzone[c] S. Greco[c]
G. Sampietro[d] S. Gallus[e]

[a]Gastrointestinal Unit and [b]Department of Internal Medicine, A. Manzoni Hospital, Lecco,
[c]Division of Gastroenterology and [d]Division of General Surgery, L. Sacco University Hospital, and
[e]Section of Medical Epidemiology, Mario Negri Pharmacological Institute, Milan, Italy

Key Words
Bowel ultrasound · Colonoscopy · Ulcerative colitis ·
Mucosal healing

Abstract

Background and Aim: Mucosal healing (MH) after short-term medical treatment is being considered as an important step in the therapeutic work-up of inflammatory bowel disorder (IBD) patients due to the potential prognostic role of MH in predicting disease outcome. However, IBD patients are reluctant to be re-endoscoped during follow-up; therefore, there is a need for non-invasive alternative index of MH which can replace endoscopy in clinical practice. We evaluated bowel ultrasound (US) as a surrogate of colonoscopy in a series of consecutive patients with active ulcerative colitis (UC). *Patients and Methods:* 83 patients with moderate to severe UC requiring high-dose steroids were initially recruited; endoscopic severity of UC was graded 0–3 according to Baron score, and US severity was also graded 0–3 according to the colonic wall thickening and the presence of vascular signal at power Doppler. 74 patients responsive to steroids and then maintained on 5-ASA compounds were followed up with repeated colonoscopy and bowel US at 3, 9 and 15 months from entry. Concordance between clinical, endoscopic and US scores at various visits was determined by kappa statistics. Multiple unconditional logistic regression models were used to assess the predictivity of Truelove, Baron and US scores measured at 3 and 9 months on the development of a UC relapse (Baron score 2–3) at 15 months. *Results:* An inconsistent concordance was found over time between 0 and I Baron scores and Truelove score (weighted κ between 0.38 and 0.94), with high and consistent concordance between 0 and I Baron scores and US scores (weighted κ between 0.76 and 0.90). On logistic regression analysis, a moderate/severe Baron score, regardless of their Truelove score, at 3 months was associated with a high risk of endoscopic activity at 15 months (OR 5.2; 95% CI: 1.6–17.6); similarly, patients with severe US scores (2–3) at 3 months had a high risk of severe endoscopic activity at 15 months (OR 9.1; 95% CI: 2.5–33.5). *Discussion:* In expert hands bowel US may be used as a surrogate of colonoscopy in evaluating the response to high-dose steroids in severe forms of UC. US score after 3 months of steroid therapy accurately predicts clinical outcome of disease at 15 months.

Copyright © 2009 S. Karger AG, Basel

Introduction

Ulcerative colitis (UC) is a chronic, relapsing-remitting, inflammatory disease of the colon. Natural history studies document that the cumulative probability of a relapse-free course decreases rapidly with time, being ap-

Fabrizio Parente, MD
Gastrointestinal Unit, A. Manzoni Hospital
IT–23900 Lecco (Italy)
Tel. +39 03 4148 9969, Fax +39 03 4148 9966
E-Mail f.parente@ospedale.lecco.it

proximately 18% at 5 years, with a colectomy rate of 24% at the same end-point [1, 2]. These studies also reveal that the course of UC has changed over the last decades, with less cumulative mortality, less severity and fewer life-threatening complications [3].

In recent years, mucosal healing, as assessed by endoscopy (ileo-colonoscopy), has emerged as an important end-point of any short-term medical therapy for inflammatory bowel disease (IBD). In particular, the most intriguing data on this matter come from the experience with biological therapies such as infliximab in Crohn's disease, where a correlation between mucosa healing and better clinical outcome has been shown [4]. Indeed, after the introduction of biologic treatment, mucosa healing has been proposed to be an important sign of efficacy in the acute stage as well as an important parameter in the individual follow-up of patients.

Since UC is a disease affecting the superficial layer of colonic mucosa, mucosa healing is, theoretically, a more achievable result of therapy compared to the transmural inflammation of Crohn's disease; thus, endoscopic response is often a target asked in clinical trials [5].

Unfortunately, patients with UC are often reluctant to be re-colonoscoped during follow-up because of the invasiveness and pain sensation during colonoscopy. Therefore, in clinical practice, response to medical therapy of patients with UC usually relies on clinical scoring systems (i.e. Truelove index, CAI or Mayo score), which are mainly based on subjective symptoms. Even the addition of serological markers of inflammation (such as the determination of C-reactive protein levels) adds little to conventional clinical scores for predicting clinical outcome, especially in UC [6, 7].

A big current debate is now arguing whether or not there is the need to achieve not only clinical response but also endoscopic remission, since direct evidences are still lacking, both concerning the ability of current treatment to induce mucosal healing, and on the clinical impact of also assessing endoscopic rather than only clinical response [8]. Thus, the key question is whether the mucosal healing itself is able to improve the outcome of the disease, and therefore if the clinical evaluation alone is not sufficient to monitor UC patients in clinical practice.

Bowel Ultrasound in Ulcerative Colitis

Bowel examination by means of transabdominal ultrasound (US) has been used in clinical practice for at least 20 years with the aim of detecting inflammatory diseases of the small and the large intestine such as appendicitis, diverticulitis, UC and Crohn's disease [9–12]. However, only during the last decade has bowel US become accepted as a primary imaging procedure in the diagnostic work-up and follow-up of inflammatory bowel disease. This has been due to the technological advancement of US equipment that has greatly improved resolution capability with good cross-sectional imaging of the gut wall and display of the surrounding mesentery, thus making it possible to detect not only bowel wall infiltrations but also peri-intestinal abnormalities. In particular, leading studies over the last few years have identified three main fields of application for bowel US in IBD: (1) the initial evaluation of patients with clinically suspected IBD; (2) the definition of the anatomic location and extension of an already diagnosed IBD (including the detection of abdominal complications), and (3) the follow-up of patients with Crohn's disease after resective or conservative surgical therapy. Some uncertainty still persists as to the potential use of bowel US in assessing disease activity and monitoring the response to medical therapy in these disorders, as very few studies have been performed in this regard.

The combination of grey scale US with the assessment of intramural blood flow by color Doppler has recently showed to be able to establish parameters predictive of clinical outcome of inflammatory bowel disease [9–14]. However, no endoscopic-controlled study has evaluated so far the usefulness of bowel US as compared to colonoscopy in monitoring response to medical therapy of patients with UC.

We have therefore evaluated the accuracy of a US activity index in assessing response to therapy as well as the risk of subsequent relapse in a defined cohort of patients with severe attack or flare-up of UC in comparison with the traditional clinical and endoscopic scores.

Patients and Methods

All patients were referred by their General Practitioners or presented as emergencies at our gastroenterological centers, and those who were diagnosed as suffering from UC were potential candidates to enter the study. Patients signed a written informed consent form to undergo endoscopic and ultrasound examination according to our institutional guidelines.

Patient Population
Patients with a first diagnosis or flare-up of UC, according to previously published criteria [15], and needing high-dose systemic steroid therapy for moderate to severe active disease, were included in the study.

Parente/Molteni/Marino/Colli/
Ardizzone/Greco/Sampietro/Gallus

For all the included patients, the following demographic and clinical data were collected at the time of enrolment: sex, familial history of IBD, smoke habitus, previous appendectomy, date of birth, age at diagnosis, duration of disease, disease extension (left, subtotal or pancolitis), clinical and endoscopic activity before starting steroid therapy, concomitant therapies. Patients with proctitis only were excluded due to the well-known difficulties of US in exploring the deep pelvis. Left colitis was defined as a colitis with extended activity up to splenic flexure, subtotal colitis was defined as activity up to the hepatic flexure, whereas extensive colitis included pancolitis.

Therapy, Assessment and Follow-Up

All patients were treated with systemic steroid (oral or parenteral) prednisolone at initial dose ranging from 40 to 60 mg/day, with tapering over a period of 3 months.

Clinical activity was evaluated by Truelove and Witts criteria [16] and classified as remission, mild disease, moderate disease and severe disease. Endoscopic activity was scored using the endoscopic index as described by Baron and classified as remission (0), mild activity (1), moderate activity (2) and severe activity (3) [17]. US severity was also graded 0–3 according to the maximum colonic wall thickening (CTW) and the degree of intramural blood flow (grade 0: CTW <4 mm and no or scarce intramural blood flow; grade 1: CTW 4–6 mm and blood flow; grade 2: CTW 6–8 mm and blood flow; grade 3: CTW >8 mm and blood flow) [18].

All patients were evaluated prospectively according to clinical and endoscopic indexes at 3, 9 and 15 months. At 3 months, the following data were collected: date of follow-up, Truelove index, Baron index, US score, added therapies, clinical and endoscopic response to steroid treatment. Then at the following visits and for the entire follow-up period, the following data were collected: date of follow-up, Truelove index, Baron index, US score and any added therapy.

Outcome Measures

Early outcome, after 3 months from the beginning of corticosteroid therapy, was used to identify patients with complete, partial response or no response using Baron score as gold standard, so that its influence on the subsequent outcome could be evaluated. Immunosuppressive treatment was started in steroid-resistant and steroid-dependent patients and included cyclosporine A, azathioprine/6-mercaptopurine and infliximab. Colectomy included proctocolectomy and ileal pouch-anal anastomosis for refractory disease. During the follow-up the following outcomes were evaluated: relapse occurrence, time to relapse (months from first steroid therapy), number of relapses, number of hospitalizations for UC, immunosuppressive treatment, colectomy.

Statistical Analysis

Concordance between clinical, endoscopic and US scores at 0, 3, 9 and 15 months was determined by kappa statistics. Multiple unconditional logistic regression models were used to assess predictivity of Truelove, Baron and US scores measured at 3 and 9 months on the development of a UC relapse (Baron score 2–3) at 15 months.

Table 1. Distribution of the 74 patients with UC who clinically responded to CS therapy at 3 months, according to age, sex and various selected covariates

Factors	n	%
Total	74	100.0
Age		
<25 years	26	35.1
25–39 years	30	40.5
≥40 years	18	24.3
Sex		
Men	46	62.2
Women	28	37.8
Family history		
No	70	94.6
Yes	4	5.4
Smoking status		
Never	47	63.5
Current	15	20.3
Ex-smokers	12	16.2
Appendectomy		
No	68	91.9
Yes	6	8.1
Colitis extension		
Left colitis	42	56.8
Extensive colitis	25	33.8
Subtotal colitis	7	9.5

Results

From 2000 to 2005, 112 patients with moderate to severe UC requiring a course of systemic corticosteroids were seen at our centers. Eighteen (16.1%) were excluded because they had already been treated with immunosuppressors – azathioprine (AZA) and/or cyclosporin A (CyA) – at the time of diagnosis, whereas 11 more patients did not satisfy all the inclusion criteria (7 had proctitis alone) or refused to enter the study, thus reducing the eligible population to 83 patients. The clinical and demographic characteristics at enrolment of the 74 patients who responded clinically to corticosteroid therapy at 3 months and were included in the final analysis are reported in table 1. Nine patients did not respond to steroids and underwent colectomy or early immunosuppressive or biological therapy. Most patients had a left colitis (56.8%) or extensive colitis (33.8%). The clinical activity was moderate in 12.2% and severe in 87.8% of patients. Endoscopic activity was moderate in 35.2% and severe in 64.8% of patients, whereas US activity was moderate in 37.8% and severe in 62.2% of patients.

Table 2. Concordance between Baron score (gold standard) and Truelove and between Baron score and US score at 3 months

a Baron score vs. Truelove score

Baron score	Truelove score			Total
	mild	moderately severe	severe	
0–I	48	3	0	51
II	7	6	0	13
III	4	6	0	10
Total	59	15	0	74

Statistics	Value	ASE	95% CI
Kappa	0.3486	0.0911	0.1700–0.5272
Weighted kappa	0.3795	0.0844	0.2140–0.5450

b Baron score vs. US score

Baron score	US score			Total
	0–1	2	3	
0–I	49	2	0	51
II	2	6	5	13
III	0	3	7	10
Total	51	11	12	74

Statistics	Value	ASE	95% CI
Kappa	0.6600	0.0774	0.5084–0.8117
Weighted kappa	0.7622	0.0578	0.6488–0.8755

Table 3. Concordance between Baron score (gold standard) and Truelove and between Baron score and US score at 15 months

a Baron score vs. Truelove score

Baron score	Truelove score			Total
	mild	moderately severe	severe	
0–I	48	1	0	49
II	6	6	1	13
III	1	5	6	12
Total	55	12	7	74

Statistics	Value	ASE	95% CI
Kappa	0.5923	0.0858	0.4242–0.7604
Weighted kappa	0.6868	0.0734	0.5430–0.8306

b Baron score vs. US score

Baron score	US score			Total
	0–1	2	3	
0–I	48	1	0	49
II	0		1	13
III	0	3	9	12
Total	48	16	10	74

Statistics	Value	ASE	95% CI
Kappa	0.8677	0.0542	0.7614–0.9740
Weighted kappa	0.9042	0.0398	0.8263–0.9821

Oral maintenance therapy was started in 68 patients who received oral salicylates (sulfasalazine or mesalazine), whereas topical mesalazine was started in the remaining patients.

Concordance between Various Scores and Long-Term Outcome

Considering endoscopy as the reference test for a good response to steroids, in the three visits we showed inconsistent concordance between 0 and I Baron scores and Truelove score (weighted κ between 0.38 and 0.94), but high and consistent concordance between 0 and I Baron scores and US scores (weighted κ between 0.76 and 0.90) (tables 2, 3).

On logistic regression analysis, a moderate to severe Truelove score at the 3rd month was associated with a high risk of endoscopic activity at the 15th month (OR 12.6; 95% CI: 2.6–61.8); similarly, patients with severe US scores (2–3) at the 3rd month regardless of their Truelove score had a high risk of severe endoscopic activity at the 15th month (OR 9.1; 95% CI: 2.5–33.5); a significant direct association, but at a lower extent has also been shown between Baron score at the 3rd and 15th months (OR 5.2; 95% CI: 1.6–17.6) (table 4).

Discussion

Systemic corticosteroids have been the mainstay of treatment for patients with active UC since the early 1960s [2]. Corticosteroids are rapidly active and highly effective, making them the drug of choice for the initial management of moderate to severe forms of UC [19, 20]. However, very few studies have assessed so far the short-term clinical outcome of steroid-treated patients, and even fewer have evaluated UC patients treated early after

Parente/Molteni/Marino/Colli/
Ardizzone/Greco/Sampietro/Gallus

Table 4. Distribution of 74 patients with UC, by Baron score at 15 months according to Baron and US score after 3 and 9 months

Factors	Baron score at 15 months				OR*	95% CI
	II–III		0–I			
	n	%	n	%		
Baron score at 3rd month						
0–I	10	40.0	41	83.7	1.00	
II	10	40.0	3	6.1	9.98	1.95–51.1
III	5	20.0	5	10.2	2.77	0.59–12.9
Ultrasound score at 3rd month						
0–1	8	32.0	43	87.8	1.00	
2	8	32.0	3	6.1	7.95	1.53–41.4
3	9	36.0	3	6.1	10.3	2.07–51.2
Baron score at 9th month						
0–I	7	28.0	43	87.8	1.00	
II	8	32.0	1	2.0	37.6	3.39–417
III	10	40.0	5	10.2	10.0	2.24–44.6
Ultrasound score at 9th month						
0–1	7	28.0	43	87.8	1.00	
2	7	28.0	3	6.1	12.3	1.89–80.0
3	11	44.0	3	6.1	16.6	3.34–83.0

* Estimated by unconditional multiple logistic regression models after allowance for smoking status and appendicectomy (backward selection).

diagnosis [16, 21–26]. Moreover, endoscopic response after corticosteroids has been analyzed in a few studies, and none used endoscopic outcome as a predictive factor for following the clinical course of the disease [16, 21, 27]. Indeed, if clinical remission is relatively common after high-dose steroid treatment, endoscopic remission is a less frequent phenomenon; data from the above-mentioned studies show that not achieving complete endoscopic remission occurs in 36–40% of patients after 2–3 months of steroid therapy. However, patients who reach endoscopic remission seem to have a more prolonged quiescent phase of disease and are less prone to develop long-term recurrence. Indeed, three studies (two of which were published in abstract form only) have shown that the 1-year relapse rate of UC patients who achieve complete endoscopic remission at the time of starting maintenance therapy with 5-ASA compounds is significantly lower as compared to those with residual endoscopic activity [28–30].

Further information on the importance of obtaining endoscopic remission after short-term medical therapy come from the recent experience with biological agents such as infliximab, which showed, both in CD and UC, a correlation between mucosal healing and better clinical outcome [4, 31]. This is the reason why after the introduction of biologic treatment, mucosal healing is being considered as an important measure of treatment efficacy, and also a main end-point in clinical trials.

Bowel US has been recently proposed as a useful tool in assessing disease activity in IBD. In particular, the combination of colonic bowel thickening determined by grey scale US along with the assessment of intramural bowel flow by power Doppler has been shown to be able to predict endoscopic activity evaluated at colonoscopy [14]. In this regard, a preliminary study of ours suggested that a consistent proportion of patients (approximately 25%) with moderate to severe UC may refer significant clinical improvement under intensive medical treatment with steroids despite a persistent endoscopic and ultrasonographic disease activity, and they are at risk of rapid recurrence after steroid withdrawal [18]. Rigorous experience in this specific setting is now provided by our results, which confirm that not achieving complete mucosal healing after short-term steroid therapy, as documented by colonoscopy or bowel US, is predictive of a negative prognosis, being associated with a higher risk of relapse at 15 months. Thus, the most important objective of any pharmacological short-term therapy for moderate to severe forms of UC should be achieving not only clinical but also, especially, endoscopic remission. In expert hands, bowel US may constitute an accurate surrogate of colonoscopy in order to assess response to treatment and may therefore be preferred to endoscopy in clinical practice, with the exclusion of diseases confined to the rectum only.

Disclosure Statement

The authors declare that no financial or other conflict of interest exists in relation to the content of the article.

References

1 Langholz E, Munkholm P, Davidsen M, et al: Course of ulcerative colitis: analysis of changes in disease activity over years. Gastroenterology 1994;107:3–11.

2 Farmer RG, Easley KA, Rankin GB: Clinical patterns, natural history, and progression of ulcerative colitis: a long term follow-up of 1116 patients. Dig Dis Sci 1993;38:1137–1146.

3 Softley A, Clamp SE, Watkinson G, et al: The natural history of inflammatory bowel disease: has there been a change in the last 20 years? Scand J Gastroenterol 1988;28(suppl 144):20–23.

4 Lichtenstein GR, Yan S, Bala M, et al: Infliximab maintenance treatment reduces hospitalizations, surgeries, and procedures in fistulizing Crohn's disease. Gastroenterology 2005;128:862–869.

5 Van Assche G, Ferrante M, Vermeire S, et al: The role and importance of endoscopic mucosal healing in Crohn's disease. Gastrointest Endosc 2004;6:138–143.

6 Vermeire S, Van Assche G, Rutgeerts P: Laboratory markers in IBD: useful, magic or unnecessary toys? Gut 2006;55:426–431.

7 Solem CA, et al: Correlation of C-reactive protein with clinical, endoscopic, histologic and radiographic activity in inflammatory bowel disease. Inflamm Bowel Dis 2005;11:707–712.

8 Rutgeerts P, Vermeire S, Van Assche G: Mucosal healing in inflammatory bowel disease: impossible ideal or therapeutic target? Gut 2007;56:453–455.

9 Simonovsky V: Ultrasound in the differential diagnosis of appendicitis. Clin Radiol 1995;50:768–773.

10 Schwerk WB, Beckh K, Raith M: A prospective evaluation of high resolution sonography in the diagnosis of inflammatory bowel disease. Eur J Gastroenterol Hepatol 1992;4:173–182.

11 Parente F, Maconi G, Bianchi Porro G: Bowel ultrasound in Crohn's disease. Current role and future applications. Scand J Gastroenterol 2002;37:871–876.

12 Pradel JA, Adell JF, Taourel P, Djafari M, Monnin-Delhom E, Bruel JM: Acute colonic diverticulitis: prospective comparative evaluation with US and CT. Radiology 1997;205:503–512.

13 Parente F, Greco S, Molteni M, Anderloni A, Maconi G, Bianchi Porro G: Bowel ultrasound in the diagnostic work-up and follow-up of inflammatory bowel disease. Inflamm Bowel Dis 2004;10:452–461.

14 Pascu M, Roznowski AB, Muller HP, Adler A, Wiedenmann B, Dignass AU: Clinical relevance of transabdominal ultrasonography and magnetic resonance imaging in patients with inflammatory bowel disease of the terminal ileum and large bowel. Inflamm Bowel Dis 2004;10:373–382.

15 Lennard-Jones JE: Classification of inflammatory bowel disease. Scand J Gastroenterol 1989;24(suppl 170):2–6.

16 Truelove SC, Witts LJ: Cortisone in ulcerative colitis: final report on a therapeutic trial. Br Med J 1955;ii:1041–1048.

17 Baron JH, Connell AM, Lennard-Jones JE, et al: Variation between observers in describing mucosal appearances in proctocolitis. Br Med J 1964;i:89–92.

18 Parente F, Ardizzone S, Greco S, Bianchi Porro G, Gallus S: Response to high-dose steroids of severe attacks of ulcerative colitis may rely on bowel ultrasound instead of colonoscopy: a preliminary study. Gut 2006;55(suppl V):A118.

19 Kornbluth A, Sachar D: Ulcerative colitis practice guidelines in adults (update): American College of Gastroenterology, Practice Parameters Committee. Am J Gastroenterol 2004;99:1371–1385.

20 Carter MJ, Lobo AJ, Travis SPL, et al: Guidelines for the management of inflammatory bowel disease in adults. Gut 2004;53:S1–S16.

21 Oshitani N, Matsumoto T, Jinno Y, et al: Prediction of short-term outcome for patients with active ulcerative colitis. Dig Dis Sci 2000;45:982–986.

22 Faubion WA, Loftus EV, Harmsen WS, et al: The natural history of corticosteroid therapy for inflammatory bowel disease: a population-based study. Gastroenterology 2001;121:255–260.

23 Ho GT, Chiam P, Drummond H, et al: The efficacy of corticosteroid therapy in inflammatory bowel disease: analysis of a 5-year UK inception cohort. Aliment Pharmacol Ther 2006;24:319–330.

24 Beattie RM, Nicholls SW, Domizio P, et al: Endoscopic assessment of the colonic response to corticosteroids in children with ulcerative colitis. J Pediatr Gastroenterol Nutr 1996;22:373–379.

25 Hyams J, Markowitz J, Lerer T, et al: The natural history of corticosteroid therapy for ulcerative colitis in children. Clin Gastroenterol Hepatol 2006;4:1118–1123.

26 Tung J, Loftus EV, Freese DK, et al: A population-based study on the frequency of corticosteroid resistance and dependence in pediatric patients with Crohn's disease and ulcerative colitis. Inflamm Bowel Dis 2006;12:1093–1100.

27 Truelove SC, Watkinson G, Draper G: Comparison of corticosteroid and sulphasalazine therapy in ulcerative colitis. Br Med J 1962;2:1708–1711.

28 Wright R, Truelove SC: Serial biopsy in ulcerative colitis during the course of a controlled therapeutic trial of various diets. Am J Dig Dis 1966;11:1854–1858.

29 Courtney MG, Nunes MB, Bergin B: Colonoscopic but not histological appearances determine likelihood of relapse of ulcerative colitis. Am J Gastroenterol 1991;86:243A.

30 Meucci G, Fasoli R, Saibeni S, et al: Prognostic significance of endoscopic remission in patients with active ulcerative colitis treated with oral and topical mesalazine: preliminary results of a prospective multicenter study. Gastroenterology 2006;130(suppl 2):A-197.

31 Rutgeerts P, Sandborn W, Feagan B, et al: Infliximab for induction and maintenance therapy of ulcerative colitis. N Engl J Med 2005;353:2462–2476.

Parente/Molteni/Marino/Colli/
Ardizzone/Greco/Sampietro/Gallus

Dig Dis 2009;27:291–296
DOI: 10.1159/000228563

Risk/Benefit Strategies Must Be Employed in the Management of Pediatric Crohn's Disease

Jeffrey S. Hyams

Division of Digestive Diseases, Hepatology, and Nutrition, Connecticut Children's Medical Center,
University of Connecticut School of Medicine, Hartford, Conn., USA

Key Words
Crohn's disease · Infliximab · Hepatosplenic T cell
lymphoma

Abstract

Clinicians caring for children with Crohn's disease must consider the long-term implications of therapeutic interventions and cumulative diagnostic studies in their patients whose disease duration will be measured in decades. There is evidence of the increased severity of pediatric Crohn's disease compared to its adult counterpart, its frequent co-morbid growth disturbances, and the frequent need for aggressive medical therapies including immunomodulators and biological agents. The initial management of most children diagnosed with Crohn's disease involves enteral nutritional support, corticosteroids, and immunomodulators. Corticosteroids, while initially helpful in decreasing signs and symptoms of disease, are occasionally ineffective, generally do not heal mucosa, impair growth, and are frequently associated with a state of corticosteroid dependency. Immunomodulators are effective maintenance therapies with corticosteroid sparing effects, but have no value in the acutely ill child. The emergence of biological therapy with its impressive record of rapid efficacy and use as maintenance therapy has prompted discussion of its incorporation into initial management, but has also raised concerns about who are the most suitable candidates, which if any medications can be used concomitantly, and long-term safety. The combined use of thiopurines and anti-TNF agents may predispose to a rare and uniformly fatal lymphoma. Identification of children at high risk for complicated disease may allow us to better evaluate risk/benefit in newly diagnosed children, and biologic agents are likely to assume an increasing role in primary therapy in those deemed at highest risk. Long-term observations will determine whether biologics will change natural history and demonstrate adequate safety.

Copyright © 2009 S. Karger AG, Basel

Introduction

Clinicians caring for children with Crohn's disease must consider the long-term implications of therapeutic interventions and cumulative diagnostic studies in their patients whose disease duration will be measured in decades. Children diagnosed with Crohn's disease will have the longest duration in which 'natural history' will be played out. At the present time, there is convincing evidence of the increased severity of pediatric Crohn's disease compared to its adult counterpart [1], its frequent co-morbid growth disturbances [2], and the frequent

Jeffrey S. Hyams, MD
Connecticut Children's Medical Center
282 Washington Street
Hartford, CT 06106 (USA)
Tel. +1 860 545 9532, Fax +1 860 545 9561, E-Mail jhyams@ccmckids.org

need for aggressive medical therapies including immunomodulators and biological agents to adequately control disease activity [3].

The past decade has witnessed a large increase in the number of drugs available to treat pediatric Crohn's disease and concomitantly an increased awareness of risk versus benefit with each new modality. Patient and family awareness of complications of treatments are easily available on the internet and this new found knowledge often frightens families about these drugs before they have been able to understand the natural history of poorly treated Crohn's disease including the high likelihood of complications requiring surgery [4] and perhaps a higher mortality rate compared to those without Crohn's disease [5].

The guiding principles of Crohn's disease treatment include induction of remission, maintenance of remission, ensuring normal growth and development, optimizing adherence, minimizing cost, and minimizing toxicity. More recently, the concept of mucosal healing has emerged as a treatment goal and appears to be more readily obtainable with aggressive therapy including biologic agents. Whether these agents change natural history has not been determined.

Current Approaches to Therapy

The initial management of most children newly diagnosed with Crohn's disease involves enteral nutritional support, 5-aminosalicylates, corticosteroids, and immunomodulators. While enteral nutritional support has found favor in some parts of the world, it is not widely utilized in others, is less successful with severe colonic involvement [6], and may be difficult to administer for extended periods of time. 5-Aminosalicylates, while commonly used in pediatric Crohn's disease, have not been subject to clinical trials in this age group. Corticosteroids, while initially very helpful in decreasing signs and symptoms of disease, are occasionally ineffective, and frequently associated with a state of corticosteroid dependency [7]. Corticosteroid therapy is generally ineffective in healing inflamed mucosa [8] and can impair growth [9]. Mood disturbances, deleterious effects on bone, and cosmetic changes limit its acceptability and it is has no maintenance efficacy. Budesonide is not as effective as prednisone and also has no demonstrated long-term efficacy [10]. Immunomodulators (azathioprine, 6-mercaptopurine, methotrexate) have convincingly been shown to be effective maintenance therapies

with corticosteroid sparing effects in children [11, 12], but are of little value in the acutely ill newly diagnosed child. Concerns about opportunistic infections and malignancy give physicians, patients, and families pause whenever their use is discussed, but they have now become standard of care for children with moderate to severe disease.

Increasing data on the use of biologic therapy in children has shown its efficacy in inducing and maintaining remission in children poorly controlled with corticosteroids and immunomodulators [13]. Clinicians are now struggling with the questions of who are the best candidates for biologic therapy, at what point in the disease course should they be given, and should they be combined with immunomodulators.

Early Use of Biologic Therapy

There are currently no clinical trials investigating the safety and efficacy of biologics as primary therapy for pediatric Crohn's disease. A recent trial in adults examined combined immunosuppression (immunomodulator plus biologic therapy, i.e., step-down therapy) versus conventional step-up therapy [14]. In this open trial patients in the step-down arm were initially treated with azathioprine plus a 3-dose induction of infliximab followed by episodic infliximab as needed, and corticosteroids as needed. The step-up group was initially treated with up to two courses of corticosteroids followed by an immunomodulator (azathioprine or methotrexate) if needed and then infliximab if needed. The primary outcome measures were remission without corticosteroids and without bowel resection at 26 and 52 weeks. Analysis was by modified intention to treat. At both weeks 26 and 52, the combined immunosuppression group had higher remission rates than the conventional group: week 26: 60 vs. 36% (p = 0.006), and week 52 62 vs. 42% (p = 0.028). Safety was comparable in the two groups. However, by 78 weeks and subsequently at 104 weeks, the proportion of each group in remission did not differ.

The second study of note is the recently presented SONIC study that randomized adult Crohn's disease patients naive to immunomodulators and biologic therapy to either azathioprine plus placebo infusions, infliximab plus placebo capsules, or infliximab plus azathioprine [15]. The primary outcome was corticosteroid-free remission without surgery at 26 weeks. Subjects needed to have a CDAI of 220–450, and be either corticosteroid dependent, have already received corticosteroids within the past year, be a budesonide failure, or be a 5-ASA failure. Corticosteroid-free remission was noted in 57% of the azathioprine/infliximab group compared to 44% receiving infliximab alone and 31% receiving azathioprine alone (all comparisons significant). Mucosal healing at week 26 was superior in the two infliximab groups compared to the azathioprine only group. When a sub-group analysis was performed looking at those subjects who had mucosal lesions on baseline endoscopy and an elevated C-reactive protein, the difference in corticosteroid-free remission at 26 weeks between the infliximab only group and the infliximab plus azathioprine group was no longer statistically different.

Concomitant Use of Immunomodulators and Biologic Therapy

Despite the intriguing results from SONIC, observations from previous anti-TNFα trials in inflammatory bowel disease have not suggested incremental efficacy by combining immunomodulator use with a biologic. Post-hoc analysis of infliximab therapy in both Crohn's disease (ACCENT 1) and ulcerative colitis (ACT 1) [16], adalimumab in Crohn's disease (CHARM) [17], and certolizumab in Crohn's disease (PRECISE) [18] showed no difference in response and remission endpoints in the respective studies when comparing patients receiving and not receiving immunomodulators when the biologic agent was started.

Further data on the potential role of concomitant immunomodulator therapy were recently presented in a study asking whether continuing an immunomodulator in a patient who has been responding to a combination of immunomodulator and infliximab for at least 6 months would add to the efficacy of scheduled maintenance infliximab compared to infliximab monotherapy [19]. In this multicenter, prospective, open-label superiority trial, patients were randomized to every 8 weeks infliximab plus their immunomodulator or infliximab alone every 8 weeks for 104 weeks. Oral prednisone or budesonide were not allowed, but 5-aminosalicylate therapy was kept stable. The primary endpoint was the proportion of patients needing early rescue infliximab due to a disease flare or interrupting further infliximab dosing due to loss of response, intolerance or intercurrent adverse event. Sixty percent of those continuing dual therapy needed to change their infliximab schedule compared to 55% of those on infliximab monotherapy

(not statistically different). Finally, a recent study examined whether concomitant methotrexate and infliximab were more effective than infliximab alone in adult patients receiving corticosteroids who initiated biologic therapy [20]. At 50 weeks, 30.6% of those on dual therapy had failed compared to 29.8% of those on infliximab alone.

Though no added efficacy has been noted with dual therapy, it has been shown that trough infliximab levels are higher in those receiving concomitant immunomodulators [19]. This has remained a theoretical reason for continuing immunomodulators, though it did not appear to have clinical significance in any of the studies preceding SONIC.

Potential Risk of Dual Therapy

So with what appears to be somewhat conflicting data the clinician needs to weigh the potential risk versus benefit of combined immunomodulator and biologic therapy. The sentinel event in this dilemma occurred in the summer of 2006 when the United States Food and Drug Administration (FDA) mandated the addition of a black box warning to the infliximab package insert describing the occurrence of hepatosplenic T cell lymphoma (HSTCL) in individuals who had received both infliximab and a thiopurine. HSTCL is a very rare and aggressive non-Hodgkin's lymphoma (NHL) that primarily targets young males and is almost uniformly fatal. In 2001, the World Health Organization (WHO) classified HSTCL as a distinct disorder under the classification of peripheral (extranodal) T cell lymphomas [21]. Commonly, subjects with HSTCL have a history of chronic antigenic stimulation in the setting of immunosuppression; it has been postulated that primary or acquired immunodeficiency can predispose to HSTCL [22]. It is thought that exposure to anti-metabolites such as azathioprine or 6-mercaptopurine cause DNA damage leading to defects in control of cellular proliferation or apoptosis resulting in malignant transformation.

To date, only about 200 cases of HSTCL have been described. The two largest series combined describe 66 patients [22, 23]. About one-third of patients have had previous organ transplantation or received immune-modifying agents for other indications. Though HSTCL has been described at all ages, the median age has been 32 years, and 70% of subjects are male. Affected individuals commonly present with fever, weight loss, hepatosplenomegaly, and abdominal pain, and lack peripheral adenopathy. The disease is always disseminated at diagnosis with involvement of liver, spleen, and bone marrow. Serum aminotransferases are commonly elevated and an erroneous diagnosis of hepatitis can be made.

As of December 2008, there have been 9 reports of subjects treated with thiopurines only and 16 reports of subjects who have been treated with infliximab and a thiopurine who have developed HSTCL [24–31] (Data on file, Centocor, Horsham, Pa., USA). For this latter group the age range has been 12–40 years (mean age 22 years) at the time of diagnosis, and all except one have been male. The mean number of infliximab infusions has been 10 (range 1–24) and 5 patients have had 3 or less infusions. There have been two cases of HSTCL in IBD patients receiving adalimumab, both of whom previously also received infliximab and a thiopurine. All cases of HSTCL in IBD patients have subsequently been fatal. There have been no cases of HSTCL developing in IBD patients treated with an anti-TNF agent without previous thiopurine exposure, in IBD patients treated with an anti-TNF agent and methotrexate, or methotrexate alone.

The relevance to IBD therapy is clearly seen when the rarity of HSTCL is examined. The incidence of non-Hodgkin's lymphoma (NHL) in subjects 10–19 years of age is approximately 20/1,000,000 (1 in 50,000) subjects per year, slightly higher for people in their 20s, and about 80/1,000,000 for individuals in their late 30s [32]. Peripheral T cell lymphomas make up about 10–15% of all NHL, and HSTCL represents about 5% of peripheral T cell lymphomas (i.e. HSTCL represents less than 1% of NHL) [21]. Thus, one would postulate an annual incidence of HSTCL in adolescents of 1/5,000,000 subjects. Given that there are likely 50,000 to 100,000 pediatric patients with IBD in the United States, one would only expect one case of HSTCL every 50 to 100 years. As noted above, there have been 25 reported cases worldwide of HSTCL in subjects with IBD. Several cases have appeared in the medical literature and the rest have been identified by reports from the pharmaceutical industry. Seven of these cases have been in patients less than 20 years of age. The common thread for all subjects with IBD who have developed HSTCL has been treatment with a thiopurine.

Clinicians should rightly ask whether current practice patterns have contributed to this apparent marked increase in such a rare malignancy. The past 20 years have seen thiopurine therapy become standard of care for moderate to severe pediatric Crohn's disease and the past decade has ushered in the era of biologic therapy with anti-TNF agents. Thiopurines can cause DNA damage and azathioprine has been classified as a human carcinogen [33]. Moreover, ionizing radiation is also a cause of DNA damage and CT scans have become frequent in the evaluation of children and adults with IBD. The potential increased likelihood of malignancy following exposure to ionizing radiation from diagnostic imaging studies, as well as the particular sensitivity of pediatric patients, has been the subject of increasing scrutiny [34–37]. Immune surveillance is impaired in the presence of thiopurines as well as with treatment with anti-TNF agents. Crohn's disease, with chronic inflammation in a mucosal surface (site of $\gamma\delta$ T cells), frequent exposure to ionizing radiation, thiopurine therapy with potential chromosomal damage, and increasing use of anti-TNFα agents would appear to combine many elements predisposing to HSTCL.

Immunomodulators or Biological Agents at Onset of Therapy?

Impressive remission rates and the potential promise of mucosal healing have clearly prompted increased consideration for biological therapy early in the disease course. For pediatric patients in particular the promise of a rapid corticosteroid-free remission prior to or during the years of rapid linear growth and sexual development are particularly inviting. For this clinician, I now consider using an anti-TNFα agent as primary therapy in the setting of extensive disease, complicated early disease, severe fistula, or disease onset in an adolescent with growth failure already showing signs of puberty in which the window for growth is short. These latter subjects also often have evidence of skeletal demineralization further complicating the potential role of corticosteroids. I do not start concomitant immunomodulator therapy in these subjects given the lack of data suggesting increased efficacy with methotrexate and the potential interaction between thiopurines and anti-TNFα agents in the pathogenesis of HSTCL.

Recent data have also suggested that antibody titers to specific microbial antigens measured at the time of diagnosis may predict the development of complicated disease requiring surgery (obstruction, perforation) [38] and may potentially play a role in helping identify subjects more likely to benefit from biological therapy at the time of diagnosis.

What Now?

Patients, families, and physicians should never lose sight of the morbidity of poorly treated Crohn's disease as they worry about the potential risks of therapeutic interventions. The reality is that poorly treated disease can lead to growth stunting, multiple surgeries, and severely impaired quality of life. As we get more natural history data on current and emerging therapies, their risks and benefits become clearer. For today it would appear that in children and adolescents minimizing exposure to ionizing radiation, and avoiding the concomitant use of thiopurines and anti-TNFα agents is prudent. Whether methotrexate should replace thiopurines as the immunomodulator of choice early in the disease course to avoid what appears to be an increased risk of HSTCL with their use is not clear. Certainly thiopurines have demonstrated efficacy in the management of pediatric and adult Crohn's disease, but whether they truly change natural history (i.e. need for surgery) remains debatable. As greater experience is gleaned with biologic agents, it is quite possible they will assume a more prominent role as primary therapy; whether they will change natural history and demonstrate a safety advantage over the current standard of care remains to be seen.

Disclosure Statement

Centocor Ortho Biotech (consultant, research support, speaker's bureau), Abbott (consultant, research support), Elan (consultant), UCB (consultant), Astra Zeneca (research support).

References

1 Van Limbergen J, Russell RK, Drummond HE, et al: Definition of phenotypic characteristics of childhood-onset inflammatory bowel disease. Gastroenterology 2008;135:1114–1122.
2 Pfefferkorn M, Burke G, Griffiths A, et al: Growth abnormalities persist in newly diagnosed children with Crohn disease despite current treatment paradigms. J Pediatr Gastroenterol Nutr 2009;48:168–174.
3 Punati J, Markowitz J, Lerer T, et al: Effect of early immunomodulator use in moderate to severe pediatric Crohn disease. Inflamm Bowel Dis 2008;14:949–954.
4 Cosnes J, Nion-Larmurier I, Beaugerie L, et al: Impact of the increasing use of immunosuppressants in Crohn's disease on the need for intestinal surgery. Gut 2005;54:237–241.
5 Card T, Hubbard R, Logan RF: Mortality in inflammatory bowel disease: a population-based cohort study. Gastroenterology 2003;125:1583–1590.
6 Griffiths AM, Ohlsson A, Sherman PM, Sutherland LR: Meta-analysis of enteral nutrition as a primary treatment of active Crohn's disease. Gastroenterology 1995;108:1056–1067.
7 Markowitz J, Hyams J, Mack D, et al: Corticosteroid therapy in the age of infliximab: acute and 1-year outcomes in newly diagnosed children with Crohn's disease. Clin Gastroenterol Hepatol 2006;4:1124–1129.
8 Modigliani R, Mary JY, Simon JF, et al: Clinical, biological, and endoscopic picture of attacks of Crohn's disease: evolution on prednisolone. Groupe d'Etude Therapeutique des Affections Inflammatoires Digestives. Gastroenterology 1990;98:811–818.

9 Hyams JS, Moore RE, Leichtner AM, et al: Relationship of type I procollagen to corticosteroid therapy in children with inflammatory bowel disease. J Pediatr 1988;112:893–898.
10 Rutgeerts P, Lofberg R, Malchow H, et al: A comparison of budesonide with prednisolone for active Crohn's disease. N Engl J Med 1994;331:842–845.
11 Markowitz J, Grancher K, Kohn N, et al: A multicenter trial of 6-mercaptopurine and prednisone in children with newly diagnosed Crohn's disease. Gastroenterology 2000;119:895–902.
12 Turner D, Grossman AB, Rosh J, et al: Methotrexate following unsuccessful thiopurine therapy in pediatric Crohn's disease. Am J Gastroenterol 2007;102:2804–2812; quiz 2803, 2813.
13 Hyams J, Crandall W, Kugathasan S, et al: Induction and maintenance infliximab therapy for the treatment of moderate-to-severe Crohn's disease in children. Gastroenterology 2007;132:863–873; quiz 1165–1166.
14 D'Haens G, Baert F, van Assche G, et al: Early combined immunosuppression or conventional management in patients with newly diagnosed Crohn's disease: an open randomised trial. Lancet 2008;371:660–667.
15 Sandborn W, Rutgeerts P, Reinisch W, et al: SONIC: a randomized, double-blind, controlled trial comparing infliximab and infliximab plus azathioprine to azathioprine in patients with Crohn's disease naïve to immunomodulators and biologic therapy. Am J Gastroenterol 2008;103(suppl):A1117.

16 Lichtenstein GR, Diamond R, Wagner C, et al: Infliximab administered as a three dose induction followed by scheduled maintenance therapy in IBD: comparable clinical outcomes with or without immunomodulators. Gastroenterology 2007;132:A504.
17 Colombel JF, Sandborn WJ, Rutgeerts P, et al: Adalimumab for maintenance of clinical response and remission in patients with Crohn's disease: the CHARM trial. Gastroenterology 2007;132:52–65.
18 Schreiber S, Khaliq-Kareemi M, Lawrance IC, et al: Maintenance therapy with certolizumab pegol for Crohn's disease. N Engl J Med 2007;357:239–250.
19 Van Assche G, Magdelaine-Beuzelin C, D'Haens G, et al: Withdrawal of immunosuppression in Crohn's disease treated with scheduled infliximab maintenance: a randomized trial. Gastroenterology 2008;134:1861–1868.
20 Feagan B, McDonald J, Panaccione R, et al: A randomized trial of methotrexate in combination with infliximab for the treatment of Crohn's disease. Gastroenterology 2008;135:294.
21 Jaffe E, Harris NL, Stein H, et al: World Health Organization Classification of Tumors/Pathology and Genetics of Tumors of Haematopoietic and Lymphoid Tissues. Lyon, International Agency for Research Press, 2001.
22 Vega F, Medeiros LJ, Gaulard P: Hepatosplenic and other gammadelta T-cell lymphomas. Am J Clin Pathol 2007;127:869–880.
23 Belhadj K, Reyes F, Farcet JP, et al: Hepatosplenic gammadelta T-cell lymphoma is a rare clinicopathologic entity with poor outcome: report on a series of 21 patients. Blood 2003;102:4261–4269.

24 Thayu M, Markowitz JE, Mamula P, et al: Hepatosplenic T-cell lymphoma in an adolescent patient after immunomodulator and biologic therapy for Crohn disease. J Pediatr Gastroenterol Nutr 2005;40:220–222.

25 Cooke CB, Krenacs L, Stetler-Stevenson M, et al: Hepatosplenic T-cell lymphoma: a distinct clinicopathologic entity of cytotoxic gamma delta T-cell origin. Blood 1996;88:4265–4274.

26 Navarro JT, Ribera JM, Mate JL, et al: Hepatosplenic T-gammadelta lymphoma in a patient with Crohn's disease treated with azathioprine. Leuk Lymphoma 2003;44:531–533.

27 Drini M, Prichard PJ, Brown GJ, Macrae FA: Hepatosplenic T-cell lymphoma following infliximab therapy for Crohn's disease. Med J Aust 2008;189:464–465.

28 Zeidan A, Sham R, Shapiro J, et al: Hepatosplenic T-cell lymphoma in a patient with Crohn's disease who received infliximab therapy. Leuk Lymphoma 2007;48:1410–1413.

29 Mackey AC, Green L, Liang LC, et al: Hepatosplenic T cell lymphoma associated with infliximab use in young patients treated for inflammatory bowel disease. J Pediatr Gastroenterol Nutr 2007;44:265–267.

30 Rosh JR, Gross T, Mamula P, et al: Hepatosplenic T-cell lymphoma in adolescents and young adults with Crohn's disease: a cautionary tale? Inflamm Bowel Dis 2007;13:1024–1030.

31 Mittal S, Milner BJ, Johnston PW, Culligan DJ: A case of hepatosplenic gamma-delta T-cell lymphoma with a transient response to fludarabine and alemtuzumab. Eur J Haematol 2006;76:531–534.

32 Surveillance Epidemiology and End Results (SEER), Cancer Statistics Review, 1975–2006, National Cancer Institute, Bethesda, http://seer.cancer.gov.

33 Karran P: Thiopurines, DNA damage, DNA repair and therapy-related cancer. Br Med Bull 2006;79–80:153–170.

34 Brody AS, Frush DP, Huda W, Brent RL: Radiation risk to children from computed tomography. Pediatrics 2007;120:677–682.

35 Brenner DJ, Hall EJ: Computed tomography: an increasing source of radiation exposure. N Engl J Med 2007;357:2277–2284.

36 Brenner DJ, Sachs RK: Estimating radiation-induced cancer risks at very low doses: rationale for using a linear no-threshold approach. Radiat Environ Biophys 2006;44:253–256.

37 Mazrani W, McHugh K, Marsden PJ: The radiation burden of radiological investigations. Arch Dis Child 2007;92:1127–1131.

38 Dubinsky MC, Kugathasan S, Mei L, et al: Increased immune reactivity predicts aggressive complicating Crohn's disease in children. Clin Gastroenterol Hepatol 2008;6:1105–1111.

Dig Dis 2009;27:297–305
DOI: 10.1159/000228564

Enteral Nutrition Should Be Used to Induce Remission in Childhood Crohn's Disease

Robert Heuschkel

Department of Paediatric Gastroenterology, Hepatology and Nutrition, Addenbrookes Hospital,
Cambridge University Hospital, Cambridge, UK

Key Words

Crohn's disease · Enteral nutrition · Inflammatory bowel disease

Abstract

Background: Exclusive enteral nutrition has been used over many years as a therapy to try and achieve a remission in adults and children presenting with acute Crohn's disease. Despite its reported efficacy at achieving clinical responses in excess of 80% in some case series, it has not been taken up widely as a first-line therapy. This is, at least in part, due to the lack of a large prospective randomised study. **Methods:** The literature is replete with small case series and anecdotal reports from units who use this therapy. Recent literature is reviewed on efficacy, application, composition and potential mechanisms of action of this therapy. **Results:** Although the evidence base remains quite limited, further data are available that suggest a clear benefit of exclusive enteral nutrition as an efficacious alternative to steroid therapy at inducing a clinical remission in Crohn's disease. Certain sub-groups are likely to benefit more, with potential benefits on growth making it particularly useful in adolescents and growing young adults. Given the lack of side effects compared to the alternative of steroid therapy, along with the clear nutritional benefits of this therapy, it remains an obvious choice for patients presenting with Crohn's disease and a degree of malnutrition. **Conclusions:** This therapy should remain a first-line therapy for children and adults presenting with mild to moderate Crohn's disease.

Copyright © 2009 S. Karger AG, Basel

Enteral Nutrition as Induction Therapy

Exclusive Enteral Nutrition

Exclusive enteral nutrition (EEN) is indicated as a first-line therapy in any child with acute Crohn's disease, provided there are no absolute contra-indications to enteral feeding per se. Nutritional treatment of Crohn's disease has been a therapeutic option since at least 1969. In the early 1970s, surgeons operating on patients with IBD sensed that nutritional intervention may have a direct effect on the disease rather than just be pre-operative nutritional support [1]. Johnson et al. [2] recently confirmed the fact that if enteral nutrition is to be used as therapy to induce remission, it must be given exclusively. Although this study showed only a 42% remission rate on exclusive elemental formula, the group receiving only 50% of their calorie requirement as enteral formula, in addition to a normal diet, only achieved a remission in 15% of cases. This also confirmed that only if a formula is given exclu-

Robert Heuschkel
Department of Paediatric Gastroenterology, Hepatology and Nutrition
Box 267, Addenbrookes Hospital, Cambridge University Hospital, Hills Rd
Cambridge CB2 0QQ (UK), Tel. +44 1223 274 827, Fax +44 1223 586 794
E-Mail robert.heuschkel@addenbrookes.nhs.uk

sively, i.e. as therapy and not as a nutritional supplement, is there a significant improvement in inflammatory markers. The issue of whether or not enteral nutrition is as effective as steroid therapy at inducing a remission has been debated for some time. However, what is clear from the paediatric literature over the last 20 years is that an exclusively nutritional therapy can be highly effective at inducing a remission from active Crohn's disease [3–5]. The best results appear to be in those children with newly diagnosed Crohn's disease, although the paediatric evidence continues to remain limited in the number of children reported [6]. Recent case series from Australia confirm efficacy in children with acute Crohn's disease, achieving 80% clinical efficacy on an intention-to-treat basis [7]. Large adult studies [8, 9], as well as some of the smaller paediatric studies [5], suggest disease distribution does not effect the efficacy of the treatment. Colonic disease appears to respond as well as terminal ileal disease, with a similar reduction in inflammatory markers, disease activity and improved mucosal histology [5]. More recent retrospective data suggests that clinical remission with isolated colonic disease may only be about 50%, compared to about 75–80% in the presence of any macroscopic ileal involvement [10]. Although there is only anecdotal evidence on the response of oral and perianal Crohn's disease to exclusive enteral nutrition [11], the authors have made use of exclusive enteral nutrition as an adjunct in treating severe perianal Crohn's disease.

Adverse effects to using EEN in Crohn's disease are very rare. However, we reported a case of refeeding syndrome in a child following her presentation with severe Crohn's colitis. A rapid loss of weight over the preceding 4 weeks, followed by treatment with exclusive polymeric nutrition, led to a dramatic fall in serum phosphate and signs of hypervolaemia in the first few days of treatment [12]. It is important to remain aware of this complication when considering the use of EEN in children with Crohn's disease who may have sub-optimal nutrition, as adequate mineral supplementation in the first few days, as well as cautious increases in calorie and protein load, can help avoid serious complications.

Elemental Diet

An elemental feed is a chemically defined diet whose protein source is amino acids or short-chain peptides, with short-chain carbohydrates and added fat, minerals and vitamins. The National Aeronautics and Space Administration (NASA) had initially designed elemental diets for astronauts [13]. This was with the intention of providing a nutritionally complete diet of which as much as

possible would be absorbed. However, whilst absorption was limited mainly to the upper small bowel, the diet did not prevent the production of stool as had been hoped.

Nutrition was initially used in inflammatory bowel disease as an adjunct in malnourished patients with growth failure. Elemental diets were developed and first used as sole therapy for IBD in adults in the 1970s [14]. It was then shown that nutrition had a beneficial effect on disease by reducing the increased gut permeability characteristic of Crohn's disease [15]. Logan et al. [15] studied 7 adults with extensive jejuno-ileal Crohn's disease. They showed a reduction in both gut protein and gut lymphocyte loss during a period of elemental feeding. This was the first report that an elemental diet could directly improve gut function, probably by reducing bowel inflammation.

In 1973, Giorgini et al. [16] reported the first successful use of enteral nutrition in treating a child with acute Crohn's disease. It was then shown that enteral nutrition was effective in treating a series of children with Crohn's disease. Successful use in combination with drug therapy led on to a further study by the same group, which first showed exclusive constant-rate elemental nutrition (CREN) to be as effective as steroid therapy at inducing a remission [17]. While both these studies had few patients, they gave the first insights into the possible benefits of nutritional therapy as treatment for childhood Crohn's disease. In addition to achieving disease remission, nutritional therapy was also found to have beneficial effects on inflammatory masses and fistulae. Simultaneously, both Morin et al. [18] and O'Morain et al. [19] documented that an elemental diet improved linear growth in several children with active Crohn's disease.

A variety of devices, formulas and regimens were then used to feed patients intra-gastrically. Continuous feeding [20, 21] and then overnight feeds predominated [22] for the induction of remission. Supplementation of an elemental diet with glutamine, a gut-specific metabolic fuel, did not further improve efficacy, although the small numbers in this study make conclusions difficult [23].

Semi-Elemental Diet

Once elemental diets had achieved their first successes, short-chain-peptide-containing diets were suggested as a better nitrogen source than amino acids [24]. Silk et al. [24] refuted previous evidence that free amino acids were better absorbed than di- and tripeptides. By using an intestinal perfusion technique in adults, they were able to demonstrate better absorption of amino acids from both casein and lactalbumin hydrolysates than from an equimolar feed of free amino acids. Not only was there a more uniform absorption of amino acids, but the hydrolysates had a beneficial effect on jejunal absorption of water and electrolytes. There followed the first small randomised study of 7–8 children in each group, in which overnight naso-gastric feeding of a semi-elemental diet was compared to prednisolone treatment in children with predominant small bowel Crohn's disease [22]. A 4- to 5-chain amino-acid-based diet was as effective as steroids at achieving a remission in active Crohn's disease. It again confirmed the North American finding that there was a clear acceleration in growth in the group not taking steroids.

Polymeric Diet

It therefore appeared that steroids may have a similar efficacy to semi-elemental feeds in the induction of remission. Several adult studies reported the efficacy of whole protein diet compared to both that of elemental diets and to steroids. Raouf et al. [25] and others all found polymeric diets to be as effective as an elemental diet at inducing remission.

Polymeric diets were also shown to be as effective as conventional steroid treatment. Gonzalez-Huix et al. [26] confirmed this in adults, and Ruuska et al. [5] and Beattie et al. [27] in children. Ruuska et al. [5], in a well-planned but small study (n = 19), showed a polymeric diet to be as effective as steroids in inducing a remission in children with acute Crohn's disease. A further great advantage in using a polymeric diet then became clear. Whilst almost all children previously required feeding by intra-gastric tube, whole protein formulas such as AL110 (Nestlé-Clintec), used by Beattie et al. [3], and Nutrison Standard (Nutricia), used by Ruuska et al. [5], were palatable enough for daily oral consumption. Children rarely required a nasogastric tube to complete their entire nutritional needs. This was confirmed in a more recent study comparing children's compliance when taking polymeric and elemental formulae [28]. In this study, there was no difference in compliance, but significantly less nasogastric tube use (33 vs. 55%) in the group taking a polymeric diet. This provided a considerable improvement in the quality of life for children on several weeks of nutritional therapy.

The most recent, and most definitive cohort study to date by Fell et al. [4] shows that a whole casein, polymeric diet (Modulen IBD, Nestlé Clinical Nutrition), rich in transforming growth factor-β (TGF-β), is well tolerated and achieves a clinical and histological remission. Twen-ty-nine consecutive patients were treated with the exclusive enteral diet for an 8-week period. Although over half had mild disease, 12 had moderate to severe disease with a paediatric Crohn's disease activity index (PCDAI) >30 [29]. A nasogastric tube was only required in one patient for the first 2 weeks of treatment. Only 2 of 29 patients failed to show any clinical response, one with severe colonic disease, the other with an inflammatory mass requiring surgery. Twenty-three of 29 patients achieved a complete remission on PCDAI scoring. The PCDAI fell dramatically within 2 weeks of starting the diet, but continued to fall until 8 weeks of treatment. There was significant macroscopic and histological improvement after treatment, with mucosal healing occurring in the terminal ileum and colon of 8 and 2 patients, respectively. Serum tumour necrosis factor-α and mucosal mRNA for IL-1β and IL-8 were significantly reduced in both the terminal ileum and the colon after treatment. Interferon-γ (IFN-γ) was significantly reduced and TGF-β was elevated in the terminal ileum alone. There is no direct evidence that the TGF-β in the enteral formula is responsible for the up-regulation of mucosal TGF-β. Nonetheless, this study strengthens the findings by Breese at al. [30] that polymeric enteral nutrition alone can achieve an improvement in histology and a complete normalisation of some of the mucosal messenger RNA of pro-inflammatory cytokines involved in tissue damage. Bannerjee et al. documented the most rapid reduction in pro-inflammatory cytokines to date, in children receiving exclusive enteral nutrition for active Crohn's disease [31]. Within 3 days of starting an exclusive polymeric diet, there was a significant reduction in IL-6 and erythrocyte sedimentation rate. This, together with improvements in C-reactive protein, IGF-1 and PCDAI by day 7, predated any measures of nutritional restitution (mid-upper arm circumference/triceps skinfold thickness). This provides further evidence that nutritional therapy in this situation is providing more than simply an optimal calorie intake.

The lipid composition of some polymeric diets has been held responsible for some of the variability in their efficacy [32]. High LCT concentrations have been associated with a poorer response in treating active Crohn's disease, with suggestions that the high linoleic acid concentration may be responsible [33], although high concentrations of MCT in the feed do not effect its short-term efficacy [34]. However, the only two randomised studies have been unable to show a difference in efficacy between formulae containing either low or high amounts of long-chain triglyceride [35]. Only one randomised study appeared to show a significant difference in remission rates depending on the fatty acid composition of the polymeric feeds. Gassull et al. [32] report a significantly better clinical remission rate in adults after 4 weeks of an exclusive enteral feed rich in n–6 fatty acids, compared to one high in monounsaturated fats (52 vs. 20%, respectively). Why this conflicts with previous evidence [26] remains unclear, although the high percentage of synthetic oleate (79% of total fat) in this study may mask beneficial effects previously seen with formulas containing different fatty acid profiles.

There is limited evidence of milk intolerance in adults with active Crohn's disease. True lactase deficiency is an unusual cause of symptoms in adults with active Crohn's disease [36]; however, up to 46% complained of gastrointestinal symptoms related to milk intake. In contrast, exclusive enteral feeding with lactose-free, whole casein diets has not been associated with intolerance in children with active disease.

Steroids versus Enteral Nutrition

Contrary to these striking paediatric findings, large adult trials [8, 37] as well as meta-analyses of the adult data have found steroids to be more effective than enteral nutrition at inducing remission in active Crohn's disease [38]. This is again confirmed in the more recent Cochrane review, where the number needed to treat with EEN compared to steroids to achieve one remission was 4 [39]. The meta-analysis by Griffiths et al. [38], whilst including both children and adults, excluded most of the smaller paediatric studies. This large review (n = 413) reported that steroids were significantly more effective at achieving a remission than enteral diets (OR 0.35; 95% CI 0.32–0.58). Like other analyses, this study also relies on clinical disease activity indices to document clinical remission rates, but these tend to favour steroid therapy by their reliance on a patient's general feeling of well-being. As a result, conclusions from these studies are frequently and inappropriately applied to children, despite there being clear differences between adult and paediatric patients. Most children have had much shorter disease duration and tend to be much more compliant with therapy. Furthermore, no comment is made on the differing adverse effects and abilities of the two treatments to heal gut mucosa, with steroids having been well documented to have limited effects on gut inflammation [40]. As yet no analysis has detected a significant difference in efficacy between elemental or polymeric diets [41].

Despite the several small paediatric studies that suggest a useful role for enteral nutrition in active Crohn's disease, the view has thus prevailed that enteral nutrition is less effective than steroid therapy. A meta-analysis of paediatric data was performed to maximise the available paediatric data [42]. Despite limited numbers of truly randomised children, sensitivity analyses allowed the authors to arrive at valid and important conclusions. The summary data clearly showed enteral nutrition to be as effective as steroids in the treatment of children with active Crohn's disease. Furthermore, to overturn this finding and demonstrate that steroids were significantly more effective than enteral nutrition would be close to impossible given the outcomes of the paediatric studies reported to date. A further attempt to meta-analyse the rather limited available paediatric data also suggest similar efficacy [43, 44]. All these studies principally address efficacy as their primary outcome measure, largely ignoring the very different side-effect profiles of each therapy. Corticosteroids have many significant adverse effects, whilst oral enteral nutrition has almost none. Prospective observational studies have also highlighted that even in the paediatric age group about 30% of children with Crohn's disease, treated with corticosteroids within 30 days of diagnosis, are corticosteroid dependent at 1 year [45].

Enteral Nutrition and Disease Distribution

There remains the further question of whether enteral nutrition is less effective at treating Crohn's colitis than Crohn's ileitis. Early use of enteral feed was limited to children with predominantly small bowel disease [46], with a suggestion that colonic disease was unresponsive to nutritional management [47]. More recent evidence from Thomas et al. [48], Ruuska et al. [5], and Fell et al. [4], however, supports the value of nutritional therapy in large bowel and small bowel disease. The improvement in colonic mucosal cytokine profiles after enteral nutrition [4] provides hard evidence that there is an effect on colonic disease. Larger studies in adults also confirm that disease location does not appear to influence the response to treatment [8, 9].

However, a more recent retrospective analysis of 60 children treated with exclusive enteral nutrition suggested disease distribution may be relevant in the response to nutritional therapy. Children with any macroscopic ileal inflammation were significantly more likely to achieve a clinical remission than those children with colonic involvement alone (75 vs. 50%) [10]. Despite this, many individuals with Crohn's colitis continue to respond extremely well, still making exclusive enteral nutrition the first choice for any child with Crohn's disease, irrespective of their disease distribution.

Food Reintroduction

There has long been uncertainty as to the best way of re-introducing adults and children onto their 'normal' diet after a period of exclusive enteral nutrition. The evidence for any of these different practices is very limited, with most approaches having been selected by experienced clinicians on the basis of theories prevalent at the time.

The best-described reintroduction program is based on the stepwise introduction foods, starting with the least allergenic [49]. One new food is introduced every 48 h and, if not tolerated, reintroduced at the end of the program. This systematic, but quite laborious program not only allows individual foods to be identified if causing immediate symptoms, but also gives the patients several more weeks on reasonable quantities of enteral nutrition while their normal diet is re-established. The most frequently implicated foods causing discomfort in adults are cereals, dairy products and yeast [49]. In a 2-year follow-up study of about 100 adults, the relapse rate was only just significantly lower in the group excluding dietary products that caused symptoms compared to those maintaining a normal diet (p = 0.048). However, in a randomised controlled trial of an exclusion diet following a remission induced with an elemental diet, subsequent rechallenge and double-blinded challenges in adults with Crohn's disease proved that specific dietary exclusions did not persist [50]. In children, only a very small minority require exclusion of specific items from their diet. A recent abstract reported less than 5% of sustained allergic reactions with graded food-reintroduction in over 100 children who completed a full food reintroduction (abstract at ESPGHAN 2007). There is thus insufficient evidence to routinely suggest exclusion of specific food items in children with Crohn's disease.

Other units use less evidence-based, but more practical reintroduction programs which range from the immediate introduction of a full diet, to a graded introduction over 3 weeks with the 'ad libitum' diet increasing by 25% each week, along with the simultaneous reduction in enteral nutrition.

Mechanism of Enteral Nutrition

Despite the wealth of information that exists about the benefits of enteral nutrition, there remain a multitude of potential mechanisms of action for EEN (table 1).

The most frequently advanced theory is that the bacterial flora within the gut lumen is modified by enteral nu-

Table 1. Mechanisms of action for EEN

Alterations in bacterial flora
Reduction in antigenic load/elimination of specific dietary components
Whole body nutritional restitution
Provision of specific nutrients/provision of enterocyte nutrition (e.g. glutamine/prebiotics)
Decreasing colonic faecal bile salt load
Direct immuno-regulatory effect
Increased concentrations of β
Reduction in total fat (linoleic acid) and fibre content

trition. The clinical evidence of any difference in flora between patients with Crohn's disease and normal controls remains slim. It was shown in the late 1970s that there are higher bacterial counts within the terminal ileum of patients with active disease [51]. Studies at that time also suggested a reduction in faecal flora after enteral nutrition [52]. More recent data from Lionetti et al. [53] confirmed that EEN leads to profound modification of gut flora, whilst gut flora in normal children remains stable over time, and supplemental enteral nutrition in Crohn's disease also led to stable changes in bacterial species over time. It is now clear that increasing severity of systemic disease is associated with an increase in the adherence of fecal bacteria to the enterocytes [54], and this does not appear to be related to the degree of local mucosal inflammation. The response of acute Crohn's disease to antibiotic therapy further implicates the bacterial flora in the disease pathogenesis [55], although antibiotics such as the quinolones and metronidazole have other immunomodulatory effects in addition to their antimicrobial actions [56]. The organisms that appear increased in the lumen of patients with Crohn's disease include Bacteroides, Eubacteria and Peptostreptococcus [57]. Elegant work on mice that develop spontaneous colitis (TCRα–/–) has confirmed that feeding with an elemental diet prevents bowel inflammation [58]. Unlike the mice fed the elemental diet, the mice fed regular chow and then develop colitis are colonised by *Bacteroides vulgatus* in >80% of the cases. Furthermore, instilling this strain into the rectum of the elementally fed mice led to development of a typical Th-2 type, T cell-induced colitis. Further animal work has shown that elemental diet may reduce progression of granulomatous enteritis by modulating the activation of T cells, the production of NO, and the generation of oxygen free radicals [59, 60].

The reduction in antigenic load that accompanies exclusive enteral nutrition may also contribute, at least in part, to bowel rest. However, a whole-protein diet, and even an ad libitum diet together with some parenteral nutrition, appear are as effective as an exclusive elemental diet at inducing a remission [3–5, 61]. The efficacy of polymeric diets and recent evidence that dietary supplementation with enteral nutrition may prolong a remission [62], suggesting that reducing luminal antigens may only play a modest role in the efficacy of this therapy.

Whether enteral nutrition per se has either a direct and/or indirect immuno-regulatory effect remains speculative. Degrees of moderate protein malnutrition have been associated with poor immune function. In rodents, protein deprivation leads to impairment of the mucosal immune response, as well as depleting a population of T cells that control oral tolerance [63, 64]. This would suggest that poor nutrition inhibit T cells that down-regulate the gut's response to foreign antigens. Enteral feeding may therefore have an indirect effect on the immune response by restoring an adequate nutritional status.

More recently, the direct influence of luminal content on immune function has been studied. Sanderson [65] provided evidence that luminal content can influence epithelial cell gene expression within the gut. Short-chain fatty acids, such as butyrate, are bacterial metabolites from unabsorbed carbohydrates. Butyrate induces secretion of insulin growth factor-binding proteins (IGFBPs) by a complex process involving histone deacetylation [66]. Butyrate has also been shown to potentiate the secretion of IL-8 by intestinal epithelial cells (Caco-2) if these are stimulated with either lipopolysaccharide (LPS) or IL-1β. LPS was only able to induce IL-8 secretion if these cells were pre-incubated with butyrate, implying direct effects of the latter on gene regulation [67]. Epithelial cell gene regulation by luminal products thus appears to be able to influence intestinal inflammation through release of inflammatory cytokines such. Up-regulation of the chemokine macrophage-inflammatory-protein-2 (MIP-2) increases local neutrophil recruitment [68].

It has also been suggested that the presence, or absence, of individual components of enteral feeds is important in immune regulation. The putative advantage of high TGF-β levels in both AL110 and CT3211 (~24 ppm) is based on the large body of experimental evidence that this cytokine has the ability to down-regulate other pro-inflammatory cytokines [69]. Fell et al. [4] demonstrated mucosal up-regulation of TGF-β within the terminal ileum after an 8-week course of TGF-β-rich CT3211. It is still unclear whether this is related to the increased luminal presence of TGF-β or is simply an epi-phenomenon of tissue repair. However, glutamine, a fuel for small bowel epithelial cells and of importance in regulating intestinal permeability, has so far failed to demonstrate any clinical benefit in randomised studies in both adults and children [23]. It has also been shown that EEN can affect the plasma antioxidant concentrations in children with acute Crohn's disease (increase in selenium, decrease in vitamins C and E), although again there was no additional effect with the addition of glutamine to the formula [70].

It may also be that enteral nutrition plays a direct role in promoting the mechanisms involved in epithelial healing. There are numerous peptides involved in the restoration of a disrupted epithelial barrier. The ulcer-associated cell lineage (UACL) [71] secretes cytoprotective peptides that promote epithelial healing. Amongst them are epidermal growth factor (EGF), TGF-α, human spasmolytic peptide (hSP) and the family of trefoil peptides. The trefoil peptides in particular have been shown to be vital in protecting against mucosal damage [72]. Enteral nutrition may contribute toward the maintenance of mucosal integrity by boosting the proliferation of the UACL [73].

Whilst the theory of 'bowel rest' has its supporters, others continue to feel it is adequate nutrition alone that could induce remission and growth in these patients [74]. Kirschner et al. [75] also demonstrated improved growth in children simply fed an extra 1,000 kcal/day. The same group later confirmed that improved nutrition not only increased linear growth, but also returned previously low levels of insulin-like growth factor-1 (IGF-1) to normal in children with active Crohn's disease [76]. Thomas et al. [77] confirmed this finding with an elemental feed, which was as effective at increasing IGF-1 as prednisolone, yet better promoted linear growth.

There are likely to be many mechanisms responsible for the clinical efficacy of enteral nutrition. It is clear, however, that the luminal environment is crucial to the expression of mucosal disease. Our ability to regulate specific aspects of this environment by nutritional or other means remains a great challenge. The multitude of variables that may be important in achieving a disease remission makes identification of single factors extremely difficult. Current attention is focused on modifying enteral formulas in line with the recent evidence on dietary fats, while continuing to ensure their clinical efficacy and tolerability.

Mucosal Healing

Attention has focused on the ability of treatments to achieve mucosal healing [78]. Breese et al. [30] gave an initial indication that enteral nutrition was able to down-regulate intestinal mucosal inflammation. Enteral nutrition was as effective as cyclosporin and steroids in reducing the percentage of IL-2-secreting cells in the terminal ileum after treatment, whilst it appeared more effective than steroids at reducing the percentage of IFN-γ-secreting cells. Furthermore, it was only the enterally fed group that showed significant histological improvement.

Despite being only a small study, Breese et al. [30] raised two important issues. Firstly that enteral nutrition may be able to heal mucosa, and secondly that mucosal cytokine analysis following treatment did not necessarily correlate with either clinical or histological indices of remission.

The mucosal cytokine responses of a much larger cohort of children were reported by Fell et al. [79]. Whilst clear clinical and histological remission was achieved in over 70% of children, cytokine profiles also dramatically improved with a polymeric diet alone. The dramatic down-regulation of the potent pro-inflammatory cytokines IL-1β, IFN-γ and IL-8 is the most concrete evidence to date that enteral nutrition acts at the mucosal level. Berni Canani et al. [80] retrospectively reviewed patients receiving EEN or corticosteroids to assess efficacy of achieving a clinical remission and also in documenting mucosal healing. Despite the lack of robust methodology, there were several children who achieved mucosal healing in the EEN-treated group compared to none in the steroid-treated group.

The issue of whether clinical, endoscopic, histological or immunological remission should be the gold standard remains a matter of personal practice. If we are to believe that the presence of chronic inflammation predisposes to long-term complications and malignancy [81], it may be a state of immunological remission at the mucosal level that should be achieved in children with a lifetime of Crohn's disease ahead of them.

Conclusions

Despite the ever-increasing choice of therapies available to children with inflammatory bowel disease, the role of nutrition remains central to their optimal management. The impact of bowel inflammation on growth and development cannot be under-estimated. As final adult height is determined during the pubertal growth spurt, it is crucial to minimise the impact that both the disease and its therapies may have on a child's growth potential.

Advances in identifying children at particular risk of growth failure may, in the future, allow specific interventions to maximise growth.

We strongly suggest that exclusive enteral nutrition remains the best primary therapy for the treatment of all children presenting with a new diagnosis of Crohn's disease, apart from those with severe perianal disease. Thereafter, the challenge is to maintain a lasting remission, particularly during puberty. This is likely to be best achieved with early use of immunosuppressants such as azathioprine/6-mercaptopurine, hoping to minimise steroid use. Continued vigilance of under-nutrition and appropriate use of dietary supplementation remains essential to an optimal outcome.

The consequences of developing a chronic inflammatory disease during childhood will be felt long after a child is handed over to our adult physician colleagues. Increased risks of osteoporotic fractures, high rates of surgery and a reduced final height are only some of the areas where nutritional therapy is vitally important. The ability of therapies to achieve healing of the gut mucosa is of utmost importance in children who have a lifetime ahead of them. Although dietary therapies do not yet play a significant therapeutic role in maintenance therapy for IBD, it is likely that evidence about potential disease-modifying dietary supplements will continue to appear. It is important that as more potent immunological agents become available to treat these diseases, we do not forget the therapeutic role of nutrition in Crohn's disease; its absence of adverse effects and its proven impact on growth and gut mucosa.

Whilst newer therapies may require less commitment from families and medical teams, their unknown long-term safety profile still makes enteral nutrition an excellent choice for children with Crohn's disease for many years to come.

Disclosure Statement

The author declares that no financial or other conflict of interest exists in relation to the content of the article.

References

1 Stephens RV, Randall HT: Use of concentrated, balanced, liquid elemental diet for nutritional management of catabolic states. Ann Surg 1969;170:642–668.

2 Johnson T, et al: Treatment of active Crohn's disease in children using partial enteral nutrition with liquid formula: a randomised controlled trial. Gut 2006;55:356–361.

3 Beattie RM, et al: Polymeric nutrition as the primary therapy in children with small bowel Crohn's disease. Aliment Pharmacol Ther 1994;8:609–615.

4 Fell JM, et al: Mucosal healing and a fall in mucosal pro-inflammatory cytokine mRNA induced by a specific oral polymeric diet in paediatric Crohn's disease. Aliment Pharmacol Ther 2000;14:281–289.

5 Ruuska T, et al: Exclusive whole protein enteral diet versus prednisolone in the treatment of acute Crohn's disease in children. J Pediatr Gastroenterol Nutr 1994;19:175–180.

6 Seidman E, et al: Semi-elemental diet vs. prednisolone in pediatric Crohn's disease. Gastroenterology 1993;104:778.

7 Day AS, et al: Exclusive enteral feeding as primary therapy for Crohn's disease in Australian children and adolescents: a feasible and effective approach. J Gastroenterol Hepatol 2006;21:1609–1614.

8 Lochs H, et al: Comparison of enteral nutrition and drug treatment in active Crohn's disease. Results of the European Cooperative Crohn's Disease Study. Part IV. Gastroenterology 1991;101:881–888.

9 Malchow H, et al: European Cooperative Crohn's Disease Study (ECCDS): results of drug treatment. Gastroenterology 1984;86:249–266.

10 Afzal NA, et al: Colonic Crohn's disease in children does not respond well to treatment with enteral nutrition if the ileum is not involved. Dig Dis Sci 2005;50:1471–1475.

11 Lim S, et al: Treatment of orofacial and ileocolonic Crohn's disease with total enteral nutrition. J R Soc Med 1998;91:489–490.

12 Afzal NA, et al: Refeeding syndrome with enteral nutrition in children: a case report, literature review and clinical guidelines. Clin Nutr 2002;21:515–520.

13 Winitz M, et al: Nature, Volume 205, 1965: Evaluation of chemical diets as nutrition for man-in-space. Nutr Rev 1991;49:141–143.

14 Voitk AJ, et al: Experience with elemental diet in the treatment of inflammatory bowel disease: is this primary therapy? Arch Surg 1973;107:329–333.

15 Logan RF, et al: Reduction of gastrointestinal protein loss by elemental diet in Crohn's disease of the small bowel. Gut 1981;22:383–387.

16 Giorgini GL, Stephens RV, Thayer WR Jr: The use of 'medical by-pass' in the therapy of Crohn's disease: report of a case. Am J Dig Dis 1973;18:153–157.

17 Navarro J, et al: Prolonged constant rate elemental enteral nutrition in Crohn's disease. J Pediatr Gastroenterol Nutr 1982;1:541–546.

18 Morin CL, et al: Continuous elemental enteral alimentation in children with Crohn's disease and growth failure. Gastroenterology 1980;79:1205–1210.

19 O'Morain C: Crohn's disease treated by elemental diet. J R Soc Med 1982;75:135–136.

20 Morin CL, et al: Continuous elemental enteral alimentation in the treatment of children and adolescents with Crohn's disease. JPEN J Parenter Enteral Nutr 1982;6:194–199.

21 O'Morain C, Segal AW, Levi AJ: Elemental diet as primary treatment of acute Crohn's disease: a controlled trial. Br Med J (Clin Res Ed) 1984;288:1859–1862.

22 Sanderson IR, et al: Remission induced by an elemental diet in small bowel Crohn's disease. Arch Dis Child 1987;62:123–127.

23 Akobeng AK, et al: Double-blind randomized controlled trial of glutamine-enriched polymeric diet in the treatment of active Crohn's disease. J Pediatr Gastroenterol Nutr 2000;30:78–84.

24 Silk DB, et al: Use of a peptide rather than free amino acid nitrogen source in chemically defined 'elemental' diets. JPEN J Parenter Enteral Nutr 1980;4:548–553.

25 Raouf AH, et al: Enteral feeding as sole treatment for Crohn's disease: controlled trial of whole protein v amino acid based feed and a case study of dietary challenge. Gut 1991;32:702–707.

26 Gonzalez-Huix F, et al: Polymeric enteral diets as primary treatment of active Crohn's disease: a prospective steroid controlled trial. Gut 1993;34:778–782.

27 Beattie RM, Walker-Smith JA: Treatment of active Crohn's disease by exclusion diet. J Pediatr Gastroenterol Nutr 1994;19:135–136.

28 Rodrigues AF, et al: Does polymeric formula improve adherence to liquid diet therapy in children with active Crohn's disease? Arch Dis Child 2007;92:767–770.

29 Hyams JS, et al: Development and validation of a pediatric Crohn's disease activity index. J Pediatr Gastroenterol Nutr 1991;12:439–447.

30 Breese EJ, et al: The effect of treatment on lymphokine-secreting cells in the intestinal mucosa of children with Crohn's disease. Aliment Pharmacol Ther 1995;9:547–552.

31 Bannerjee K, et al: Anti-inflammatory and growth-stimulating effects precede nutritional restitution during enteral feeding in Crohn disease. J Pediatr Gastroenterol Nutr 2004;38:270–275.

32 Gassull MA, et al: Fat composition may be a clue to explain the primary therapeutic effect of enteral nutrition in Crohn's disease: results of a double blind randomised multicentre European trial. Gut 2002;51:164–168.

33 Miura S, et al: Modulation of intestinal immune system by dietary fat intake: relevance to Crohn's disease. J Gastroenterol Hepatol 1998;13:1183–1190.

34 Sakurai T, et al: Short-term efficacy of enteral nutrition in the treatment of active Crohn's disease: a randomized, controlled trial comparing nutrient formulas. JPEN J Parenter Enteral Nutr 2002;26:98–103.

35 Leiper K, et al: A randomised controlled trial of high versus low long chain triglyceride whole protein feed in active Crohn's disease. Gut 2001;49:790–794.

36 von Tirpitz C, et al: Lactose intolerance in active Crohn's disease: clinical value of duodenal lactase analysis. J Clin Gastroenterol 2002;34:49–53.

37 Malchow H, et al: Feasibility and effectiveness of a defined-formula diet regimen in treating active Crohn's disease. European Cooperative Crohn's Disease Study III. Scand J Gastroenterol 1990;25:235–244.

38 Griffiths AM, et al: Meta-analysis of enteral nutrition as a primary treatment of active Crohn's disease. Gastroenterology 1995;108:1056–1067.

39 Zachos M, Tondeur M, Griffiths AM: Enteral nutritional therapy for induction of remission in Crohn's disease. Cochrane Database Syst Rev 2007;1:CD000542.

40 Modigliani R, et al: Clinical, biological, and endoscopic picture of attacks of Crohn's disease: evolution on prednisolone. Groupe d'Etude Therapeutique des Affections Inflammatoires Digestives. Gastroenterology 1990;98:811–818.

41 Zachos M, Tondeur M, Griffiths AM: Enteral nutritional therapy for inducing remission of Crohn's disease. Cochrane Database Syst Rev 2001;3:CD000542.

42 Heuschkel RB: Enteral nutrition in children with Crohn's disease. J Pediatr Gastroenterol Nutr 2000;31:575.

43 Dziechciarz P, et al: Meta-analysis: enteral nutrition in active Crohn's disease in children. Aliment Pharmacol Ther 2007;26:795–806.

44 Day AS, et al: Systematic review: nutritional therapy in paediatric Crohn's disease. Aliment Pharmacol Ther 2008;27:293–307.

45 Markowitz J, et al: Corticosteroid therapy in the age of infliximab: acute and 1-year outcomes in newly diagnosed children with Crohn's disease. Clin Gastroenterol Hepatol 2006;4:1124–1129.

46 Murch SH, Walker-Smith JA: Nutrition in inflammatory bowel disease. Baillieres Clin Gastroenterol 1998;12:719–738.

47 Rigaud D, et al: Controlled trial comparing two types of enteral nutrition in treatment of active Crohn's disease: elemental versus polymeric diet. Gut 1991;32:1492–1497.

48 Thomas AG, Taylor F, Miller V: Dietary intake and nutritional treatment in childhood Crohn's disease. J Pediatr Gastroenterol Nutr 1993;17:75–81.

49 Riordan AM, et al: Treatment of active Crohn's disease by exclusion diet: East Anglian multicentre controlled trial. Lancet 1993;342:1131–1134.

50 Pearson M, et al: Food intolerance and Crohn's disease. Gut 1993;34:783–787.

51 Peac S, et al: Mucosal-associated bacterial flora of the intestine in patients with Crohn's disease and in a control group. Gut 1978;19:1034–1042.

52 Axelsson CK, Justesen T: Studies of the duodenal and fecal flora in gastrointestinal disorders during treatment with an elemental diet. Gastroenterology 1977;72:397–401.

53 Lionetti P, et al: Enteral nutrition and microflora in pediatric Crohn's disease. JPEN J Parenter Enteral Nutr 2005;29(4 suppl):S173–S175; discussion S175–S178, S184–S188.

54 Swidsinski A, et al: Mucosal flora in inflammatory bowel disease. Gastroenterology 2002;122:44–54.

55 Rutgeerts P, et al: Controlled trial of metronidazole treatment for prevention of Crohn's recurrence after ileal resection. Gastroenterology 1995;108:1617–1621.

56 Pourtaghi N, et al: The effect of subgingival antimicrobial therapy on the levels of stromelysin and tissue inhibitor of metalloproteinases in gingival crevicular fluid. J Periodontol 1996;67:866–870.

57 Linskens RK, et al: The bacterial flora in inflammatory bowel disease: current insights in pathogenesis and the influence of antibiotics and probiotics. Scand J Gastroenterol Suppl 2001;234:29–40.

58 Kishi D, et al: Alteration of V beta usage and cytokine production of CD4+ TCR beta beta homodimer T cells by elimination of *Bacteroides vulgatus* prevents colitis in TCR alpha-chain-deficient mice. J Immunol 2000;165:5891–5899.

59 Tanaka S, et al: Amelioration of chronic inflammation by ingestion of elemental diet in a rat model of granulomatous enteritis. Dig Dis Sci 1997;42:408–419.

60 Tanaka S, et al: Elemental diet reduces progression of chronic inflammation and alters nitric oxide metabolism in a rat model of granulomatous colitis. Gastroenterology 1999 (abstract).

61 Greenberg GR, et al: Controlled trial of bowel rest and nutritional support in the management of Crohn's disease. Gut 1988;29:1309–1315.

62 Wilschanski M, et al: Supplementary enteral nutrition maintains remission in paediatric Crohn's disease. Gut 1996;38:543–548.

63 Koster F, Pierce NF: Effect of protein deprivation on immunoregulatory cells in the rat mucosal immune response. Clin Exp Immunol 1985;60:217–224.

64 Lamont AG, Gordon M, Ferguson A: Oral tolerance in protein-deprived mice. II. Evidence of normal 'gut processing' of ovalbumin, but suppressor cell deficiency, in deprived mice. Immunology 1987;61:339–343.

65 Sanderson IR: Dietary regulation of genes expressed in the developing intestinal epithelium. Am J Clin Nutr 1998;68:999–1005.

66 Nishimura A, et al: Short-chain fatty acids regulate IGF-binding protein secretion by intestinal epithelial cells. Am J Physiol 1998;275:E55–E63.

67 Fusunyan RD, et al: Butyrate enhances interleukin (IL)-8 secretion by intestinal epithelial cells in response to IL-1beta and lipopolysaccharide. Pediatr Res 1998;43:84–90.

68 Ohtsuka Y, et al: MIP-2 secreted by epithelial cells increases neutrophil and lymphocyte recruitment in the mouse intestine. Gut 2001;49:526–533.

69 Kulkarni AB, et al: Transforming growth factor beta 1 null mutation in mice causes excessive inflammatory response and early death. Proc Natl Acad Sci USA 1993;90:770–774.

70 Akobeng AK, et al: Effect of exclusive enteral nutritional treatment on plasma antioxidant concentrations in childhood Crohn's disease. Clin Nutr 2007;26:51–56.

71 Wright NA, et al: Trefoil peptide gene expression in gastrointestinal epithelial cells in inflammatory bowel disease. Gastroenterology 1993;104:12–20.

72 Babyatsky MW, et al: Oral trefoil peptides protect against ethanol- and indomethacin-induced gastric injury in rats. Gastroenterology 1996;110:489–497.

73 Beattie RM, Bentsen BS, MacDonald TT: Childhood Crohn's disease and the efficacy of enteral diets. Nutrition 1998;14:345–350.

74 Kirschner BS: Nutritional consequences of inflammatory bowel disease on growth. J Am Coll Nutr 1988;7:301–308.

75 Kirschner BS, et al: Reversal of growth retardation in Crohn's disease with therapy emphasizing oral nutritional restitution. Gastroenterology 1981;80:10–15.

76 Kirschner BS, Sutton MM: Somatomedin-C levels in growth-impaired children and adolescents with chronic inflammatory bowel disease. Gastroenterology 1986;91:830–836.

77 Thomas AG, et al: Insulin like growth factor-I, insulin like growth factor binding protein-1, and insulin in childhood Crohn's disease. Gut 1993;34:944–947.

78 Walker-Smith JA: Mucosal healing in Crohn's disease. Gastroenterology 1998;114:419–420.

79 Fell JM, et al: Normalisation of mucosal cytokine mRNA in association with clinical improvement in children with Crohn's disease treated with polymeric diet. J Paediatr Gastroenterol 1998;26:544.

80 Berni Canani R, et al: Short- and long-term therapeutic efficacy of nutritional therapy and corticosteroids in paediatric Crohn's disease. Dig Liver Dis 2006;38:381–387.

81 Munkholm P, et al: Intestinal cancer risk and mortality in patients with Crohn's disease. Gastroenterology 1993;105:1716–1723.

Dig Dis 2009;27:306–311
DOI: 10.1159/000228565

Top-Down Therapy: Is the Evidence Strong Enough?

Eugeni Domènech   Míriam Mañosa   Eduard Cabré

Department of Gastroenterology and Hepatology, IBD Unit, Hospital Universitari Germans Trias i Pujol,
Badalona and Centro de Investigaciones Biomédicas en Red de Enfermedades Hepáticas y Digestivas (CIBEREHD),
Barcelona, Spain

Key Words
Crohn's disease · Inflammatory bowel disease · Top-down
therapy · Immunomodulators · Biologicals · Anti-TNF ·
Mucosal healing

Abstract
Crohn's disease (CD) has usually been managed in an escalation manner, introducing more powerful (and toxic) drugs
only once those with a better safety profile had failed. However, the natural history of CD under conventional therapeutic strategies results in high intestinal resection requirements and high rates of clinical relapse and steroid
dependence. Indirect data seem to point at an improved efficacy of drugs when they are introduced early after disease
diagnosis. The spreading use of immunomodulators and the
appearance of biological agents prompted the idea of their
early introduction in order to change the natural history of
the disease. By now, only thiopurines have been shown to
reduce steroid requirements, relapse rates, and even surgical requirements, at least in pediatric CD. However, many
other 'top-down' treatment strategies have not yet been
evaluated. In addition, there is a risk of overtreating those
10–30% of patients that will have a benign course of the disease; that's the reason why the implementation of top-down
strategies remains as a matter of debate.

Copyright © 2009 S. Karger AG, Basel

Introduction

The increasing knowledge in both the pathophysiology and the natural history of Crohn's disease (CD) has
led to important changes in its management. Symptom
abatement was the main treatment goal some decades
ago, and the severity of clinical presentation prompted
the use of one drug or another depending on their therapeutic efficacy and potential side effects. Treatment goals
progressively evolved to a more strict control of the disease; symptom relief was not the only objective, and nor-
malization of biological markers (ESR, anemia, C-reactive protein) became another important therapeutic target. With the spreading use of immunomodulators and,
specially, with the appearance of biological agents, it became apparent that a wider use of more powerful drugs
might result beneficial despite a likely increase in the risk
of severe side effects. In the last years, the idea of changing the natural history of the disease by early introducing
these therapies has been raising, leading to consider the
possibility of preventing (if not avoiding) recurrent relapses, disease complications, and intestinal resections,
in order to improve and maintain the patient's quality of
life. The aim of this article is to review the current evidence for the use of what has been called 'top-down' therapy, and also to revisit the definition of 'top-down' itself
and their possible variations.

Eugeni Domènech, MD, PhD
Hospital Universitari Germans Trias i Pujol, 5ª planta, edifici general
Gastroenterology Department, Carretera del Canyet s/n
ES–08916 Badalona, Catalonia (Spain)
Tel. +34 93 497 8909, E-Mail edomenech.germanstrias@gencat.cat

Natural History of Crohn's Disease under Conventional Therapy

Conventional therapy of CD is based on the escalation of drugs, from those with a better safety profile but a lower efficacy (antibiotics, mesalazine) to those with improved efficacy but a greater risk of side effects (steroids, immunomodulators, biologicals, surgery). Most of the available studies assessing long-term CD evolution come from series of patients managed in a conventional manner; thus, there is enough information to evaluate which is the long-term efficacy of this treatment strategy.

The development of intestinal stenosis and penetrating disease-related complications (such as intra-abdominal masses or abscesses, entero-organic fistulae, perianal disease) are considered to be the major disabling situations in the evolution of CD. These complications are usually managed surgically and, except for perianal disease, intestinal resection is required. Recently, Vienna's and Montreal's classification of CD allowed to distinguish different disease behaviors; by means of this useful categorization, two large, retrospective studies agreed in showing that up to 50% of patients will develop stenosing or penetrating complications within the first 5 years from disease diagnosis, and that this will increase up to 70% after 10 years [1, 2]. These figures correlate with the rates of intestinal resection that were reported to be around 40 and 60%, at 5 and 10 years after diagnosis, respectively, in a large Portuguese series from a hospital cohort by the end of the nineties [3]. Despite the spreading (but not earlier) use of immunomodulators, the proportion of patients requiring intestinal resection has not decreased, as shown in a recently published Dutch study in which resectional requirements were evaluated in an incident population-based cohort of CD patients [4].

Nevertheless, quality of patient's life in CD is not only disabled by the development of these complications, but also by the need of repeated hospital admissions, courses of steroids (with their annoying and constant side effects), or uncontrolled inflammatory activity (a frequent cause of anemia, malnutrition, and malaise). This has also been evaluated in several studies. Ho et al. [5] and Faubion et al. [6] evaluated the mid-term outcome (1 year) after a first course of steroids in two cohorts of CD patients. Briefly, about 25% of the initial responders became steroid-dependent and one third required surgery. It could be argued that these disabling outcomes only occur in that subset of patients with a more aggressive disease. However, when looking at those patients with mild disease, it seems that this is not the case. For instance, in a RCT performed by Hanauer et al. [7] in patients entering remission with oral budesonide for a mild-to-moderate activity flare, only 40–50% of them remained in remission after 1 year. Romberg-Camps et al. [4] recently showed that the probability to remain free of any relapse of the disease (treated medically or surgically) was as low as 10%, ten years after diagnosis.

Drug Efficacy May Depend on Disease Duration

Some indirect data suggest that drug efficacy may vary depending on disease duration. Kugathasan et al. [8] evaluated the response to a single infusion of infliximab in pediatric luminal CD, and stated that those children with shorter disease duration (less than 2 years) had a prolonged response to the drug. Post-hoc analysis of large RCTs that evaluated the efficacy of different biological agents reached similar conclusions, but this could be biased by several factors such as inclusion/exclusion criteria, or even marketing interests. Another way to assess this issue is to compare the results of studies with similar designs but with different population in terms of disease duration (fig. 1). When comparing the efficacy of thiopurines to maintain steroid-induced disease remission, the Markowitz study achieved a 91% of success after 18 months in new-onset pediatric CD [9], whereas in the study by Candy et al. [10] with adult CD (median time of disease duration of 2.6 years) only 42% remained in remission after 15 months, and in the GETAID study with steroid-dependent disease (median duration of disease 4 years) the success rate was as low as 32% after 1 year [11]. Similar findings are obtained when assessing the rate of clinical remission after the administration of three infliximab infusions for luminal CD. In the step-up/top-down study by D'Haens et al. [12], the median disease duration at inclusion was 2 weeks; the remission rate at week 10 in the 'top-down' arm resulted in 64%. In the REACH study, which included children with active luminal CD, the median duration of disease was 1.4 years. After the initial 3 scheduled infusions, the remission rate resulted in 59% [13]. Finally, in the ACCENT-I trial that included adult CD patients with active luminal disease with a median duration of the disease of 8 years, the remission rate in the infliximab arms (those who received 3 infusions) was 42% [14]. It has to be taken into account that these comparisons may also be biased by several factors such as smoking (a deleterious factor in CD evolution) that is not present in childhood but affects 50% or even more of adult CD patients, or the proportion of pa-

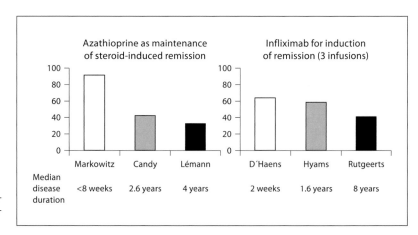

Fig. 1. Different drug efficacy in the setting of RCTs depending on disease duration.

tients treated with concomitant immunomodulators that was not the same in all these studies.

There is a biological explanation for this different response to a drug in different time settings. Kugathasan et al. [15] demonstrated that the production of IFN-γ in response to IL-12 modulation is increased in early stages of the disease but lost with progression to late CD. In addition, T cell production of IL-4 and IL-10 is lower in early disease as compared to late CD. This change in the cytokine pattern of the inflamed mucosa and different immunologic response could explain a different efficacy of a same drug depending on disease duration.

This pathophysiological consideration would also explain the relevance of the rapidity in achieving clinical remission. Veloso [3], in a retrospective study with a large series of CD patients, suggested that an earlier control of inflammatory activity could be associated to a lower rate of relapses later on.

Keeping in mind that the earlier the inflammation is controlled, the longer the patient will remain in remission, and that at least some drugs work better when used early in the disease evolution, it seems reasonable to consider early introduction of those drugs with proven efficacy in order to prevent a disabling disease course in the future.

Early Introduction of Thiopurines or Biologic Agents

To date, only one RCT has evaluated the efficacy of early introduction of thiopurines in CD. Markowitz et al. [9] included 55 pediatric patients who had been diagnosed of CD within the previous 8 weeks and presented moder-ate-to-severe activity. All children were treated with prednisone 40 mg/day and randomized to receive placebo or mercaptopurine 1.5 mg/kg/day for 18 months. At the end of follow-up, patients in the mercaptopurine group had a significantly higher probability to remain in remission and a significantly lower cumulative dose of steroids. Unfortunately, the study was not powered and follow-up was not long enough to find differences in both the development of stenosing or penetrating complications and the surgery requirements. This study became a cornerstone in the management of pediatric CD, and some years later a retrospective series of similar characteristics reproduced the results with azathioprine after a successful course of systemic steroids in clinical practice [16].

In another classical study, Cosnes et al. [17] evaluated retrospectively the use of immunomodulators and its clinical impact in a large cohort of adult CD patients who were diagnosed from the late 1970s to the end of the 1990s. Although the authors noted an increasing use of thiopurines throughout the study period and a parallel significant decrease in 'large' intestinal resections, this was not associated to a reduction in the total rate of intestinal resection. However, most patients receiving thiopurines started them once disease complications had developed or even after surgery, leading the authors to conclude that these drugs were introduced too late in the evolution of the disease to have a relevant clinical impact. Recently, a French study in a population-based incident cohort of pediatric CD showed for the first time that the stenosing disease behavior and the use of steroids were the only factors associated to a higher risk for surgery, whereas the use of azathioprine was the only protective factor [18].

By now, no study has assessed the early introduction of biologicals for both inducing and maintaining disease remission. D'Haens et al. [12] recently reported the results of the so-called 'step-up/top-down' trial in which patients with CD who were naïve of steroids, immunomodulators, and biologicals were randomized to be managed by means of a conventional therapeutic algorithm (initially with steroids and introducing thiopurines only in case of refractoriness or more than two relapses, and biologicals if immunomodulators failed) or an early intensive strategy (induction of remission with 3 infliximab infusions and initial introduction of thiopurines, and infliximab on demand if the patient relapsed). It has to be pointed out that the included patients had a median time of disease duration of only 2 weeks. Briefly, the main conclusions of the study were: (1) patients in the 'top-down' group achieved clinical remission earlier than those in the conventional management; (2) immunomodulators were introduced in almost 70% of patients in the conventional management group after 1 year, and (3) a greater proportion of patients achieved mucosal healing as measured by endoscopic monitoring two years after inclusion in the 'top-down' group. Once again, the study was not powered enough and follow-up was too short to find differences in the development of stenosing/penetrating complications or in surgical requirements between the two groups.

The Importance of Mucosal Healing in Crohn's Disease

As mentioned above, studies with a long follow-up period (5–10 years) are needed if a change in the natural history of CD is to be evaluated. This is unlikely to occur in the setting RCTs, but the mid- and long-term outcome of CD may be predicted by monitoring endoscopic (mucosal) lesions. Early studies on postoperative natural history of CD showed that the development of new mucosal lesions in the neoterminal ileum preceded clinical relapse; moreover, the severity of these mucosal lesions seen at ileocolonoscopy correlated with the risk of clinical recurrence in the follow-up [19]. Under this perspective, it seems logical that those drugs or treatment strategies with lower relapse rates should also achieve the disappearance of mucosal lesions in a higher proportion of patients. Reciprocally, if those treatments that achieve higher rates of mucosal healing were associated to a lower probability of disease complications and surgical requirements, then, monitoring mucosal healing should predict a more favor-

able course of disease. Several studies have reported a rate of mucosal healing of around 30% of patients after inducing clinical remission with steroids [20], enteral nutrition [21], or infliximab [22]. However, as far as the relevance of mucosal healing lies on its impact of long-term outcome, it should be assessed during maintenance therapies rather than after short-term treatments. In that setting, D'Haens et al. [23] retrospectively analyzed 20 patients responding to azathioprine, and reported 70% of mucosal healing in colonic disease and 54% in the terminal ileum. Rutgeerts et al. [22], in a sub-study of the ACCENT-I trial, found mucosal healing in 50% of 26 patients receiving scheduled infliximab therapy for 1 year. In view of these data and, as expected, the 'top-down' strategy achieved mucosal healing in 73% patients 2 years after starting therapy; moreover, Baert et al. [24] reported that those patients who achieved mucosal healing after 2 years of treatment had a significantly higher probability to remain in clinical remission for the following 2 years.

Definition of 'Top-Down' Strategy

In a recent review, Shergill and Terdiman [25] defined 'top-down' strategy as the 'early introduction of immunomodulators and biologicals'. Armuzzi et al. [26], in a wider definition, included the 'use of highly effective, but potentially more toxic, treatment strategies early in the course of a chronic disease, in order to prevent disease progression and complications'. Reasonably, any therapeutic strategy in Crohn's disease must include two regimens: induction and maintenance of remission. Under this perspective, any 'top-down' regimen should use those drugs/treatments that have proven efficacy in inducing disease remission such as enteral nutrition, steroids, biologic agents, and even surgery. In fact, a recent study reported that ileocecal resection in CD patients naïve of immunomodulators and biologicals was followed by a symptomatic relapse rate of only 50% after 10 years [27]. Whichever of these induction treatments are, they should be followed by those therapies proven to be effective in the long-term maintenance of remission: immunomodulators or biologicals. However, 'top-down' philosophy is not limited to the use of some treatments and it also includes the concept of *early introduction* (right from diagnosis) of these therapies. By now, only the combination of steroids + thiopurines [9], and biologicals + thiopurines [12] have been evaluated. In this sense, RCTs are warranted and maybe every possible 'top-down' combination will have its own 'patient profile'.

Conclusions

The natural history of CD under conventional therapeutic strategies results in high intestinal resection requirements and a high rate of clinical relapse or steroid dependence. Indirect data and biological studies point at the earlier effective treatments are introduced, the better they work. However, 10–30% of CD patients will present a benign course. Although still far from conclusively demonstrating that this strategy can change the natural history of the disease, thiopurines have shown to reduce steroid requirements, relapse rates, and even surgical requirements, at least in paediatric CD. The question is, while good indicators of poor prognosis in the mid-term are still lacking, whether immunomodulators, biologicals or surgery must be introduced at the time of CD diagnosis in all patients.

Acknowledgement

CIBEREHD is funded by the Instituto de Salud Carlos III, from the Spanish Ministry of Health.

Disclosure Statement

E. Domènech has been an advisor and has lectured for Centocor, Schering-Plough, Abbott, UCB Pharma and Ferring.

References

1 Louis E, Collard A, Oger AF, Degroote E, Aboul Nasr El Yafi FA, Belaiche J: Behaviour of Crohn's disease according to the Vienna classification: changing pattern over the course of the disease. Gut 2001;49:777–782.

2 Cosnes J, Cattan S, Blain A, Beaugerie L, Carbonnel F, Parc R, Gendre JP: Long-term evolution of disease behavior of Crohn's disease. Inflamm Bowel Dis 2002;8:244–250.

3 Veloso FT, Ferreira JT, Barros L, Almeida S: Clinical outcome of Crohn's disease: analysis according to the Vienna classification and clinical activity. Inflamm Bowel Dis 2001;7: 306–313.

4 Romberg-Camps MJ, Dagnelie PC, Kester AD, Hesselink-van de Kruijs MA, Cilissen M, Engels LG, Van Deursen C, Hameeteman WH, Wolters FL, Russel MG, Stockbrügger RW: Influence of phenotype at diagnosis and of other potential prognostic factors on the course of inflammatory bowel disease. Am J Gastroenterol 2009;104:371–383.

5 Ho GT, Chiam P, Drummond H, Loane J, Arnott ID, Satsangi J: The efficacy of corticosteroid therapy in inflammatory bowel disease: analysis of a 5-year UK inception cohort. Aliment Pharmacol Ther 2006;24: 319–330.

6 Faubion WA Jr, Loftus EV Jr, Harmsen WS, Zinsmeister AR, Sandborn WJ: The natural history of corticosteroid therapy for inflammatory bowel disease: a population-based study. Gastroenterology 2001;121:255–260.

7 Hanauer S, Sandborn WJ, Persson A, Persson T: Budesonide as maintenance treatment in Crohn's disease: a placebo-controlled trial. Aliment Pharmacol Ther 2005;21:363–371.

8 Kugathasan S, Werlin SL, Martinez A, Rivera MT, Heikenen JB, Binion DG: Prolonged duration of response to infliximab in early but not late pediatric Crohn's disease. Am J Gastroenterol 2000;95:3189–3194.

9 Markowitz J, Grancher K, Kohn N, Lesser M, Daum F: A multicenter trial of 6-mercaptopurine and prednisone in children with newly diagnosed Crohn's disease. Gastroenterology 2000;119:895–902.

10 Candy S, Wright J, Gerber M, Adams G, Gerig M, Goodman R: A controlled double blind study of azathioprine in the management of Crohn's disease. Gut 1995;37:674–678.

11 Lémann M, Mary JY, Duclos B, Veyrac M, Dupas JL, Delchier JC, Laharie D, Moreau J, Cadiot G, Picon L, Bourreille A, Sobahni I, Colombel JF; Groupe d'Etude Therapeutique des Affections Inflammatoires du Tube Digestif (GETAID): Infliximab plus azathioprine for steroid-dependent Crohn's disease patients: a randomized placebo-controlled trial. Gastroenterology 2006;130: 1054–1061.

12 D'Haens G, Baert F, van Assche G, Caenepeel P, Vergauwe P, Tuynman H, De Vos M, van Deventer S, Stitt L, Donner A, Vermeire S, Van de Mierop FJ, Coche JC, van der Woude J, Ochsenkühn T, van Bodegraven AA, Van Hootegem PP, Lambrecht GL, Mana F, Rutgeerts P, Feagan BG, Hommes D; Belgian Inflammatory Bowel Disease Research Group; North-Holland Gut Club: Early combined immunosuppression or conventional management in patients with newly diagnosed Crohn's disease: an open randomised trial. Lancet 2008;371:660–667.

13 Hyams J, Crandall W, Kugathasan S, Griffiths A, Olson A, Johanns J, Liu G, Travers S, Heuschkel R, Markowitz J, Cohen S, Winter H, Veereman-Wauters G, Ferry G, Baldassano R, REACH Study Group: Induction and maintenance infliximab therapy for the treatment of moderate-to-severe Crohn's disease in children. Gastroenterology 2007; 132:863–873.

14 Rutgeerts P, Feagan BG, Lichtenstein GR, Mayer LF, Schreiber S, Colombel JF, Rachmilewitz D, Wolf DC, Olson A, Bao W, Hanauer SB: Comparison of scheduled and episodic treatment strategies of infliximab in Crohn's disease. Gastroenterology 2004; 126:402–413.

15 Kugathasan S, Saubermann LJ, Smith L, Kou D, Itoh J, Binion DG, Levine AD, Blumberg RS, Fiocchi C: Mucosal T-cell immunoregulation varies in early and late inflammatory bowel disease. Gut 2007;56:1696–1705.

16 Jaspers GJ, Verkade HJ, Escher JC, de Ridder L, Taminiau JA, Rings EH: Azathioprine maintains first remission in newly diagnosed pediatric Crohn's disease. Inflamm Bowel Dis 2006;12:831–836.

17 Cosnes J, Nion-Larmurier I, Beaugerie L, Afchain P, Tiret E, Gendre JP: Impact of the increasing use of immunosuppressants in Crohn's disease on the need for intestinal surgery. Gut 2005;54:237–241.

18 Vernier-Massouille G, Balde M, Salleron J, Turck D, Dupas JL, Mouterde O, Merle V, Salomez JL, Branche J, Marti R, Lerebours E, Cortot A, Gower-Rousseau C, Colombel JF: Natural history of pediatric Crohn's disease: a population-based cohort study. Gastroenterology 2008;135:1106–1113.

19 Rutgeerts P, Geboes K, Vantrappen G, Beyls J, Kerremans R, Hiele M: Predictability of the postoperative course of Crohn's disease. Gastroenterology 1990;99:956–963.

20 Landi B, Anh TN, Cortot A, Soule JC, Rene E, Gendre JP, Bories P, See A, Metman EH, Florent C; and The Groupe d'Etudes Thérapeutiques des Affections Inflammatoires Digestives: Endoscopic monitoring of Crohn's disease treatment: a prospective, randomized clinical trial. Gastroenterology 1992;102:1647–1653.

21 Fell JM, Paintin M, Arnaud-Battandier F, Beattie RM, Hollis A, Kitching P, Donnet-Hughes A, MacDonald TT, Walker-Smith JA: Mucosal healing and a fall in mucosal pro-inflammatory cytokine mRNA induced by a specific oral polymeric diet in paediatric Crohn's disease. Aliment Pharmacol Ther 2000;14:281–289.

22 Rutgeerts P, Diamond RH, Bala M, Olson A, Lichtenstein GR, Bao W, Patel K, Wolf DC, Safdi M, Colombel JF, Lashner B, Hanauer SB: Scheduled maintenance treatment with infliximab is superior to episodic treatment for the healing of mucosal ulceration associated with Crohn's disease. Gastrointest Endosc 2006;63:433–442.

23 D'Haens G, Geboes K, Rutgeerts P: Endoscopic and histologic healing of Crohn's (ileo-) colitis with azathioprine. Gastrointest Endosc 1999;50:667–671.

24 Baert P, Moortgat L, Van Assche GA, Caenepeel P, Vergauwe PL, De Vos M, Stokkers PC, Hommes DW, Vermeire S, Rutgeerts PJ, Feagan B, D'Hanes G: Mucosal healing predicts sustained clinical remission in early Crohn's disease. Gastroenterology 2008;134(suppl 1):A-640.

25 Shergill AK, Terdiman JP: Controversies in the treatment of Crohn's disease: the case for an accelerated step-up treatment approach. World J Gastroenterol 2008;14:2670–2677.

26 Armuzzi A, De Pascalis B, Fedeli P, De Vincentis F, Gasbarrini A: Infliximab in Crohn's disease: early and long-term treatment. Dig Liver Dis 2008;40(suppl 2):S271–S279.

27 Cullen G, O'Toole A, Keegan D, Sheahan K, Hyland JM, O'Donoghue DP: Long-term clinical results of ileocecal resection for Crohn's disease. Inflamm Bowel Dis 2007; 13:1369–1373.

Dig Dis 2009;27:312–314
DOI: 10.1159/000228566

Immunomodulation with Methotrexate: Underused and Undervalued?

Frank M. Ruemmele

University Paris-Descartes, Faculty of Medicine, INSERM U793, Hôpital Necker Enfants Malades, Paediatric Gastroenterology, Paris, France

Key Words

Inflammatory bowel disease · Crohn's disease · Azathioprine · Methotrexate · Clinical remission

Abstract

Therapeutic options for the treatment of inflammatory bowel disease (IBD) are multiple. There are excellent clinical trials showing in patients with IBD that immunomodulatory therapy is highly efficacious in the disease control in moderate active to severe forms. Most clinical experience was gained over the last years with the purine analogues azathioprine (AZA)/6-mercaptopurine (6-MP). These drugs are now considered as gold standard in the treatment of severe Crohn's disease (CD). However, for patients who fail to respond or who do not tolerate AZA/6-MP therapy, methotrexate is an interesting alternative drug. Two initial clinical trials validated the use of MTX in adult CD cohorts. There are now two retrospective analyses in pediatric cohorts available which nicely demonstrate the efficacy of MTX to maintain long-term remission in CD patients with active and severe disease progression. The remission rates are close to 50% in long-term follow-up, an efficacy comparable to purine analogues. Overall tolerance of MTX was good, with about 10% of adverse events in either study. Taken together, there are first data indicating that MTX might play a role comparable to AZA in the treatment of CD; however, to date it seems to be underused in the routine care of IBD patients.

Copyright © 2009 S. Karger AG, Basel

Immunosuppressive or immunomodulatory strategies are now integral part of the treatment of patients with Crohn's disease (CD). Since the precise molecular basis of CD remains still unclear, different treatment strategies were tested in the past. Best experience was gained with drugs that are able to block or down-regulate the inflammatory cascade within the intestinal mucosa [1–3]. There is good experimental evidence that active induction of effector T cell apoptosis is a major anti-inflammatory mechanism, allowing to control the inflammatory reactions within the intestinal mucosa of patients [3–5]. Two well-known drugs with pro-apoptotic effects on T cells are purine analogues and methotrexate (MTX).

Most clinical experience was gained over the last years with the purine analogues azathioprine (AZA)/6-mercaptopurine (6-MP). These drugs are now considered as the gold standard in the treatment of severe CD [2, 6]. Two recent Cochrane-based meta-analyses (five studies including 319 adult CD patients in remission and eight studies analyzing adult CD patients with active disease) clearly underlined the efficacy of AZA/6-MP to induce (after a treatment interval of at least 17 weeks) and to maintain remission [6, 7]. One single randomized placebo-controlled pediatric study confirmed the efficacy of AZA/6-MP in children with CD [8]: A total of 55 pediatric CD patients with moderate to severe disease activity were randomized to receive either 6-mercaptopurine or placebo in parallel to steroid induction therapy. In the

Prof. Dr. Dr. med. Frank M. Ruemmele
University Paris-Descartes, Faculty of Medicine, INSERM U793
Hôpital Necker Enfants Malades, Paediatric Gastroenterology
149, rue de Sèvres, FR–75015 Paris (France)
Tel. +33 144 492 516, Fax +33 144 492 501, E-Mail frank.ruemmele@nck.aphp.fr

6-MP group, withdrawal from steroids was faster and the number of patients who come into and maintained in steroid-free remission was significantly higher compared to patients on placebo. The remission rate in the 6-MP group was 91% at the 18-month visit compared to 53% in the placebo group [8]. These impressive data may probably give a somewhat overoptimistic view of the efficacy of AZA/6-MP in the treatment of pediatric CD. In fact, controlled trials in adult CD populations indicate that the use of purine analogues allows maintaining remission in approximately 1 of 2 patients on a prolonged manner [6, 7]. This is in keeping with our recent retrospective analysis, indicating that the efficacy of AZA to maintain remission in pediatric CD patients with a severe disease activity is below 50% after 24 months of evolution [Riello et al., submitted].

For patients who do not tolerate or escape therapy with (AZA)/6-MP, there is a marked need for alternative immunosuppressive drugs. Two recent retrospective studies indicate that MTX might be a good second-line choice for AZA/6-MP failures or intolerant pediatric patients [9, 10]. The recent French multicenter study [9] showed that MTX improved the clinical course in 49 of 61 CD patients with a clinical remission rate of 39, 49 and 45% at 3, 6 and 12 months, respectively. Follow-up over at least 24 months confirmed a sustained remission on MTX monotherapy up to 40 months. However, close to 30% of patients experienced a relapse after 13 ± 10 months of treatment in this analysis. The median MTX dose used in this study was 17.0 mg/m^2 (range: 11.9–22.5 mg/m^2). All children received MTX parenterally, either via subcutaneous or intramuscular injections. Adverse reactions were observed in 14 patients (24%) requiring MTX discontinuation in 6 children (10%) (liver enzyme elevation n = 2, varicella zoster n = 1, nausea n = 3). MTX allowed definitive corticosteroid discontinuation in 36 patients.

Comparable results were observed in the study of Turner et al. [10]. In this North American four-center retrospective cohort study, the efficacy of methotrexate in maintaining remission was assessed based on PCDAI measurements, the need for steroids, and height velocity. Patients served as their own historical controls. Forty-two percent of 60 children treated with methotrexate were in clinical remission without steroids at both 6 and 12 months. A strong steroid sparing effect was observed compared with the year prior to methotrexate (p < 0.001). Success rates were similar in previously thiopurine-intolerant and -refractory patients. Height velocity increased from –1.9 to –0.14 SDS (p = 0.004) in the year following therapy. In a median 3-year follow-up, a third of the patients did not require escalation of therapy; the others required step-up therapy with infliximab or surgery. Eight children (13%) stopped methotrexate due to adverse events, including, most commonly, elevated liver enzymes, and one serious episode of sepsis. The mean induction dose of MTX used was 0.44 ± 0.1 mg/kg/week or 13.8 ± 2.7 mg/m^2/week (range 9.1–17.9 mg/m^2/week); all but 17 children (28% of total cohort) were treated with subcutaneous MTX. Seventeen patients at the Philadelphia IBD clinics received oral MTX, 12 of whom following 3–4 months of initial subcutaneous dosing.

These data are in keeping with two placebo-controlled studies in adult CD patients [11, 12]: MTX was shown to be successful in inducing and maintaining remission after steroid tapering in 39 versus 19% of a total of 141 patients with steroid-resistant CD. In the second study, MTX' potential to maintain remission was about 65% at 40 weeks compared to 39% with placebo. Comparable trials in pediatric CD patients are still missing. Parenteral MTX application (s.c., i.v. or i.m.) seems to be more efficacious in maintaining remission compared to oral MTX.

The experience of immunomodulatory therapy in maintaining remission in pediatric CD has to be evaluated in comparison to the efficacy of anti-TNF drugs, as well as other biologics. This comparison has not only to be based on efficacy but also safety data [13]. There are observational studies indicating and confirming that the prolonged used of AZA/6-MP clearly enhances the risk of CD patients to develop a lymphoma, mainly EBV-induced B cell lymphomas [Beaugerie et al., submitted]. This has to be taken into account when considering long-term maintenance therapy with immunomodulators. Concerning prolonged MTX therapy, there are less good data, since MTX was markedly less frequently used in the past compared to thiopurine analogues. On the other hand, biologics, mainly anti-TNF drugs, are now used for a little more than ten years. And their use including adverse events is extremely well studied and documented. There is no doubt on the efficacy of anti-TNF drugs to induce and also to maintain remission particularly in severe pediatric CD [14, 15]. The available safety data on the prolonged used of anti-TNF therapy in CD are rather reassuring, however, no sufficient long-term data on pediatric CD exist so far. Therefore, no clear recommendations can be given at this time point if immunomodulatory therapy or treatment with biologics should be considered as treatment of choice in particularly severe as well as moderate active CD in children.

In summary, MTX seems to be an alternative immunomodulatory drug to AZA/6-MP with reasonable good results in the treatment of pediatric CD. Altogether, about 50% of patients respond and remain in prolonged remission under MTX monotherapy. In approximately 10% of patients, the short-time toxicity of MTX leads to drug discontinuation, indicating an overall acceptable tolerance profile. MTX might be used as first-line therapy in the future. However, there is a great need to perform well-powered placebo-controlled trials as well as trials comparing the efficacy of AZA/6-MP to MTX and to compare these immunomodulators to biologics before definitive recommendations can be given for pediatric CD.

Disclosure Statement

The author declares that no financial or other conflict of interest exists in relation to the content of the article.

References

1 Targan SR: Current limitations of IBD treatment: where do we go from here? Ann NY Acad Sci 2006;1072:1–8.
2 Baumgart DC, Sandborn WJ: Inflammatory bowel disease: clinical aspects and established and evolving therapies. Lancet 2007; 369:1641–1657.
3 Sturm A, de Souza HS, Fiocchi C: Mucosal T cell proliferation and apoptosis in inflammatory bowel disease. Curr Drug Targets 2008;9:381–387.
4 Atreya R, Mudter J, Finotto S, Müllberg J, Jostock T, Wirtz S, Schütz M, Bartsch B, Holtmann M, Becker C, Strand D, Czaja J, Schlaak JF, Lehr HA, Autschbach F, Schürmann G, Nishimoto N, Yoshizaki K, Ito H, Kishimoto T, Galle PR, Rose-John S, Neurath MF: Blockade of interleukin 6 trans signaling suppresses T-cell resistance against apoptosis in chronic intestinal inflammation: evidence in crohn disease and experimental colitis in vivo. Nat Med 2000; 6:583–588.
5 Doering J, Begue B, Lentze MJ, Rieux-Laucat F, Goulet O, Schmitz J, Cerf-Bensussan N, Ruemmele FM: Induction of T lymphocyte apoptosis by sulphasalazine in patients with Crohn's disease. Gut 2004;53:1632–1638.
6 Sandborn W, Sutherland L, Pearson D, May G, Modigliani R, Prantera C: Azathioprine or 6-mercaptopurine for inducing remission of Crohn's disease. Cochrane Database Syst Rev 2000;2:CD000545.

7 Prefontaine E, Sutherland LR, Macdonald JK, Cepoiu M: Azathioprine or 6-mercaptopurine for maintenance of remission in Crohn's disease. Cochrane Database Syst Rev 2009;1:CD000067.
8 Markowitz J, Grancher K, Kohn N, Lesser M, Daum F: A multicenter trial of 6-mercaptopurine and prednisone in children with newly diagnosed Crohn's disease. Gastroenterology 2000;119:895–902.
9 Uhlen S, Belbouab R, Narebski K, Goulet O, Schmitz J, Cézard JP, Turck D, Ruemmele FM: Efficacy of methotrexate in pediatric Crohn's disease: a French multicenter study. Inflamm Bowel Dis 2006;12:1053–1057.
10 Turner D, Grossman AB, Rosh J, Kugathasan S, Gilman AR, Baldassano R, Griffiths AM: Methotrexate following unsuccessful thiopurine therapy in pediatric Crohn's disease. Am J Gastroenterol 2007;102:2804–2812.
11 Feagan BG, Rochon J, Fedorak RN, Irvine EJ, Wild G, Sutherland L, Steinhart AH, Greenberg GR, Gillies R, Hopkins M, et al: Methotrexate for the treatment of Crohn's disease. The North American Crohn's Study Group Investigators. N Engl J Med 1995;332:292–297.

12 Feagan BG, Fedorak RN, Irvine EJ, Wild G, Sutherland L, Steinhart AH, Greenberg GR, Koval J, Wong CJ, Hopkins M, Hanauer SB, McDonald JW: A comparison of methotrexate with placebo for the maintenance of remission in Crohn's disease. North American Crohn's Study Group Investigators. N Engl J Med 2000;342:1627–1632.
13 Cucchiara S, Escher JC, Hildebrand H, Amil-Dias J, Stronati L, Ruemmele FM: Pediatric inflammatory bowel diseases and the risk of lymphoma: should we revise our treatment strategies? J Pediatr Gastroenterol Nutr 2009;48:257–267.
14 Hyams J, Crandall W, Kugathasan S, Griffiths A, Olson A, Johanns J, Liu G, Travers S, Heuschkel R, Markowitz J, Cohen S, Winter H, Veereman-Wauters G, Ferry G, Baldassano R; REACH Study Group: Induction and maintenance infliximab therapy for the treatment of moderate-to-severe Crohn's disease in children. Gastroenterology 2007; 132:863–873.
15 Ruemmele FM, Lachaux A, Cézard JP, Morali A, Maurage C, Giniès JL, Viola S, Goulet O, Lamireau T, Scaillon M, Breton A, Sarles J; Groupe Francophone d'Hépatologie, Gastroentérologie et Nutrition Pédiatrique: Efficacy of infliximab in pediatric Crohn's disease: a randomized multicenter open-label trial comparing scheduled to on demand maintenance therapy. Inflamm Bowel Dis 2009;15:388–394.

Dig Dis 2009;27:315–321
DOI: 10.1159/000228567

Treatment of Severe Ulcerative Colitis: Differences in Elderly Patients?

Stephan R. Vavricka   Gerhard Rogler

Division of Gastroenterology and Hepatology, University Hospital Zurich, Zurich, Switzerland

Key Words
Ulcerative colitis · Cyclosporine · Infliximab

Abstract
Almost as many as 10% of patients with ulcerative colitis have late onset with the first flare occurring at 60–70 years of age. The course of the disease and the basic principles of management in geriatric populations do not differ from those in younger patients. However, elderly patients pose distinct problems in therapy choice. In middle-aged patients untreated severe ulcerative colitis has been reduced to <1% in specialized centers at the present time but is still high in the elderly. In general, the management requires close collaboration between gastroenterologists and surgeons. In adult patients, current evidence supports initial treatment with intravenous steroids. However, only 40% of patients show complete response after corticosteroid therapy and almost 30% come to colectomy. Cyclosporine still has a first place as salvage therapy because of its short half-life and its established short-term efficacy in about 70% of patients who fail steroids. The drug should be avoided in frail or elderly patients (especially over 80 years old) with significant comorbidity, and also where colectomy is likely to be necessary in the short to medium term. The long-term benefit of this therapy remains unsatisfactory as colectomy is often only delayed. Infliximab is the choice for those patients with a less severe colitis and less likelihood of urgent colectomy. Tacrolimus has only been used in one randomized controlled trial with similar results to cyclosporine. Surgery is still the definitive procedure for the treatment of ulcerative colitis in adult patients, and its timing is of paramount importance.

Copyright © 2009 S. Karger AG, Basel

Introduction

Ulcerative colitis (UC) exhibits bimodality in age-specific incidence rates with the second peak occurring at 60–70 years of age [1–5]. Almost as many as 10% of patients with UC have late onset [6]. The course of the disease and the basic principles of management in geriatric populations do not differ from those in younger patients. However, elderly patients pose distinct problems in therapy choice. Since patients older than 60 years are excluded from most therapeutic trials on severe UC, the treating physician is left with many open questions for the elderly patient with UC. Unfortunately, even the current ECCO guidelines on UC do not live up to expectations [7–9]. Guidelines appear most necessary where evidence is limited, and therefore such guidelines should cover more special situations such as treatment of the elderly patient. The aim of this article is to summarize the literature on medical treatment of severe UC focusing on (1) the age of the patients included in the respective studies, and (2) finding age-specific characteristics in current medical trials.

KARGER

Fax +41 61 306 12 34
E-Mail karger@karger.ch
www.karger.com

© 2009 S. Karger AG, Basel
0257–2753/09/0273–0315$26.00/0

Accessible online at:
www.karger.com/ddi

Stephan R. Vavricka, MD
Division of Gastroenterology and Hepatology, University Hospital
Raemistrasse 100
CH-8091 Zurich (Switzerland)
Tel. +41 44 255 21 24, Fax +41 44 255 94 97, E-Mail stephan.vavricka@usz.ch

Table 1. Therapy options in patients with moderate and severe UC

Author	Drug	Regime	Study type	Year	Patients	Response/remission	Age (range)	Study period
Intensive intravenous steroid treatment (IIVST)								
Truelove [10]	IIVST	cortisone 100 mg/day i.v.	Controlled trial, pc	1955	210 (109 cortisone, 101 P)	remission 45/109 = 41% (vs. 16% in P) response 30/109 = 27% (vs. 24% in P) no change/worse 34/109 = 31% (vs. 60% P)	NA	6 weeks
Truelove [11]	IIVST	prednisolone 60 mg/day i.v. hydrocortisone 100 mg rectally/day	Case series	1974	49	remission 36/49 = 73% response 4/49 = 8% no change/worse 9/49 = 18%	NA	5 days
Truelove [12]	IIVST	prednisolone 60 mg/day i.v. hydrocortisone 100 mg rectally/day	Case series	1978	100	remission 60/100 = 60% response 15/100 = 15% no change/worse 25/100 = 25%	5–84	5 days
Meyers [23]	IIVST	hydrocortisone 300 mg/day vs. cortico-tropin 120 U/day i.v.	RCT, db	1983	66	remission 28/66 = 42%		10 days
Cyclosporine A (CyA)								
Lichtiger [14]	CyA	4 mg/kg vs. placebo	RCT, db	1994	20 (11 CyA, 9 P)	response CyA: 9/11 = 82% P: 0/9 = 0%	34 (18–60)	7 days
D'Haens [15]	CyA	4 mg/kg vs. 40 mg M-pred	RCT, db	2001	30 (14 CyA, 15 M-pred, 1 DA)	response: CyA: 9/14 = 64% M-pred: 8/15 = 53%	36 (20–67)	8 days
Infliximab (IFX)								
Järnerot [17]	IFX	1 × 5 mg/kg	RCT, db	2005	45 (24 IFX, 21 P)	colectomy rate IFX: 7/24 = 29% P: 14/21 = 67%	37 (19–61)	3 months
Ochsenkühn [38]	IFX	5 mg/kg week 0/2/6 vs. prednisolone 1.5 mg/kg	RCT, db	2004	13 (6 IFX, 7 pred-nisolone)	response: IFX: 5/6 = 83% prednisolone: 6/7 = 85%	31 (21–44)	13 weeks
Probert [39]	IFX	5 mg/kg week 0/2	RCT, pc	2003	43 (23 IFX, 20 P)	remission: IFX 9/23 = 39% P 6/20 = 30%	41 (29–50)	8 weeks
Rutgeerts [36]	IFX	5 mg/kg, 10 mg/kg, placebo at week 0/2/6 then every 8 weeks	RCT, db	2005	364 (ACT1) 364 (ACT2): 121 P, 121 IFX 5 mg/kg, 121 IFX 10 mg/kg	ACT1 week 8 response: IFX 69% 5 mg/kg vs. 37% placebo ACT2 week 8: IFX 64% 5 mg/kg vs. 29% placebo	42	ACT 1: 46 weeks ACT 2: 22 weeks
Sands [40]	IFX	5 mg/kg, 10 mg/kg, 20 mg/kg, placebo	RCT, db	2001	11 8 IFX, 3 P	response: IFX 4/8 = 50% P: 0/3 = 0%	37 31–63	2 weeks
Armuzzi [37]	IFX	5 mg/kg at week 0/2/6 then every 8 weeks; M-pred 0.7–1 mg/kg/day	RCT, open-label	2004	20 10 IFX, 10 M-pred	remission	24–53	2 weeks
Tacrolimus (Tacro)								
Ogata [18]	Tacro	0.05 mg/kg/day	RCT, db	2006	65 21 high conc. (10–15 ng/ml) 22 low conc. (5–10 ng/ml), 20 P	response: high conc.: 13/19 = 68% low conc.: 8/21 = 38% P: 2/20 = 10%	33	2 weeks

IIVST = Intensified intravenous steroid therapy; CyA = cyclosporine A; IFX = infliximab; Tacro = tacrolimus; RCT = randomized controlled trial; db = double-blind; pc = placebo-controlled; DA = drop-out; P = placebo; M-pred = methylprednisone.

Medical Treatment of Uncomplicated Severe Ulcerative Colitis

Patients with severely active UC can be treated initially with oral corticosteroids. Those patients failing may require hospitalization for administration of intravenous corticosteroids [10–12]. In patients who present as steroid-refractory UC or treatment failure, CMV colitis has to be excluded by sigmoidoscopy with biopsies. It is believed that CMV colitis might be responsible for treatment failures in UC patients in up to 10% [13]. Cyclosporine, infliximab, and tacrolimus are used as rescue therapy in patients with severe UC who fail intravenous corticosteroids [14–18]. All three therapies are graded as evidence level EL1b in intravenous-steroid resistant UC of any extent in the new ECCO guidelines [8]. The different medical treatment modalities (steroids, cyclosporine, infliximab, and tacrolimus) will be discussed in the following section and a summary of those studies can be found in table 1. A special focus was posed on the age range of patients who have been included in the respective studies. Table 2 summarizes the most relevant statements regarding elderly patients with severe UC.

Steroids

Steroids are efficacious in UC and severe attacks of UC are treated with intensified intravenous steroid therapy (IIVST). The first placebo-controlled trial on steroid therapy in severe UC was reported by Truelove and Witts [10] in 1955. In this trial, remission was achieved in 41%, response in 27% and no change/worse outcome was noted in 31% of patients, respectively (table 1). Despite this established treatment, severe flares of UC have a high colectomy rate varying from 38 to 47% [11, 19]. Of patients with UC affecting the entire colon, up to 60% have been reported to have surgery within three months [19]. However, this may vary from country to country. Colectomy rates especially in northern Europe are higher as compared to central and southern Europe. Clearly colectomy rates in Switzerland are lower in newly diagnosed pancolitis.

In 1974, Truelove and Jewell [11] described the Oxford regimen for the treatment of severe UC (table 1). This regime is essentially based on the use of intravenous cortocosteroids (hydrocortisone 100 mg 4×/day or methylprednisone 60–80 mg/day with hydrocortisone 100 mg rectally/day), the meticulous monitoring of patients and clear decision making concerning surgery [11, 12]. It was reported that 60% of patients had a complete response

Table 2. Statements regarding elderly patients with UC

UC patients present with an age-specific incidence rate with a second peak occurring at 60–70 years [1]
In elderly patients with UC, there is a higher rate of corticosteroid-dependent patients leading to an increased requirement of immunosuppressive treatment [25]
UC patients older than 50 years need renal function tests before starting cyclosporine therapy [30]
Elderly UC patients either tend to have proctitis or limited left-sided colitis [1, 26] or present with a severe initial episode with toxic megacolon [6]
Early surgical interventions are recommended for elderly patients with severe UC [1, 2]

and 15% showed improvement to this therapy [12]. The lack of improvement to this intensive therapy by day 5 is considered an absolute indication for emergency colectomy [11–12, 20]. In a systematic review of 32 trials of steroid therapy for acute severe UC involving 1,991 patients from 1974 to 2006, the overall response to steroids (intravenous hydrocortisone, methylprednisolone, or betamethasone) was 67% [21]. The ECCO consensus on UC grades intravenous steroid therapy as evidence level EL1b [8].

Studies conducted to compare different types of steroids and adrenocorticotropic hormone did not demonstrate any clear advantage of one type versus the others [22–24]. Regarding elderly patients, there is only one case-control Spanish study, which included patients older than 60 years (8 patients with CD and 25 patients with UC). The authors found a higher rate of corticosteroid-dependent patients leading to an increased requirement of immunosuppressive treatment in the elderly group [25]. The Italian Colon-Rectum Study group reported on 1,705 patients with UC. In this cohort 436 patients were under 25 years old and 386 patients were over 50 years old. Interestingly, younger patients tended to have a greater anatomical-clinical severity with greater use of steroids in the acute phase of UC [26].

Cyclosporine A

Promising results from uncontrolled trials [27, 28] were substantiated by a two-center, randomized, placebo-controlled trial from North America in which intravenous cyclosporine at a dose of 4 mg/kg was given to UC patients not responding to intravenous steroids. An initial response rate of 82% was described within a mean time to response of 7 days, versus 0% in the group that received steroids alone (table 1) [14]. In the past decade, a few controlled trials and many case series confirmed that intravenous cyclosporine at a dose of 2–4 mg/kg/day induces clinical remission in over 50% of the patients in the short term so that colectomy can often be avoided [14–16, 29]. Cyclosporine has been shown to be at least as effective as corticosteroids in a double-blind controlled trial comparing i.v. cyclosporine with i.v. corticosteroids as monotherapy for a severe attack of UC [15]. The same group also reported a randomized, double-blind study comparing 4 versus 2 mg/kg intravenous cyclosporine. The study showed that the higher-dose cyclosporine has no additional clinical benefit over lower-dose cyclosporine in the treatment of severe attacks of UC. Although differences in adverse events were not observed, it was concluded that because most cyclosporine-associated adverse events are dose dependent, the use of 2 mg/kg should improve the long-term toxicity profile of the agent [16]. Although the value of cyclosporine for the management of severe UC has been accepted in most referral centers, concerns about toxicity have prevented its use in many hospitals. Cyclosporine can lead to side effects such as hypertension, renal failure, hypertrichosis and neurotoxicity, which lead to death in some patients, thus limiting its use. However, with the continuous i.v. treatment over 24 h such deleterious events have never been reported. Especially patients older than 50 years are more likely to have impaired renal function and must therefore have an accurate quantification of creatinine clearance before cyclosporine therapy is started [30]. The benefit of avoiding colectomy therefore needs to be balanced against the risk of inducing profound immunosuppression and severe side effects.

Long-term prognosis with cyclosporine therapy is reported to be improved by the introduction of azathioprine or mercaptopurine on discharge from the hospital in association with oral cyclosporine as bridging therapy [31]. Cyclosporine is typically discontinued after 3–4 months, the time window which azathioprine needs to start its delayed action [32]. It is even debatable if cyclosporine treatment should be given to a patient who has proven azathioprine resistance or intolerance. A recent systematic Cochrane review on severe UC has shown that the evidence indicating that cyclosporine is more effective than standard corticosteroid therapy is weak, and that cyclosporine does not avoid the overall need for colectomy [33]. This Cochrane analysis states that 'the long-term benefit is unclear, when adverse events such as cy-

closporine-induced nephrotoxicity may become more obvious'. Most institutions have therefore restricted the use of cyclosporine to patients whose disease is refractory to corticosteroids, given the important risk of toxicity and the high cost of cyclosporine. Although there is a risk of relevant drug toxicity, most patients will opt for cyclosporine if offered, rather than undergo colectomy. A study from Cohen et al. [34] assessed 42 patients who received cyclosporine during an acute severe relapse. They found that patients who retained their colon felt physically and psychologically healthier with a significantly better quality of life compared with those who had undergone colectomy. On the basis of these observations, the systematic use of cyclosporine in severe UC is still debated. Moreover, retrospective series showed that, despite an initial response to cyclosporine, many patients would eventually undergo proctocolectomy a few years down the line [35].

Infliximab
More than 15 years ago, the potent anti-inflammatory effects of anti-tumor necrosis factor (TNF) therapy with the chimeric antibody infliximab were shown in Crohn's disease, in rheumatoid arthritis and later also in UC. Six randomized controlled trials were performed to the present date for evaluation of induction of remission in patients with UC [17, 36–40]. Four studies compared infliximab to placebo [17, 36, 39, 40], one study compared infliximab to oral steroids [38] and the other to intravenous corticosteroids [37]. A small placebo-controlled trial reported in 2001 [40] recruited 11 patients failing 5 days of i.v. steroids to receive a single dose of infliximab or placebo. Four of the eight patients receiving infliximab were deemed treatment success at 2 weeks versus none of the three patients given placebo. The trial was not continued because of recruitment difficulty. A Scandinavian multicenter randomized placebo-controlled trial has recently shown that infliximab given as a single 5 mg/kg infusion was significantly more effective than placebo. In this study, 29% (7/24) of the patients in the infliximab group had a colectomy within 90 days (primary end point), compared with 67% (14/21) in the placebo group, and this is a statistically significant difference (p = 0.017) [17]. The study, however, refers to a follow-up of 3 months and provides no information on the long-term follow-up. Two large studies, called ACT1 and ACT2, evaluated each 364 patients with active UC. Patients were randomized to intravenous infusions of infliximab at 5 mg/kg, 10 mg/kg or placebo. Response rates were reported to 69% (ACT1) and 64% (ACT2) at week 8

[36]. It should however be noted that hospitalized patients with severe colitis represent a very different population to the outpatients in the ACT1 and ACT2 studies and large controlled trials are needed as described in the ECCO guidelines [7–9].

In summary, the use of infliximab as a treatment for severe UC seems promising, but is not yet clearly defined. In particular, whether early use of infliximab will prevent colectomy is uncertain.

Tacrolimus

Only one double-blind randomized placebo-controlled study has been performed so far [8]. This trial showed after 2 weeks of treatment clinical remission in 19% (4/21) of patients in the high target serum concentration group, and in 5% (1/20) in the placebo group. Further, a statistically significant dose-dependent rate of clinical improvement at 2 weeks and a colectomy-free survival of all patients at week 10 were demonstrated. Tacrolimus may be effective for short-term clinical improvement in patients with refractory UC. It carries many of the risks including nephrotoxicity of cyclosporine.

Special Age-Related Situations in Severe Ulcerative Colitis

Toxic Megacolon

It has been suggested that UC tends to be less extensive when it develops later in life; the majority of elderly patients have proctitis or limited left-sided involvement [1, 26]. On the other hand, it has been claimed that older patients appear to be more likely to present with a severe initial episode and to develop toxic megacolon, both of which are associated with a high fatality rate. In a community-based study from Aberdeen, Scotland, 14% of patients aged over 70 had severe initial episodes, compared with 7% of younger patients [6]. The excess of severe first episodes in older patients accounted for an increased mortality rate of 19% compared with 1.7% for the entire study population.

Surgery

Early surgical intervention has been recommended for elderly patients with severe UC, because postoperative complications such as toxic megacolon, free perforation, massive hemorrhage, and mortality are more common in the elderly when surgery is delayed and performed when they are critically ill [1, 2]. It is unclear whether the higher mortality rate in elderly patients with UC, reaching 19% in some reports, is due to the disease process itself or the adverse effects of concomitant illnesses [1]. Postponing surgery on the basis of advanced age alone may increase mortality, whereas prompt surgical intervention has been associated with dramatic reductions in mortality in elderly patients with severe colitis [41]. Nevertheless, surgery is still the definitive procedure for the treatment of UC in adult and older patients, and its timing is of paramount importance. Morbidity of severe UC results from prolonged ineffective medical treatment and therefore a delay in surgical treatment should be avoided. The surgical procedure most commonly performed in adult and older patients is a subtotal abdominal colectomy and ileostomy, followed about 3 months later (when the patient is off steroids with an improved nutritional state) by completion proctectomy and the formation of an ileal-pouch anal anastomosis (IPAA).

Conclusion

Severe UC occurring in the elderly is an important issue in the field of gastroenterology, considering that the proportion of elderly persons is increasing in our society. Sometimes, however, stoicism of the elderly patient is a formidable obstacle to early diagnosis. Severe UC must be considered a medical emergency especially in the elderly patient, even if the mortality rate for this disease is decreasing. Several factors might have contributed to the reduction in mortality that has been observed over the past 30 years, such as the widespread use of the Oxford (corticosteroid) regimen, which has now been integrated with the administration of cyclosporine and infliximab, the early detection of complications, the careful timing of surgery and the improved anesthesiological and surgical techniques. Key issues remain as to what should be first- and second-line therapies in different age groups, when surgery should be undertaken, and the risk of switching between immunosuppressants in these critically ill patients. As about 30% of severe UC cases continue to need colectomy, the timing of surgery and the collaboration between gastroenterologist and surgeon remain the most important goals in the management especially in older patients. More studies in different age groups in patients with severe UC are desperately needed and the management needs to be defined according to those studies.

Acknowledgements

This study was supported by a research grant from the Swiss National Science Foundation grant 320000-114009/1 (to S.R.V.), 3347CO-108792 (Swiss IBD Cohort) and a grant of the Zurich Center of Integrative Human Physiology.

Disclosure Statement

The authors declare that no financial or other conflict of interest exists in relation to the content of the article.

References

1 Grimm IS, Friedman LS: Inflammatory bowel disease in the elderly. Gastroenterol Clins North Am 1990;19:361–389.

2 Brandt LJ, Dickstein G: Inflammatory bowel disease: specific concerns in the elderly. Geriatrics 1989;44:107–111.

3 Sedlack RE, Nobrega FT, Kurland LT, Sauer WG: Inflammatory colon disease in Rochester, Minnesota, 1935–1964. Gastroenterology 1972;62:935–941.

4 Bonnevie O, Riis P, Anthonisen P: An epidemiological study of ulcerative colitis. Scand J Gastroenterol 1968;3:432–438.

5 De Dombal Fr, Burch PR, Watkinson G: Aetiology of ulcerative colitis. Gut 1969;10:270–277.

6 Sinclair TS, Brunt PW, Mowat NA: Nonspecific proctocolitis in northeastern Scotland: a community study. Gastroenterology 1983;85:1–11.

7 Stange EF, Travis SP, Vermeire S, Reinisch W, Geboes K, Barakauskiene A, Feakins R, Fléjou JF, Herfarth H, Hommes DW, Kupcinskas L, Lakatos PL, Mantzaris GJ, Schreiber S, Villanacci V, Warren BF: European evidence-based consensus on the diagnosis and management of ulcerative colitis: definitions and diagnosis. J Crohns Colitis 2008;2:1–23.

8 Travis SP, Stange EF, Lémann M, Oresland T, Bemelman WA, Chowers Y, Colombel JF, D'Haens G, Ghosh S, Marteau P, Kruis W, Mortensen NJ, Penninckx F, Gassull M: European evidence-based consensus on the management of ulcerative colitis: current management. J Crohns Colitis 2008;2:24–62.

9 Biancone L, Michetti P, Travis S, Escher JC, Moser G, Forbes A, Hoffmann JC, Dignass A, Gionchetti P, Jantschek G, Kiesslich R, Kolacek S, Mitchell R, Panes J, Soderholm J, Vucelic B, Stange E: European evidence-based consensus on the management of ulcerative colitis: special situations. J Crohns Colitis 2008;2:63–92.

10 Truelove SC, Witts LJ: Cortisone in ulcerative colitis. Br Med J 1955;ii:1041–1048.

11 Truelove SC, Jewell DP: Intensive intravenous regimen for severe attacks of ulcerative colitis. Lancet 1974;i:1067–1070.

12 Truelove SC, Willoughby CP, Lee EG, Kettlewell MG: Further experience in the treatment of severe attacks of ulcerative colitis. Lancet 1978;ii:1086–1088.

13 Hommes DW, Sterringa G, van Deventer SJ, Tytgat GN, Weel J: The pathogenicity of cytomegalovirus in inflammatory bowel disease: a systematic review and evidence-based recommendations for future research. Inflamm Bowel Dis 2004;10:245–250.

14 Lichtiger S, Present DH, Kornbluth A, Gelernt I, Bauer J, Galler G, Michelassi F, Hanauer S: Cyclosporine in severe acute ulcerative colitis refractory to steroid therapy. N Engl J Med 1994;330:1841–1845.

15 D'Haens G, Lemmens L, Geboes K, Vandeputte L, Van Acker F, Mortelmans L, Peeters M, Vermeire S, Penninckx F, Nevens F, Hiele M, Rutgeerts P: Intravenous cyclosporine versus intravenous corticosteroids as single therapy for severe attacks of ulcerative colitis. Gastroenterology 2001;120:1323–1329.

16 Van Assche G, D'Haens G, Noman M, Vermeire S, Hiele M, Asnong K, Arts J, D'Hoore A, Penninckx F, Rutgeerts P: Randomized double-blind controlled comparison of 4 mg/kg versus 2 mg/kg intravenous cyclosporine in severe ulcerative colitis. Gastroenterology 2003;125:1025–1031.

17 Järnerot G, Hertervig E, Friis-Liby I, Blomquist L, Karlen P, Grännö C, Vilien M, Ström M, Danielsson A, Verbaan H, Hellström PM, Magnuson A, Curman B: Infliximab as rescue therapy in severe to moderately severe ulcerative colitis: a randomized, placebo-controlled study. Gastroenterology 2005;128:1805–1811.

18 Ogata H, Matsui T, Nakamura M, Iida M, Takazoe MM, Suzuki Y, Hibi T: A randomized dose finding study of oral tacrolimus (FK506) therapy in refractory ulcerative colitis. Gut 2006;55:1255–1262.

19 Järnerot G, Rolny P, Sandberg-Gertzén H: Intensive intravenous treatment of ulcerative colitis. Gastroenterology 1985;89:1005–1013.

20 Meyers S, Janowitz HD: Systemic corticosteroid therapy of ulcerative colitis. Gastroenterology 1985;89:1189–1191.

21 Turner D, Walsh CM, Steinhart AH, Griffiths AM: Response to corticosteroids in severe ulcerative colitis: a systematic review of the literature and a meta-regression. Clin Gastroenterol Hepatol 2007;5:103–110.

22 Powell-Tuck J, Buckell NA, Lennard-Jones JE: A controlled comparison of corticotrophin and hydrocortisone in the treatment of severe proctocolitis. Scand J Gastroenterol 1977;12:971–975.

23 Meyers S, Sachar DB, Goldberg JD, Janowitz HD: Corticotropin versus hydrocortisone in the intravenous treatment of ulcerative colitis. A prospective, randomized, double-blind clinical trial. Gastroenterology 1983;85:351–357.

24 Meyers S, Lerer PK, Feuer EJ, Johnson JW, Janowitz HD: Predicting the outcome of corticoid therapy for acute ulcerative colitis. Results of a prospective, randomized, double-blind clinical trial. J Clin Gastroenetrol 1987;9:50–54.

25 Rodriguez-D'Jesus A, Casellas F, Malagelada JR: Epidemiology of inflammatory bowel disease in the elderly. Gastroenterol Hepatol 2008;31:269–273.

26 Riegler G, Tartaglione MT, Carratu R, D'Inca R, Valpiani D, Russo MI, Papi C, Fiorentini MT, Ingrosso M, Andreoli A, Vecchi M: Age-related clinical severity at diagnosis in 1705 patients with ulcerative colitis: a study by GISC (Italian Colon-Rectum Study Group). Dig Dis Sci 2000;45:462–465.

27 Sandborn WJ: A critical review of cyclosporine therapy in inflammatory bowel disease. Inflamm Bowel Dis 1995;1:48–63.

28 Actis GC, Ottobrelli A, Pera A, Barletti C, Ronti V, Pinna-Pintor M, Verme G: Continuously infused cyclosporine at low dose is sufficient to avoid emergency colectomy in acute attacks of ulcerative colitis without the need for high-dose steroids. J Clin Gastroenterol 1993;17:10–13.

29 Carbonnel F, Boruchowicz A, Duclos B, Soulé JC, Lerebours E, Lémann M, Belaiche J, Colombel JF, Cosnes J, Gendre JP: Intravenous cyclosporine in attacks of ulcerative colitis: short-term and long-term responses. Dig Dis Sci 1996;41:2471–2476.

30 Kornbluth A, Present DH, Lichtiger S, Hanauer S: Cyclosporine for severe ulcerative colitis: a user's guide. Am J Gastroenterol 1997;92:1424–1428.

31 Campbell S, Travis S, Jewell D: Cyclosporine use in acute ulcerative colitis: a long term experience. Eur J Gastroenterol Hepatol 2005;17:79–84.

32 Fernandez-Banares F, Bertran X, Esteve-Comas M, Cabre E, Menacho M, Humbert P, Planas R, Gassull MA: Azathioprine is useful in maintaining long-term remission induced by intravenous cyclosporine in steroid-refractory severe ulcerative colitis. Am J Gastroenterol 1996;91:2498–2499.

33 Shibolet O, Regushevskaya E, Brezis M, Soares-Weiser K: Cyclosporine A for induction of remission in severe ulcerative colitis. Cochrane Database Syst Rev 2005;1: CD004277.

34 Cohen RD, Brodsky AL, Hanauer SB: A comparison of the quality of life in patients with severe ulcerative colitis after total colectomy versus medical treatment with intravenous cyclosporine. Inflamm Bowel Dis 1999;5:1–10.

35 Arts J, D'Haens G, Zeegers M, Van Assche G, Hiele M, D'Hoore A, Penninckx F, Vermeire S, Rutgeerts P: Long-term outcome of treatment with intravenous cyclosporine in patients with severe ulcerative colitis. Inflamm Bowel Dis 2004;10:73–78.

36 Rutgeerts P, Sandborn WJ, Feagan BG, Reinisch W, Olson A, Johanns S, Travers S, Rachmilewitz D, Hanauer SB, Lichtenstein GR, de Villiers WJ, Present D, Sands BE, Colombel JF: Infliximab for induction and maintenance therapy for ulcerative colitis. N Engl J Med 2005;353:2462–2476.

37 Armuzzi A, De Pascalis B, Lupascu A, Fedeli P, Leo D, Mentella MC, Vincenti F, Melina D, Gasbarrini G, Pola P, Gasbarrini A: Infliximab in the treatment of steroid-dependent ulcerative colitis. Eur Rev Med Pharmacol Sci 2004;8:231–233.

38 Ochsenkühn T, Sackmann M, Göke B: Infliximab for acute, not steroid-refractory ulcerative colitis: a randomized pilot study. Eur J Gastroenterol Hepatol 2004;16:1167–1171.

39 Probert CS, Hearing SD, Schreiber S, Kuhbacher T, Ghosh S, Arnott ID, Forbes A: Infliximab in moderately severe glucocorticoid resistant ulcerative colitis: a randomized controlled trial. Gut 2003;52:998–1002.

40 Sands BE, Tremaine WJ, Sandborn WJ, Rutgeerts PJ, Hanauer SB, Mayer L, Targan SR, Podolsky DK: Infliximab in the treatment of severe, steroid-refractory ulcerative colitis: a pilot study. Inflamm Bowel Dis 2001;7:83–88.

41 Condie JD Jr, Laslie KO, Smiley DF: Surgical treatment for inflammatory bowel disease in the older patient. Surg Gynecol Obstet 1987;165:135–142.

Dig Dis 2009;27:322–326
DOI: 10.1159/000228568

Severe Acute Ulcerative Colitis: The Pediatric Perspective

Dan Turner

Pediatric Gastroenterology Unit, Shaare Zedek Medical Center, The Hebrew University of Jerusalem, Jerusalem, Israel

Key Words

Ulcerative colitis · Pediatric ulcerative colitis activity index · Corticosteroids · Infliximab

Abstract

Many features of pediatric ulcerative colitis (UC) are similar to adult-onset disease, but the rate of extensive disease is doubled in children. It is, therefore, not surprising that the admission rate for severe UC is higher in childhood-onset UC, reaching 28% by the age of 16 years. Approximately 30–40% of children will fail corticosteroids and require second-line medical therapy or colectomy. A pediatric UC activity index (PUCAI) score of >65 indicates severe disease and the index can assist in determining the need and timing of second-line medical therapy or colectomy early during the admission. A PUCAI score of >45 points on day 3 identify patients likely to fail corticosteroids (negative predictive value 90–95%), and a score >70 points on day 5 identify patients who will require short-term treatment escalation (positive predicting value 95–100%). Data in children are limited, but it seems that cyclosporine, tacrolimus and infliximab achieve a similar short-term response rate, in the range of 60–80%. Infliximab has the advantage that it may be given for a prolonged period of time while calcineurin inhibitors should not be used for more than 3–4 months, bridging to a thiopurine regimen. Colectomy is indicated in toxic megacolon or in cases refractory to one salvage therapy. The choice of colectomy in other cases should carefully consider its effect on the patient's quality of life, its impact on the physical and emotional development at a critical age of personality development, and its association with a high infertility rate in females undergoing pouch procedure before childbearing age.

Copyright © 2009 S. Karger AG, Basel

Review

Severe acute ulcerative colitis (UC) remains a therapeutic challenge to both pediatric and adult gastroenterologists. Until recently, little progress had been made since 1974 when Truelove and coworkers [1, 2] established intravenous corticosteroids as the mainstay of treatment in severe exacerbations, reducing mortality rate from 24% to eventually less than 1%. A meta-regression reported a weighted 33% steroid-failure rate in pooled data concerning 29 different studies of 1991 adult patients hospitalized with acute UC [3]. These figures remained stable over the last three decades despite the introduction of calcineurin inhibitors as salvage therapy. More recently, clinical controlled trials have shown that infliximab is successful in inducing remission in adults with steroid-refractory severe UC [4, 5]. Most severe UC studies have been conducted in adults, but childhood inflammatory bowel disease (IBD) may not be similar to adult-onset disease. Children with UC suffer more frequently from disease extending proximal to the splenic flexure [6–8], a condition prone to a less favorable outcome. On the other hand, studies in children with IBD of remicade

Dan Turner, MD, PhD
Pediatric Gastroenterology and Nutrition Unit
The Hebrew University of Jerusalem, Shaare Zedek Medical Center, POB 3235
Jerusalem 91031 (Israel)
Tel. +972 2 655 5111, Fax +972 2 655 5756, E-Mail turnerjd2001@yahoo.com

[9, 10], thiopurines [11, 12], and nutritional therapy [13] often show a better response to therapy than similar studies performed in adults. In addition, children may present with slightly different symptoms than adults [14, 15] and have age-related psychological and organic concerns. Management of pediatric severe UC, therefore, may differ from adults. This review aims to highlight these differences and to offer a management approach in children.

The definition of severe UC has not been consistent in both pediatrics and adults. The most widely used criteria to define severity of UC is the Truelove and Witts' criteria, published in 1955 [2]. Of 28 published cohort studies of severe UC [3], 20 defined severity according to the Truelove and Witts' criteria [2], three according to Lichtiger [16] and one according to the Seo index [17]. Among the studies that utilized the Truelove and Witts' classification, 12 required the fulfillment of all five items and eight applied a more liberal definition. These inconsistencies are pronounced in children where some of the variables are not as frequent compared with adults. For instance, fever and tachycardia, important variables in adults [18–23], are not frequently found in children [7, 24]. Therefore, an index developed exclusively for children may be of greater value than the existing adult measures. As such, the Pediatric UC Activity Index (PUCAI) has been shown to be valid and reliable in prospective and retrospective cohorts [7, 25]. A PUCAI score of at least 65 points was found to be highly associated with physicians' global assessment of severe disease and correlated well with constructs of severe disease [24].

The incidence of severe acute attacks in childhood UC is considerably higher than in adults. While it is estimated that only 15% of adults will be admitted at least once for a severe UC attack during their lifetime, in pediatric-onset disease, 30–40% of patients will require at least one admission during childhood [24, 26]. This figure may reflect a more severe disease phenotype in children with UC, possibly due to a stronger genetic factor as reflected by the higher prevalence of extensive disease.

No comparative study has evaluated the optimal administration of intravenous corticosteroids in severe pediatric UC. In adults, no regimen or dose was found to be superior to the others. No advantage was found for using a daily dose of more than 60 mg methylprednisolone equivalent [3]. It is a common practice to initiate 1–1.5 mg/kg/day methylprednisolone up to 40–60 mg, while the higher dose is reserved for the more severe cases. Gradual tapering of the steroid dose should be attempted over 10–12 weeks.

Colonic width on radiography can predict outcome of acute severe UC in adults [27]. Age- and size-related variations in radiographic appearance make this variable less accurate in children. Nonetheless, the distribution of transverse colonic dilatation in children over 11 years of age generally follows that of adults, in which a width over 55–60 mm is associated with more severe disease and, in the appropriate clinical setting, toxic megacolon [14, 24].

Approximately 30–40% of children will not respond to steroid therapy and will require treatment escalation [3, 24]. Although some advocate using intravenous steroids for an extended length of time in refractory cases, most agree that second-line therapy should be offered after 3–10 days of lack of response to intravenous steroids [27–32]. Accurate identification of children failing steroid therapy early in the admission is important to reduce complication rate and unnecessary admission days. Several adult studies examined variables able to predict response to corticosteroid therapy in acute severe UC [3]. Three predictive indices in adults and one in children have been developed to evaluate therapy failure on the third day of corticosteroid treatment [18, 27, 33, 34]. In a prospective analysis by Travis et al. [33], stool frequency of >8/day or 3–8/day and C-reactive protein (CRP) >45 mg/l on the third day of therapy had a PPV of 85% for colectomy. Lindgren et al. [18] developed the fulminant colitis index (stool frequency/day + 0.14X CRP mg/l) with a PPV of ~70% at a cutoff score of >8 at day 3 of therapy. Ho et al. [27] developed an index based on stool frequency, albumin level and colonic dilatation.

We have previously suggested a two-stage protocol, in which children are screened after 3 days of steroid therapy for their risk of failing intravenous corticosteroids. Second-line therapy may then be introduced 2 days later following repeated evaluation. The 2-day time interval allows close monitoring, discussion with the family, surgical consultation and preparation for medical therapy (e.g. infectious screening before anti-TNF therapy). A PUCAI score of >45 on the third day of corticosteroid therapy should dictate planning of second-line therapy and >70 points on the fifth day indicate that the likelihood of future response to corticosteroids is slim and thus execution of the planned therapy is warranted. Using these cutoff values yielded a negative predictive value (NPV) of 94% and a positive predictive value (PPV) of 43% on day 3, and PPV of 100% and NPV of 87% on day 5 [24, 35]. In a pediatric study of a head-to-head comparison between this approach, the fulminant colitis index and the Seo index, the PUCAI-based approach performed

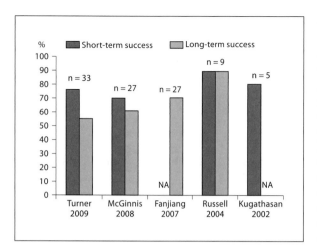

Fig. 1. Outcome of infliximab in severe pediatric UC in published cohorts and case series. Long-term follow-up was very heterogeneous in follow-up time (6 months to 2.5 years) and in the way infliximab was used. References to studies in figure [35, 53–56]. NA = Not applicable.

best with an area under the ROC curve of 0.82 (95% CI 0.75–0.90) [35]. Those who do not meet the day-5 criteria but still have moderately to severe disease (i.e. PUCAI ≥35) may be slow responders and should be treated with corticosteroids for several more days until making a final decision. The PUCAI may be easily scored based on history taking alone without the need for endoscopy, bloodletting or physical examination.

Several unique considerations in children influence the choice of treatment escalation when corticosteroids are unsuccessful in inducing clinical remission. An open discussion with the family stressing the pros and cons of each option is fundamental to any plan. Colectomy is a potentially lifesaving procedure that may dramatically improve quality of life of children with ongoing severely active disease [36]. In view of the cumulative toxic effect of medications over many future years in childhood disease, the option of colectomy should be considered when the disease course requires prolonged intense therapy to maintain remission. On the other hand, colectomy has several disadvantages that are pronounced in children. First, the idea of ileostomy at a critical time of physical and emotional development often deters children and their parents from this option. Second, colectomy and ileal pouch anal anastomosis (IPAA), while curing the colitis per se, is not without complications and concerns. Meagher et al. [37] found that 10% of patients after colec-

tomy experienced incontinence, 48% had at least one episode of pouchitis, and 9% had pouch failure. Data from children reflect similar findings [36]. Moreover, females undergoing IPAA will experience reduced fertility which is a particular problem before childbearing age [38]. Finally, disease location in young children with Crohn's disease is more often confined to the colon, making the differentiation between Crohn's disease and UC difficult. In some pediatric institutions, any colitis phenotype under the age of 5 years is termed IBD-U (IBD type unclassified). Since pouch construction in Crohn's disease is associated with poor surgical outcome, colectomy is less appealing in this age group. Even when colectomy is required, pouch formation should be delayed until the diagnosis of the underlying disease is established with as much certainty as possible. These considerations lead to the common practice in children with refractory severe UC to favor second-line medical therapy before proctocolectomy.

Cyclosporine has been used for many years [39], with reported short-term success rate in real-life adult cohorts of 51% [3] and up to 80% in specialized sub-cohorts [40]. In several very small pediatric cohorts and case series, the short-term success rate of cyclosporine was 60–87% [41–47]. However, 30–50% of the initial responders will eventually require colectomy. A thiopurine regimen should be prescribed concomitantly while using cyclosporine as a bridge to thiopurine maintenance therapy [41]. The concomitant use of an immunomodulator dramatically improves the long-term success rate. This is also true when using tacrolimus (FK-506), which has a better bioavailability than cyclosporine thus allowing for oral treatment. A clinical trial in adults found that drug levels of 10–15 ng/ml achieved a higher success rate than lower levels [48]. Although in adults tacrolimus seems to be as effective as cyclosporine, the data in children are restricted to two case series that showed short-term success rate of 89% [49] and 55% [50].

Both tacrolimus and cyclosporine should be discontinued after 3–4 months of treatment, to minimize adverse effects. Approximately 15% of patients treated with cyclosporine experience significant adverse events including nephrotoxicity, serious infection, seizures, anaphylaxis, and very rarely death. Minor adverse events are common including paresthesias, hypomagnesemia, hypertension, hypertrichosis, headache, minor nephrotoxicity, abnormal liver enzymes, minor infections, hyperkalemia, and gingival swelling [51]. In children, tacrolimus was associated with tremor, convulsions, hypomagnesemia, hypertension, hyperglycemia and headaches

[49, 50]. Therefore, these parameters and renal function should be closely monitored. Extrapolating from organ transplantation literature, it seems that tacrolimus may have a more appealing toxicity profile than cyclosporine.

Anti-TNF therapy is effective in inducing clinical and endoscopic remission in UC, as shown in clinical trials performed in adults [4, 5, 52]. Infliximab may be at least as effective as calcineurin inhibitors used as salvage therapy in severe pediatric UC (fig. 1). Long-term use of infliximab is customary in adults and children, which is an advantage over cyclosporine and tacrolimus, especially in those who flared when already treated with an effective thiopurine dose. In thiopurine-naïve children, the data are insufficient to support the use of one therapy over the other. Nonetheless, the toxicity profile of infliximab may be more appealing than those of cyclosporine and tacrolimus.

Despite the paucity of data, decision making in acute severe pediatric UC deserves special considerations, especially when determining the timing and type of second-line therapy. Identifying a subset of children who are at high risk to fail corticosteroid therapy during the first 5 days of treatment is an achievable goal using the PUCAI score. This approach can successfully identify on the fifth day of steroid therapy some of the patients who will require second-line therapy. An open discussion with the family while reflecting the consequences, risks and benefit of each option is paramount in determining the therapeutic strategy. Dealing with the consequences of treatment is easier for children of all ages who feel that they were part of the decision making process.

Acknowledgements

The author would like to thank Drs. Anne M. Griffiths and Ari Silbermintz for their worthwhile comments on this review.

Disclosure Statement

The author declares that no financial or other conflict of interest exists in relation to the content of the article.

References

1 Truelove SC, Jewell DP: Intensive intravenous regimen for severe attacks of ulcerative colitis. Lancet 1974;i:1067–1070.
2 Truelove SC, Witts LJ: Cortisone in ulcerative colitis; final report on a therapeutic trial. Br Med J 1955;29:1041–1048.
3 Turner D, Walsh CM, Steinhart AH, Griffiths AM: Response to corticosteroids in severe ulcerative colitis: a systematic review of the literature and a meta-regression. Clin Gastroenterol Hepatol 2007;5:103–110.
4 Jarnerot G, Hertervig E, Friis-Liby I, Blomquist L, Karlen P, Granno C, et al: Infliximab as rescue therapy in severe to moderately severe ulcerative colitis: a randomized, placebo-controlled study. Gastroenterology 2005;128:1805–1811.
5 Sandborn WJ: Is there a role for infliximab in the treatment of severe ulcerative colitis?: The American experience. Inflamm Bowel Dis 2008;14:S232–S233.
6 Griffiths AM: Specificities of inflammatory bowel disease in childhood. Best Pract Res Clin Gastroenterol 2004;18:509–523.
7 Turner D, Otley AR, Mack D, et al: Development and evaluation of a Pediatric Ulcerative Colitis Activity Index (PUCAI): a prospective multicenter study. Gastroenterology 2007;133:423–432.

8 Moum B, Ekbom A, Vatn MH, Elgjo K: Change in the extent of colonoscopic and histological involvement in ulcerative colitis over time. Am J Gastroenterol 1999;94: 1564–1569.
9 Hyams J, Crandall W, Kugathasan S, et al: Induction and maintenance infliximab therapy for the treatment of moderate-to-severe Crohn's disease in children. Gastroenterology 2007;132:863–873; quiz 1165–1166.
10 Hanauer SB, Feagan BG, Lichtenstein GR, et al: Maintenance infliximab for Crohn's disease: the ACCENT I randomised trial. Lancet 2002;359:1541–1549.
11 Markowitz J, Grancher K, Kohn N, Lesser M, Daum F: A multicenter trial of 6-mercaptopurine and prednisone in children with newly diagnosed Crohn's disease. Gastroenterology 2000;119:895–902.
12 Candy S, Wright J, Gerber M, Adams G, Gerig M, Goodman R: A controlled double blind study of azathioprine in the management of Crohn's disease. Gut 1995;37:674–678.
13 Zachos M, Tondeur M, Griffiths AM: Enteral nutritional therapy for induction of remission in Crohn's disease. Cochrane Database Syst Rev 2007;1:CD000542.

14 Benchimol EI, Turner D, Mann EH, et al: Toxic megacolon in children with inflammatory bowel disease: clinical and radiographic characteristics. Am J Gastroenterol 2008;103:1524–1531.
15 Langholz E, Munkholm P, Krasilnikoff PA, Binder V: Inflammatory bowel diseases with onset in childhood. Clinical features, morbidity, and mortality in a regional cohort. Scand J Gastroenterol 1997;32:139–147.
16 Lichtiger S, Present DH: Preliminary report: cyclosporin in treatment of severe active ulcerative colitis. Lancet 1990;336:16–19.
17 Seo M, Okada M, Yao T, Ueki M, Arima S, Okumura M: An index of disease activity in patients with ulcerative colitis. Am J Gastroenterol 1992;87:971–976.
18 Lindgren SC, Flood LM, Kilander AF, Lofberg R, Persson TB, Sjodahl RI: Early predictors of glucocorticosteroid treatment failure in severe and moderately severe attacks of ulcerative colitis. Eur J Gastroenterol Hepatol 1998;10:831–835.
19 Gulati R, Rawal KK, Kumar N, et al: Course of severe ulcerative colitis in northern India. Trop Gastroenterol 1995;16:19–23.
20 Lennard-Jones JE, Ritchie JK, Hilder W, Spicer CC: Assessment of severity in colitis: a preliminary study. Gut 1975;16:579–584.

21 Benazzato L, D'Inca R, Grigoletto F, et al: Prognosis of severe attacks in ulcerative colitis: effect of intensive medical treatment. Dig Liver Dis 2004;36:461–466.

22 Daperno M, Sostegni R, Scaglione N, et al: Outcome of a conservative approach in severe ulcerative colitis. Dig Liver Dis 2004;36:21–28.

23 Spicer CC: The prediction of success or failure of medical treatment for acute colitis. J R Coll Physicians Lond 1975;9:252–256.

24 Turner D, Walsh CM, Benchimol EI, et al: Severe paediatric ulcerative colitis: incidence, outcomes and optimal timing for second-line therapy. Gut 2008;57:331–338.

25 Turner D, Hyams J, Markowitz J, et al: Appraisal of the pediatric ulcerative colitis activity index (PUCAI). Inflamm Bowel Dis 2009;15:1218–1223.

26 Barabino A, Tegaldo L, Castellano E, et al: Severe attack of ulcerative colitis in children: retrospective clinical survey. Dig Liver Dis 2002;34:44–49.

27 Ho GT, Mowat C, Goddard CJ, et al: Predicting the outcome of severe ulcerative colitis: development of a novel risk score to aid early selection of patients for second-line medical therapy or surgery. Aliment Pharmacol Ther 2004;19:1079–1087.

28 Meyers S, Lerer PK, Feuer EJ, Johnson JW, Janowitz HD: Predicting the outcome of corticoid therapy for acute ulcerative colitis. Results of a prospective, randomized, double-blind clinical trial. J Clin Gastroenterol 1987;9:50–54.

29 Jakobovits SL, Travis SP: Management of acute severe colitis. Br Med Bull 2006;75–76:131–144.

30 Kugathasan S, Dubinsky MC, Keljo D, et al: Severe colitis in children. J Pediatr Gastroenterol Nutr 2005;41:375–385.

31 Werlin SL, Grand RJ: Severe colitis in children and adolescents: diagnosis, course, and treatment. Gastroenterology 1977;73:828–832.

32 Kornbluth A, Sachar DB: Ulcerative colitis practice guidelines in adults (update): American College of Gastroenterology, Practice Parameters Committee. Am J Gastroenterol 2004;99:1371–1385.

33 Travis SP, Farrant JM, Ricketts C, et al: Predicting outcome in severe ulcerative colitis. Gut 1996;38:905–910.

34 Seo M, Okada M, Yao T, Matake H, Maeda K: Evaluation of the clinical course of acute attacks in patients with ulcerative colitis through the use of an activity index. J Gastroenterol 2002;37:29–34.

35 Turner D, Mack D, Uusoue K, et al (ed): A prospective multicenter study of outcomes and predictors of response in severe pediatric ulcerative colitis. World Congr Gastroenterol Hepatology and Nutrition, Brazil, 2008.

36 Ceriati E, Deganello F, De Peppo F, et al: Surgery for ulcerative colitis in pediatric patients: functional results of 10-year follow-up with straight endorectal pull-through. Pediatr Surg Int 2004;20:573–578.

37 Meagher AP, Farouk R, Dozois RR, Kelly KA, Pemberton JH: J ileal pouch-anal anastomosis for chronic ulcerative colitis: complications and long-term outcome in 1,310 patients. Br J Surg 1998;85:800–803.

38 Cornish JA, Tan E, Teare J, et al: The effect of restorative proctocolectomy on sexual function, urinary function, fertility, pregnancy and delivery: a systematic review. Dis Colon Rectum 2007;50:1128–1138.

39 Shibolet O, Regushevskaya E, Brezis M, Soares-Weiser K: Cyclosporine A for induction of remission in severe ulcerative colitis. Cochrane Database Syst Rev 2005;1:CD004277.

40 Durai D, Hawthorne AB: Review article: how and when to use ciclosporin in ulcerative colitis. Aliment Pharmacol Ther 2005;22:907–916.

41 Castro M, Papadatou B, Ceriati E, et al: Role of cyclosporin in preventing or delaying colectomy in children with severe ulcerative colitis. Langenbecks Arch Surg 2007;392:161–164.

42 Barabino A, Torrente F, Castellano E, et al: The use of ciclosporin in paediatric inflammatory bowel disease: an Italian experience. Aliment Pharmacol Ther 2002;16:1503–1507.

43 Ramakrishna J, Langhans N, Calenda K, Grand RJ, Verhave M: Combined use of cyclosporine and azathioprine or 6-mercaptopurine in pediatric inflammatory bowel disease. J Pediatr Gastroenterol Nutr 1996;22:296–302.

44 Treem WR, Cohen J, Davis PM, Justinich CJ, Hyams JS: Cyclosporine for the treatment of fulminant ulcerative colitis in children. Immediate response, long-term results, and impact on surgery. Dis Colon Rectum 1995;38:474–479.

45 Benkov KJ, Rosh JR, Schwersenz AH, Janowitz HD, LeLeiko NS: Cyclosporine as an alternative to surgery in children with inflammatory bowel disease. J Pediatr Gastroenterol Nutr 1994;19:290–294.

46 Treem WR, Davis PM, Hyams JS: Cyclosporine treatment of severe ulcerative colitis in children. J Pediatr 1991;119:994–997.

47 Kirschner BS, Whitington PF, Malfeo-Klein R: Experience with cyclosporine A (CyA) in severe non-specific ulcerative colitis. Pediatr Res 1989;25:A117.

48 Ogata H, Matsui T, Nakamura M, et al: A randomised dose finding study of oral tacrolimus (FK506) therapy in refractory ulcerative colitis. Gut 2006;55:1255–1262.

49 Ziring DA, Wu SS, Mow WS, Martin MG, Mehra M, Ament ME: Oral tacrolimus for steroid-dependent and steroid-resistant ulcerative colitis in children. J Pediatr Gastroenterol Nutr 2007;45:306–311.

50 Bousvaros A, Kirschner BS, Werlin SL, et al: Oral tacrolimus treatment of severe colitis in children. J Pediatr 2000;137:794–799.

51 Sternthal MB, Murphy SJ, George J, Kornbluth A, Lichtiger S, Present DH: Adverse events associated with the use of cyclosporine in patients with inflammatory bowel disease. Am J Gastroenterol 2008;103:937–943.

52 Lawson MM, Thomas AG, Akobeng AK: Tumour necrosis factor alpha blocking agents for induction of remission in ulcerative colitis. Cochrane Database Syst Rev 2006;3:CD005112.

53 McGinnis JK, Murray KF: Infliximab for ulcerative colitis in children and adolescents. J Clin Gastroenterol 2008;42:875–879.

54 Fanjiang G, Russell GH, Katz AJ: Short- and long-term response to and weaning from infliximab therapy in pediatric ulcerative colitis. J Pediatr Gastroenterol Nutr 2007;44:312–317.

55 Russell GH, Katz AJ: Infliximab is effective in acute but not chronic childhood ulcerative colitis. J Pediatr Gastroenterol Nutr 2004;39:166–170.

56 Kugathasan S, Prajapati DN, Kim JP, et al: Infliximab outcome in children and adults with ulcerative colitis. Gastroenterology 2002;122:A615.

Dig Dis 2009;27:327–334
DOI: 10.1159/000228569

Treatment of Ulcerative Colitis in the Elderly

Ashwin N. Ananthakrishnan[a]   David G. Binion[b]

[a]Division of Gastroenterology and Hepatology, Medical College of Wisconsin, Milwaukee, Wisc., and
[b]Division of Gastroenterology, Hepatology and Nutrition, University of Pittsburgh School of Medicine, Pittsburgh, Pa., USA

Key Words

Ulcerative colitis · Inflammatory bowel disease · Thromboembolism

Abstract

Ulcerative colitis (UC) has a bimodal age distribution, with the majority of patients being diagnosed between the second and fourth decades of life. However, a second peak in diagnosis occurs in older patients and an estimated 15% of patients present after age 65. Caring for older UC patients who have either presented later in life or who have carried an inflammatory bowel disease (IBD) diagnosis for multiple decades may pose additional challenges in management. Recent studies using nationwide administrative databases from the USA have demonstrated that older IBD patients are challenged by worse hospital outcomes. This pattern, seen for both UC and Crohn's disease, demonstrated increased rates of vascular complications (i.e. venous thrombosis), worse post-operative outcomes and increased rates of complicated and prolonged clinical courses compared to younger IBD patients. This article provides an overview of caring for elderly patients with UC, including diagnostic and therapeutic considerations. Copyright © 2009 S. Karger AG, Basel

Ulcerative Colitis Demographics: The Aging Colitis Population

The percentage of inflammatory bowel disease (IBD) patients who meet the criteria for geriatric age, being 65 years of age or older, is not precisely defined. A review of the previously described Medical College of Wisconsin's IBD Center database demonstrated that approximately 11.8% of 382 UC patients were over the age of 65, while 9% of 916 Crohn's disease patients were in the geriatric age group. Among the elderly ulcerative colitis (UC) patients, 16 of 45 (36%) were diagnosed at age ≥65, while 29 of 83 (34.9%) elderly Crohn's disease patients presented at age ≥65.

Reviews from population-based samples of patients, including the Olmsted County IBD Database, also demonstrated approximately 10% of their cohort being geriatric [1]. Analysis of the National Hospital Ambulatory Medical Care Survey and National Ambulatory Medical Care Survey (NHAMCS/NAMCS) maintained by the National Center for Health Statistics (NCHS) revealed an increasing proportion of ambulatory visits for IBD (both UC and CD) being constituted by the elderly population, suggesting rising burden of disease related to IBD in the elderly [2]. In addition, one quarter of US hospital admissions related to IBD occurred in patients older than age 65.

David G. Binion, MD, Division of Gastroenterology, Hepatology and Nutrition
University of Pittsburgh Medical Center Presbyterian Hospital
University of Pittsburgh School of Medicine, Mezzanine Level – C Wing
200 Lothrop Street, Pittsburgh, PA 15216 (USA)
E-Mail binion@pitt.edu

Differential Diagnosis of Colitis in Older Patients: Infection, Ischemia and SCAD

UC typically presents with symptoms such as abdominal pain, fecal urgency and bloody diarrhea. However, these symptoms are not specific to UC, and similar to the younger IBD patient, it is important to consider a variety of differential diagnoses.

Infectious Colitis

Similar to younger IBD patients, the majority of cases of bloody diarrhea result from infectious pathogens, with organisms associated with bacterial food poisoning (i.e. *Campylobacter, Escherichia coli* O157H7, *Salmonella, Shigella*) being most common. Enteric infection with *E. coli* O157H7 will often produce more severe illness in elderly individuals and may be associated with renal failure. It is important to perform stool studies to identify and distinguish this pathogen prior to initiating immunosuppressive therapy appropriate for UC.

Clostridium difficile

An additional enteric pathogen which will mimic an IBD colitis flare which is particularly relevant to the elderly UC population is *C. difficile* [3]. This spore-forming anaerobe is classically associated with antibiotic exposure and disturbance in the enteric flora, which will lead to expansion of this organism. *C. difficile* has doubled in incidence in North America over the past 10 years. This infection has classically been associated with patients from high-risk environments, specifically long-term care facilities (i.e. nursing homes) and hospitals. Recent research suggests that IBD patients are at high-risk of acquiring *C. difficile* infection, and an elderly IBD population may represent one of the highest-risk individuals for acquiring this infection [4]. Stool analysis for the presence of *C. difficile* toxins A and B is the most frequent employed modality for diagnosis, but the sensitivity of this assay is fairly low. In IBD patients infected with *C. difficile* in 2005, 54% of patients were diagnosed on the initial stool analysis, and 4 stool samples were required to reach a diagnostic accuracy above 90% suggesting that repeat testing may be indicated in patients where there is a high index of suspicion for this infection [5]. IBD patients with *C. difficile* rarely demonstrated pseudomembranes, which are found in approximately half of *C. difficile*-infected patients with no prior history of colitis. The majority of IBD patients who contracted *C. difficile* had pre-existing diagnoses of UC or Crohn's colitis, and 10% of patient presented with concomitant *C. difficile* infection at the time of the IBD diagnosis. *C. difficile* super-infection will lead to an exacerbation of colitis, and over half of infected IBD patients will require hospitalization. Treatment of the hospitalized IBD patient with *C. difficile* represents a high-risk scenario, as high rates of colectomy have been identified in this setting. Use of oral vancomycin as the primary antibiotic regimen targeting *C. difficile* has resulted in improved rates of medical treatment success for hospitalized IBD patients. Rapidly decreasing oral corticosteroid dosing has also improved clinical outcomes, as the ability to mount an antibody response to toxin A is felt to be the critical mechanism for clearing an infection. In severely ill patients, infliximab has been used in conjunction with oral vancomycin and lower dosages of corticosteroids with overall reduced rates of colectomy.

Ischemic Colitis

A particularly important differential diagnosis to be considered in the setting of colitis in the elderly is ischemic colitis. This is the most common vascular injury seen in the human gastrointestinal tract, occurring at rates varying from 5 to 44 cases per 100,000 person-years [6]. Ischemic colitis is caused by compromised vascular flow to the large bowel, and may range from mild transient injury to potentially life-threatening transmural infarction [7]. The classic findings of ischemic colitis include the triad of acute abdominal pain, bloody stool and low blood pressure. The classic patient with ischemic colitis is an elderly female older than age 65 [8, 9], but other subsets of individuals can also manifest injury, with long-distance runners being one example [10], while drug-induced ischemic colitis can also affect seemingly low-risk individuals (i.e. use of serotonin-modulating agents in patients with irritable bowel syndrome) [11, 12].

Multiple etiologies underlie ischemic colitis, but all share the mechanism of decreased perfusion of the large bowel. Key contributing mechanisms include decreased cardiac output, chronic renal failure [13], cardiac arrhythmia, shock [14, 15], arterial thrombosis, embolism, complications of surgery (i.e. failed re-implantation of the inferior mesenteric artery following abdominal aortic aneurysm repair) [16], colonic obstruction with increased luminal pressure leading to impaired mucosal perfusion [12], hypercoagulability [17, 18], vasculitis [19], intra-abdominal inflammation or infection or complications of drugs [17, 20, 21].

The clinical presentation of ischemic colitis depends on the severity of vascular injury and the anatomic segment affected by the ischemic insult [22]. The most commonly affected vascular territory involved with inferior mesenteric artery which supplies blood to the left colon. Ischemic colitis involving the left colon will typically result in abdominal pain, increased bowel movements and rectal bleeding. Ischemic injury to the right colon may manifest with a broader range of presentations including more subtle abdominal symptoms, or conversely more dramatic symptoms in patients with transmural injury to the thinner right colon wall. Mild right colonic ischemia may present with abdominal pain in the absence of bloody diarrhea or altered bowel function.

Physical findings of ischemic colitis are variable, but will frequently present with mild tenderness and/or abdominal distention. More severe injury will present with peritonitis, and this has been estimated to occur in up to 20% of patients experiencing ischemic colitis.

Diagnostic testing is often non-specific in ischemic colitis. In the majority of cases routine laboratories (i.e. blood counts, creatinine phosphokinase, amylase, serum lactate and lactate dehydrogenase) are all normal. Severe ischemic colitis may demonstrate an elevated white blood count and acidosis. Radiologic findings in ischemic colitis are variable, paralleling the severity of the ischemic injury. Most commonly, non-specific radiographic findings are present, which will include bowel dilation, ileus and mural thickening. Thumbprinting, the classic, pathognomonic radiographic finding in ischemic colitis, is identified in only 20% cases. CT scanning is helpful in the evaluation of ischemic colitis, as it will help to define the extent of the colonic injury. The diagnosis of ischemic colitis is confirmed by colonoscopy and biopsy, but the decision to evaluate the entire colon must be carefully weighed given the severity of injury and the propensity of the ischemic colon to perforate. The endoscopic appearance of ischemic colitis will manifest a sequence of appearances ranging from friability, petechial hemorrhages and pale appearing mucosa early in the disease. The later appearance of the evolving colitis may demonstrate a hemorrhagic and sloughing mucosa. The most severe ischemic colonic injury demonstrates gangrene, with a bluish-black, dusky mucosal appearance. Histopathology will also demonstrate an evolving tissue injury, with the early process showing mucosal hemorrhage, edema and tissue necrosis and later injury showing leukocytic infiltration, sloughing of the surface epithelium and mucosal ulceration. During the resolution of ischemic colitis, histology will demonstrate repair with granulation tissue and scarring which may ultimately lead to stricture formation.

Treatment of ischemic colitis is supportive, emphasizing dietary limitation and antibiotics which cover bowel flora [23]. Patients with moderate to severe ischemic colitis, which will manifest radiographic changes, require hospitalization to facilitate bowel rest, administration of intravenous antibiotics and pain control. Restriction of diet is recommended as bacterial translocation can occur in the injured bowel, and avoiding the physiologic demand for increased enteric blood flow required during digestion may also limit further ischemic injury. Likewise, medications which may adversely effect perfusion including non-steroidal anti-inflammatory drugs and aspirin should be avoided during the acute period of bowel injury.

The majority of patients with moderate-to-severe ischemic colitis requiring hospital admission will recover within 48 h. Complete resolution of ischemic colitis may require multiple week for resolution to occur. Colectomy and diverting ileostomy should be considered in patients who have failed to resolve over a 2-week time period, or in the setting of impending sepsis. It is estimated that up to 20% of patients with ischemic colitis will experience this protracted clinical course, and these individuals are at risk for the development of strictures should they finally resolve the injury. The surgical management of ischemic colitis requires a conservative approach, favoring the use of diverting ostomies and avoiding creation of anastomoses which may involve ischemic tissues, due to high rates of anastomotic failure and intra-abdominal sepsis. Close surgical management is necessary in patients with refractory disease, as overt gangrene can emerge in patients who fail to re-establish circulation, which will lead to perforation and high rates of perioperative mortality.

Segmental Colitis Associated with Diverticula (SCAD)

Diverticulosis is an extremely common clinical finding in Western countries, occurring in 5–10% of the population over age 45, and rising in incidence to 80% of individuals over age 85 [24]. Diverticula are typically asymptomatic, but episodes of acute diverticulitis may affect up to 20% of patients during their lifetime. Acute diverticulitis is felt to be a microperforation of the bowel wall with associated peritonitis, occurring most commonly where the vasa recta will penetrate across the bowel wall. In distinction from this well-characterized acute inflammatory complication, a form of chronic inflammation involving a colonic segment involved with diverticula has also been described. Segmental colitis associated with diverticular disease (SCAD) was initially described in the 1980s and 1990s [25], and this typically resembles IBD at both the endoscopic and histologic levels. SCAD will occur in individuals with a normal rectum and proximal colon [26], and will typically demonstrate a segment of colitis in a field of diverticula. Patients presenting with SCAD are typically over age 60, are more frequently male and will present with symptoms ranging from painless hematochezia to lower abdominal cramps or altered bowel habits. Occasionally patients with SCAD will demonstrate fever, leukocytosis, nausea and/or weight loss.

Endoscopy is essential to establish a diagnosis of SCAD, and findings will typically include mucosal erythema, granularity and/or friability of the sigmoid colon with sparing of the rectum and more proximal colon. Histology will range from a chronic colitis similar to IBD, to non-specific findings, often similar to mucosal prolapse.

Therapy of SCAD will initially follow the treatment approach for acute diverticulitis [27]. After ruling out potential infectious pathogens with stool testing, including analysis for the presence of *C. difficile* toxin, SCAD patients are typically treated with a regimen of oral broad-spectrum antibiotics for 7–10 days, which will include coverage for bowel flora. Following completion of this antibiotic regimen, long-term management of SCAD emphasizes treatment with oral fiber supplementation [28]. The majority of patients with SCAD respond to conservative treatment. Patients who fail to respond to antibiotics can receive mesalamine compounds as well as topical steroid enemas. There is a small subgroup of patients with SCAD who develop more aggressive chronic inflammation, similar to Crohn's disease, manifesting with noncaseating granulomas and fissuring ulcers or fistulae. These individuals will often require segmental resection, and follow-up studies evaluating SCAD patients for the subsequent 6–12 months have demonstrated that the majority of individuals do not progress to overt Crohn's disease.

The etiopathogenesis of SCAD may represent an overlap with either classic IBD or pouchitis, the complication associated with increased mucosal bacterial counts in patients who have undergone ileoanal pouch reconstruction following colectomy. SCAD patients share histologic findings with pouchitis and the initial treatment for both of these conditions employs antibiotics targeting bowel flora. Bacterial stasis in diverticula may represent a critical etiologic component for the development of diverticular colitis, which drives the development of chronic bowel inflammation in this form of IBD.

Treatment of UC in Elderly Patients

Medical Treatment Options

Elderly UC patients are candidates for treatment with all of the therapeutic options available for younger IBD patients. Following induction with corticosteroids, elderly UC patients with mild UC can receive maintenance therapy with agents such as the 5-ASA compounds [29, 30]. Disease of moderate severity may require immunosuppressive drugs such as azathioprine and 6-mercaptopurine [31], with severe, or steroid-refractory disease requiring the most potent class of maintenance treatment, the biologic agent infliximab [32].

All of the major trials for 5ASA compounds as well as infliximab did include elderly UC patients in their study populations, with no specific upper limit for age restriction amongst elderly patients for the majority of the 5ASA trials as well as infliximab (www.clinicaltrials.gov). However, none of these trials have been specifically analyzed to compare the rates of response and remission in elderly patients with those in younger IBD patients. Also importantly, adverse effects of these agents have also not been evaluated specifically in the elderly IBD population. All of the major trials for 5ASA compounds as well as infliximab included elderly UC patients in their study populations, with no specific upper limit for age restriction amongst elderly patients for the majority of the 5ASA trials as well as infliximab (www.clinicaltrials.gov). Data regarding the use of azathioprine and 6-mercaptopurine for the treatment of UC is limited [31], and did not specifically evaluate response rates in elderly patients. Case reports from tertiary referral centers demonstrated clinical efficacy in elderly patients for immunosuppressive agents, and use of these agents should be considered in elderly UC patients.

An important consideration in the management of elderly UC patients is the loss of physical reserve which accompanies aging. Elderly patients who present with severe colitis flare should have consideration for earlier inpatient management. The rationale for this more aggressive strategy is multiple and includes both pragmatic and therapeutic implications. The ability to handle fecal urgency and multiple nocturnal trips to the bathroom, which are hallmark features of UC flare, may not be readily handled by an elderly individual without assistance. As discussed in the next section, elderly patients may not be able to tolerate the stress of colitis flare and this may translate into worse clinical outcomes. The ability to rapidly induce remission with more potent agents (i.e. intravenous steroids, initiation of biologic therapy with infliximab) compared with a course of oral corticosteroids, can often be more readily initiated in the inpatient setting. Our IBD center recommends immediate assessment of tuberculosis exposure status at the time of admission with either the placement of a PPD skin test or sending the in vitro interferon gamma release assay (i.e. Quantiferon Gold TB), so that patients not exhibiting a rapid clinical response can be initiated on infliximab [33]. Our center has emphasized the use of infliximab as an outpatient treatment strategy for refractory UC patients, so the extension of this strategy for early in-hospital initiation follows this paradigm [34].

Hospitalization Outcomes

Use of all of these treatment modalities for elderly UC patients who are experiencing significant flare is an even more important issue when one considers that hospitalized older IBD patients are at increased risk for worse clinical outcome. Ananthakrishnan et al. [2] used the Nationwide Inpatient Sample, an administrative database of approximately 1,000 short-stay hospitals in the US, which is maintained by the Healthcare Cost Utilization Project (HCUP) to determine the impact of age on IBD inpatient outcome. In 2004, there were 105,423 IBD admissions, of which 25% occurred in patients who were over the age of 65. A majority of the elderly IBD patients carried a UC diagnosis.

When the patient populations were adjusted for the presence of co-morbidity, it became apparent that age is an independent predictor of mortality in IBD inpatient admissions. The oldest patients had the highest mortality, even when adjusting for co-morbidities. Factors which were associated with mortality in the oldest cohort of IBD patients included malnutrition and the requirement for bowel surgery during the inpatient stay, while female sex was found to be associated with diminished mortality. In UC, elderly age was predictive of mortality with an odds ratio of 2.84 (1.43–5.63).

Surgical Outcomes for Elderly UC Patients

UC patients who have failed to respond to medical treatment will require surgical management with colectomy with either permanent ileostomy or pouch reconstructive surgery. The concern regarding elderly UC patients failing medical therapy is their overall lack of reserve, and the impact of co-morbid illness which may worsen their surgical outcome. Two studies have evaluated surgical outcomes in elderly UC patients. Almogy et al. [35] reviewed the surgical experience in elderly UC

patients at the Mt. Sinai Hospital in New York, and identified 113 consecutive UC patients who underwent surgery between 1960 and 1999 and were age 65 years or older. The authors found that the indication for colectomy changed during the four decades evaluated, as toxic megacolon was significantly decreased in the more recent time period and surgery for dysplasia has replaced adenocarcinoma as the leading reason for colectomy in elderly UC patients. These authors found that surgery-associated adverse outcomes decreased significantly from 50% of cases during the 1960–1984 time period (13% deaths, 37% major complications) to 27% in the most recent time period evaluated (1994–1999; with 3% deaths, 24% major complications). These authors further defined that male sex, albumin level ≤2.8 g/dl and need for urgent surgery were independent predictors of poor outcome.

Page et al. [36] evaluated factors affecting surgical risk in elderly IBD patients, using a case-control approach comparing surgical outcome in patients 60 years or older compared with younger individuals using multivariate models. The dataset included 30 IBD patients age 60 or older and 75 IBD patients younger than age 60. These authors found that elderly IBD patients had an increased rate of postoperative complications along with an increased length of hospital stay and increased operating room time. The effect of elderly age persisted after adjustment for co-morbidity and use of immunosuppressive therapy. A similar longer duration of post-operative stay was found in the study using a nationwide sample by Ananthakrishnan et al. [2] who also identified a higher incidence of post-operative cardiovascular (OR 2.26, 95% CI 1.13–4.54) and pulmonary (OR 1.66, 95% CI 1.12–2.48) complications in the elderly. As such, it is important to accurate risk stratify elderly patients who may be particularly at a high risk for these complications and institute early appropriate interventions to minimize the occurrence of these complications.

UC patients who have undergone colectomy may be candidates for ileoanal reconstruction procedures. The ability to successfully rebuild a pouch reservoir for fecal continence and take down of the end-ileostomy has represented an important advance in the surgical options available for patients with severe/refractory UC requiring total colectomy. However, the prevalence of anorectal dysfunction in the aging population may make the outcome of these procedures less successful. Delaney et al. [37] from the Cleveland Clinic Foundation prospectively evaluated the effect of age on surgical results, functional outcome and quality of life after ileal pouch anal anastomosis (IPAA). Among 1,895 patients who underwent the reconstructive procedure, 42 patients were older than age 65. Patients were assessed 1, 3, 5 and 10 years after surgery. The majority of elderly pouch patients had UC (81%). Within 1 year of surgery, elderly UC patients were experiencing on average 1.5 nocturnal bowel movements and 6 daily bowel movements. Nocturnal seepage was described in 44% of elderly patients, and 44% described never being incontinent. These results were slightly worse than those in younger cohorts of patients, but these differences did not achieve statistical significance. When elderly UC patients were asked to describe whether having undergone the ileoanal pouch anastomosis had an impact on their quality of life, 28% said that social restrictions were imposed as a result of surgery, 33% had experienced sexual restrictions, which was significantly higher than in younger age groups. On the positive side, 89% of elderly UC patients stated that they would opt to undergo the pouch reconstruction again, and 96% would recommend the surgery to others. These authors concluded that ileo-anal pouch anastomosis could be safely performed with acceptable results in elderly UC patients.

It is important for physicians and surgeons involved in the management of these elderly IBD patients to discuss the risk benefits of these procedures with the patients prior to surgery so that a fully informed decision may be taken prior to reconstructive surgery. Patients with pre-existing diagnosis of anorectal dysfunction or incontinence may not be candidates for such reconstructive surgery and may have better function and quality of life outcomes with permanent ileostomy.

Special Scenarios Relevant to the Elderly UC Population

Thrombotic Complications in Elderly UC Patients Requiring Hospitalization

IBD is now recognized as a hypercoagulable state [38]. One of the highest risk time period for clotting complications to occur is during inpatient IBD management. Medical admissions for UC are typically focused on the management of severe colitis, where patients experience multiple clinical factors which predispose to clotting. Among these are dehydration, thrombocytosis, and increased inflammatory activity, all of which may contribute to activation of clotting cascades. Surgical management is also associated with increased rates of clotting for

all of the above-listed reasons, as well as the activation of tissue factor which occurs during the operation itself and decreased mobility in the postoperative period.

In a recent review of clotting complications in IBD patients, Nguyen et al. [39] demonstrated that elderly IBD patients were at significantly increased risk of developing venous clotting complications which rose in a linear relationship to age. Using the Nationwide Inpatient Sample dataset, elderly UC patients demonstrated the highest rates of venous thromboembolism, which occurred in 25% or more of the hospitalizations in patients who were 50 years and older. Approximately 1/3 of the UC patients who were older than age 80 experienced a venous clotting complication during a hospitalization in the year 2004. These high rates of clotting complications suggest that prophylaxis strategies using heparin compounds should be considered in elderly UC patients during hospitalization for medical or surgical management.

Comorbid Illnesses

Elderly UC patients are more likely to have co-morbid illness compared to those of a younger age group. In the study of the Nationwide Inpatient Sample by Ananthakrishnan et al. [2], 9.6% of elderly IBD patients had 3 or more comorbid conditions compared to 2.6% of the <65-year-old IBD patients. In concert with this was the finding that fewer elderly IBD patients had no comorbid conditions (46%) compared with younger IBD patients (79%). As such, it is important to take into account the effect of both disease and therapy on underlying co-morbid illness in these patients. Long-term use of corticosteroids may be associated with worsening of diabetes control. Steroid use may also be associated with fluid retention, which may be significant in patients with underlying hypertension, congestive heart failure or renal disease. Elderly patients may also have underlying ocular problems such as glaucoma which may be worsened by steroids. Osteoporosis and osteopenia are prevalent in the older population making it important to consider preventative and treatment measures with use of calcium, vitamin D, and bisphosphonates as indicated. Elderly patients may also be at a higher risk for infectious complications with steroids and the immunosuppressive agents such as azathioprine or infliximab, though such analysis has not been specifically performed from large treatment registries. Elderly patients may also have a lower reserve to withstand complications from disease such as blood loss and may merit from more active therapy than the younger patient.

Drug Interactions, Polypharmacy and Medication Adherence

In line with the higher co-morbid burden in the elderly, it is important to consider the fact that these patients are more likely to be on multiple medications raising concerns for both drug interactions and medication adherence [40]. Higher pill burden has been associated with non-adherence. Elderly patients with underlying cognitive defects or with limited functional ability may be especially prone to non-adherence with regimens involving multiple pills spread out over varying times of the day. Visiting nurse programs or other social support mechanisms may be important in this cohort to ensure adherence with therapy and optimal outcomes.

Preservation of Functional Independence and Quality of Life

A particularly important issue in the management of the elderly UC patient is the importance of preserving quality of life and functional independence. Multiple nocturnal bowel movements or frequency and urgency of bowel movements may be particularly disabling in this population which is also likely to have impaired mobility. Cautious use of antimotility agents may be warranted in this cohort to maximize continence and maintain independence in activities of daily living. According to estimates from the HCUP-NIS, less than 1% of patients aged 18–45 years with a primary discharge diagnosis of UC or Crohn's required discharged to a nursing home or rehab facility compared to 15.7% of those aged 65–84 years and 35.7% aged 85+ years [2]. Similarly, the proportion requiring home health care on discharge was 4.7% for those aged 18–44 years compared to 12.6% for those between the ages of 65 and 84 years.

Directions for Future Research

There are several areas in the management of the elderly UC patients that merit future investigation. It is not yet known if the response rates to treatments as well the susceptibility to adverse effects are different between elderly and younger adult UC patients. The impact of disease activity as well as treatment on quality of life outcomes in the elderly also merits special attention.

Conclusions

Elderly UC patients constitute an increasing proportion of patients with IBD. Although they share many similarities with younger IBD patients in regards to treatment options, elderly patients are at risk for worse outcomes related to medical or surgical hospitalizations if they become severely ill. This implies that elderly UC patients have less reserve, and may not tolerate the stress of colitis flare, as well as physiologic challenges of abdominal surgery. Elderly UC patients who are hospitalized are at markedly increased risk for venous thrombotic complications. For all of these reasons, elderly UC patients warrant an aggressive medical approach to achieve and maintain remission. Elderly UC patients are at risk of ischemic and infectious complications, including *C. difficile* colitis, which may complicate their underlying IBD. Future studies are warranted to define the optimal treatment algorithms for the optimal elderly UC population.

Disclosure Statement

The authors declare that no financial or other conflict of interest exists in relation to the content of the article.

References

1 Jess T, et al: Survival and cause specific mortality in patients with inflammatory bowel disease: a long term outcome study in Olmsted County, Minnesota, 1940–2004. Gut 2006;55:1248–1254.
2 Ananthakrishnan AN, McGinley EL, Binion DG: Inflammatory bowel disease in the elderly is associated with worse outcomes: a national study of hospitalizations. Inflamm Bowel Dis 2009;15:182–189.
3 Issa M, Ananthakrishnan AN, Binion DG: *Clostridium difficile* and inflammatory bowel disease. Inflamm Bowel Dis 2008;14:1432–1442.
4 Ananthakrishnan AN, McGinley EL, Binion DG: Excess hospitalisation burden associated with *Clostridium difficile* in patients with inflammatory bowel disease. Gut 2008;57:205–210.
5 Issa M, et al: Impact of *Clostridium difficile* on inflammatory bowel disease. Clin Gastroenterol Hepatol 2007;5:345–351.
6 Gandhi SK, et al: Ischemic colitis. Dis Colon Rectum 1996;39:88–100.
7 Guttormson NL, Bubrick MP: Mortality from ischemic colitis. Dis Colon Rectum 1989;32:469–472.
8 Binns JC, Isaacson P: Age-related changes in the colonic blood supply: their relevance to ischaemic colitis. Gut 1978;19:384–390.
9 Brandt LJ, Boley SJ, Mitsudo S: Clinical characteristics and natural history of colitis in the elderly. Am J Gastroenterol 1982;77:382–386.
10 Lucas W, Schroy PC 3rd: Reversible ischemic colitis in a high endurance athlete. Am J Gastroenterol 1998;93:2231–2234.
11 Friedel D, Thomas R, Fisher RS: Ischemic colitis during treatment with alosetron. Gastroenterology 2001;120:557–560.

12 Chang L, et al: Incidence of ischemic colitis and serious complications of constipation among patients using alosetron: systematic review of clinical trials and post-marketing surveillance data. Am J Gastroenterol 2006; 101:1069–1079.

13 Flobert C, et al: Right colonic involvement is associated with severe forms of ischemic colitis and occurs frequently in patients with chronic renal failure requiring hemodialysis. Am J Gastroenterol 2000;95:195–198.

14 Lambert M, de Peyer R, Muller AF: Reversible ischemic colitis after intravenous vasopressin therapy. JAMA 1982;247:666–667.

15 Byrd RL, Cunningham MW, Goldman LI: Nonocclusive ischemic colitis secondary to hemorrhagic shock. Dis Colon Rectum 1987; 30:116–118.

16 Seeger JM, et al: Routine reimplantation of patent inferior mesenteric arteries limits colon infarction after aortic reconstruction. J Vasc Surg 1992;15:635–641.

17 Mann DE Jr, et al: Ischemic colitis and acquired resistance to activated protein C in a woman using oral contraceptives. Am J Gastroenterol 1998;93:1960–1962.

18 Yee NS, Guerry Dt, Lichtenstein GR: Ischemic colitis associated with factor V Leiden mutation. Ann Intern Med 2000;132:595–596.

19 Kistin MG, Kaplan MM, Harrington JT: Diffuse ischemic colitis associated with systemic lupus erythematosus: response to subtotal colectomy. Gastroenterology 1978;75:1147–1151.

20 Niazi M, et al: Spectrum of ischemic colitis in cocaine users. Dig Dis Sci 1997;42:1537–1541.

21 Charles JA, et al: Ischemic colitis associated with naratriptan and oral contraceptive use. Headache 2005;45:386–389.

22 Scharff JR, et al: Ischemic colitis: spectrum of disease and outcome. Surgery 2003;134: 624–629; discussion 629–630.

23 Medina C, et al: Outcome of patients with ischemic colitis: review of fifty-three cases. Dis Colon Rectum 2004;47:180–184.

24 Ferzoco LB, Raptopoulos V, Silen W: Acute diverticulitis. N Engl J Med 1998;338:1521–1526.

25 Peppercorn MA: Drug-responsive chronic segmental colitis associated with diverticula: a clinical syndrome in the elderly. Am J Gastroenterol 1992;87:609–612.

26 Harpaz N, Sachar DB: Segmental colitis associated with diverticular disease and other IBD look-alikes. J Clin Gastroenterol 2006; 40(suppl 3):S132–S135.

27 Lamps LW, Knapple WL: Diverticular disease-associated segmental colitis. Clin Gastroenterol Hepatol 2007;5:27–31.

28 Makapugay LM, Dean PJ: Diverticular disease-associated chronic colitis. Am J Surg Pathol 1996;20:94–102.

29 Schroeder KW, Tremaine WJ, Ilstrup DM: Coated oral 5-aminosalicylic acid therapy for mildly to moderately active ulcerative colitis: a randomized study. N Engl J Med 1987;317:1625–1629.

30 Levine DS, et al: A randomized, double blind, dose-response comparison of balsalazide (6.75 g), balsalazide (2.25 g), and mesalamine (2.4 g) in the treatment of active, mild-to-moderate ulcerative colitis. Am J Gastroenterol 2002;97:1398–1407.

31 Jewell DP, Truelove SC: Azathioprine in ulcerative colitis: final report on controlled therapeutic trial. Br Med J 1974;iv:627–630.

32 Rutgeerts P, et al: Infliximab for induction and maintenance therapy for ulcerative colitis. N Engl J Med 2005;353:2462–2476.

33 Schoepfer AM, et al: Comparison of interferon-gamma release assay versus tuberculin skin test for tuberculosis screening in inflammatory bowel disease. Am J Gastroenterol 2008;103:2799–2806.

34 Jarnerot G, et al: Infliximab as rescue therapy in severe to moderately severe ulcerative colitis: a randomized, placebo-controlled study. Gastroenterology 2005;128:1805–1811.

35 Almogy G, et al: Surgery for ulcerative colitis in elderly persons: changes in indications for surgery and outcome over time. Arch Surg 2001;136:1396–1400.

36 Page MJ, et al: Factors affecting surgical risk in elderly patients with inflammatory bowel disease. J Gastrointest Surg 2002;6:606–613.

37 Delaney CP, et al: Prospective, age-related analysis of surgical results, functional outcome, and quality of life after ileal pouch-anal anastomosis. Ann Surg 2003;238:221–228.

38 Hatoum OA, Binion DG: The vasculature and inflammatory bowel disease: contribution to pathogenesis and clinical pathology. Inflamm Bowel Dis 2005;11:304–313.

39 Nguyen GC, Sam J: Rising prevalence of venous thromboembolism and its impact on mortality among hospitalized inflammatory bowel disease patients. Am J Gastroenterol 2008;103:2272–2280.

40 Cross RK, Wilson KT, Binion DG: Polypharmacy and Crohn's disease. Aliment Pharmacol Ther 2005;21:1211–1216.

Dig Dis 2009;27:335–340
DOI: 10.1159/000228570

Surgery in Ulcerative Colitis: Indication and Timing

Peter Andersson   Johan D. Söderholm

Department of Surgery, Linköping University Hospital, Linköping, Sweden

Key Words

Inflammatory bowel disease · Acute colitis ·
Reconstructive surgery · Ileal pouch-anal anastomosis ·
Ileorectal anastomosis · Dysplasia

Abstract

Surgery continues to play an important role in the therapeutic arsenal in ulcerative colitis. In acute colitis, close collaboration between the gastroenterologist and the surgeon is pertinent. Absolute indications for surgery include toxic megacolon, perforation, and severe colorectal bleeding. In addition, surgery should always be considered upon deterioration during medical therapy. The recommended operation in acute colitis is colectomy and ileostomy, with the rectum left in situ; reconstruction is not an option in the acute setting. In chronic continuous colitis, often with long-term steroid therapy, healing conditions are poor. A staged procedure is preferred also in these cases. In cases with dysplasia, surgery should be done after verifying the dysplasia since these patients often have little symptoms from their colitis. The proctocolectomy should in these cases include total mesorectal excision. Ileal pouch-anal anastomosis is the standard bowel reconstruction in ulcerative colitis. The various options should, however, always be thoroughly discussed, considering the pros and cons in each individual patient, before a choice is made. Ileorectal anastomosis is a temporary alternative in select cases (e.g. young women not having had children). Reconstructive surgery is best done approximately 6 months after primary surgery. Surgery for ulcerative colitis should be seen as complementary to medical treatment and may prevent complications, improve the patients' quality of life and occasionally be life-saving. Correct assessment and optimised medical treatment are prerequisites for surgery on accurate indications and good surgical results. Therefore, close interactions between gastroenterologists and colorectal surgeons are mandatory for optimal patient outcome.

Copyright © 2009 S. Karger AG, Basel

Introduction

Although medical therapy has advanced during the past decades and colectomy rates may be decreasing [1], surgery continues to play an important role in the therapeutic arsenal in ulcerative colitis (UC). In most epidemiological studies, cumulative risks for bowel surgery of 25–30% were found [2–4], with higher numbers for extensive and active disease [5]. As much as 10% of the patients will need surgery during the first year of illness [3], in many cases as emergency procedures. The patients with UC therefore need combined careful attention from the gastroenterologist and the colorectal surgeon. It is also important to see surgery as an additional therapeutic alternative and not as a 'failure of medical therapy' to achieve optimal outcome over the lifetime of the individuals hit with UC.

The four main groups of indications for surgery in UC remain: (1) acute colitis with severe complications or not responding to medical therapy; (2) chronic continuous disease causing steroid dependency in adults or impaired

KARGER

Fax +41 61 306 12 34
E-Mail karger@karger.ch
www.karger.com

© 2009 S. Karger AG, Basel
0257–2753/09/0273–0335$26.00/0

Accessible online at:
www.karger.com/ddi

Prof. Johan D. Söderholm, MD, PhD
Department of Clinical and Experimental Medicine and Colorectal Surgery Unit
Department of Surgery, Linköping University Hospital
SE–581 85 Linköping (Sweden)
Tel. +46 13 22 46 02, Fax +46 13 22 35 70, E-Mail johan.d.soderholm@liu.se

growth and/or delayed puberty in children and adolescents; (3) dysplasia and/or cancer of the colon, and (4) reconstruction after previous colectomy. The timing of the surgery is always essential, with the time span ranging from hours to days in acute colitis, weeks in continuous disease, to weeks to months in the cases of dyplasia/cancer. In reconstructive surgery, the timing and the choice of method of reconstruction have to take into account the whole life situation of the affected individual.

Acute Colitis

In the cases of acute colitis, a close collaboration between the medical gastroenterologist and the colorectal surgeon is pertinent. Preferentially, the surgical team should be contacted in every case of severe colitis admitted to the hospital to be able to evaluate the patient and follow the course of the attack. The patient should at an early stage be informed that colectomy is an alternative should the colitis be refractory to medical treatment. To be able to make the correct decision about colectomy, the colorectal surgeon *must* be consulted at any deterioration during i.v. steroid therapy and/or before rescue treatment with anti-TNF or ciclosporin is started.

The absolute indications for surgery are toxic megacolon, perforation, and severe colorectal bleeding. However, in most acute cases surgery will be performed because of non-response to i.v. steroids and rescue therapy and/or deterioration during medical treatment. It is recommended that the response is assessed objectively on day 3–4 [6] by stool frequency, CRP levels and abdominal imaging (plain abdominal or CT scan) and using for example the Oxford index [7] or Sweden index (no. of daily stools + 0.14 × CRP (mg/l) on day 4; Index ≥8: predictor of need for colectomy) [8]. By using these indices on day 3–4, it is possible to make an evidence-based decision for early introduction of rescue therapy. The ECCO guidelines advocate colectomy if there is no improvement within a further 4–7 days [6]. Thereby, an appropriate assessment for need of colectomy can and should be done within 7–10 days of medical therapy [9], a treatment period shown not to be associated with increased postoperative morbidity [10, 11]. A third line of medical therapy (rescue of rescue) was recently shown to be associated with a high risk of severe complications [12] and should normally not be considered in front of colectomy in acute UC.

The recommended operation in acute colitis is colectomy and ileostomy, with the rectum left in situ [6]. In the trained surgeon's hands this operation is quick, easy and safe [13], and leaves all options open for reconstruction. There is some controversy about the handling of the rectal stump in the severely inflamed colo-rectum. The alternative techniques are division of the rectum at the level of the promontory (warrants transanal rectal drainage to prevent blowout due to retention) or to bring the recto-sigmoid up through the abdominal fascia (closed in the subcutaneous fat or as a mucous fistula). The latter options are considered very safe as no closed bowel is left within the abdomen [14, 15]. Colectomy with an ileostomy allows the patients to recover from the colitis, with quick return of health and nutritional status, and allows tapering of steroids. The operation can however seldom be considered as a final solution, and to optimize bowel function the patients will have to go through additional surgery with additional risks and costs.

Chronic Continuous Colitis

In chronic continuous colitis, i.e. active disease despite optimized maintenance therapy and often involving steroid dependency, the conditions for healing are far from optimal. Even if these patients are usually in a better general condition than the acute colitis cases, they have often been under steroid therapy for along time period, incurring a high risk of septic complications and poor conditions of anastomotic healing [16, 17]. Because of the compromised healing, a staged procedure is preferred also in these cases [6], i.e. primary surgery with colectomy and ileostomy, leaving the rectum intact (preferentially with the stump brought up through the abdominal fascia because of the impaired healing) to consider the options of reconstruction at a later stage. Pending surgery attempts should be made to optimize the patient from a nutritional point of view and the steroid dose should be kept at a minimum.

Dysplasia and Cancer

A diagnosis of cancer of the colon or rectum in a patient with UC is an absolute indication for surgery, which implies proctocolectomy and usually ileal pouch-anal anastomosis (IPAA). The case of dysplasia in UC is, however, often a more delicate situation. Dysplasia, both high-grade and low-grade, does entail an increased risk for cancer development [18] that warrants action, but the diagnosis of dysplasia in UC is sometimes difficult, and interobserver variation is a significant concern [19]. Moreover, these patients often have little or no symptoms from their colitis, and proctocolectomy with IPAA is a procedure with not negligible risks of postoperative morbidity and impact on quality of life (see below). Surgery for dysplasia should therefore be done only after dysplasia can be confirmed by at least two experienced GI pathologists [20], and decision-making in multidisciplinary teams is pertinent. With a single finding of low-grade dysplasia, a more vigorous colonoscopy follow-up program is often suggested as an acceptable compromise [21, 22].

Proctectomy for cases with dysplasia and cancer should include total mesorectal excision [20], which increases the risk for pelvic nerve damage compared to the technique usually used for proctectomy in IBD. There is some debate about the best modus operandi for the pouch-anal anastomosis. Mucosectomy of the rectal mucosa with a hand-sewn anastomosis to the dentate line is often recommended. However, this procedure is technically difficult and might damage the anal transitional zone, which is important for anal function, and does not guarantee removal of all rectal mucosa. Therefore the double-stapled technique, often leaving a rectal cuff, is acceptable because of its better functional results [23], even in the presence of inflammation in the remaining anorectal cuff [24]. The remaining rectal cuff should, however, be no more than 1–2 cm above the dentate line to minimize the mucosal surface at risk of malignant transformation. Although the risk for development of dysplasia (<5% after 10 years) and cancer (only case reports) of the cuff and pouch mucosa is low [25, 26], it is advocated that patients operated for dysplasia/cancer should be kept under endoscopic surveillance [26], irrespective of the technique used for the pouch-anal anastomosis.

Reconstructive Surgery

Ileal pouch-anal anastomosis (IPAA) has been the standard bowel reconstruction in ulcerative colitis for the last 25 years. IPAA offers the patients an unchanged body image since no permanent stoma is needed and is in most cases a very good way out, but it is not always the ideal solution. The pouch is most commonly constructed as a J-pouch of the distal ileum anastomosed to the anal canal. In recent years, laparoscopic surgery has been shown to be feasible for pouch surgery [27, 28], but with no proven benefits so far [29–31]. It is generally recommended to do the restorative surgery as a two-stage procedure with a temporary covering loop ileostomy during the healing period of the pouch [6]. A temporary ileostomy adds a second operation with complication risks [32], but severe septic complications from anastomotic leaks from the pouch are avoided [33–35]. The anal route of defecation is preserved by using the IPAA. However, function is often less than perfect, with incontinence to flatus and soiling in 10–20% during daytime and in 50–60% at nighttime [36], often requiring pads. Moreover, there is a considerable risk of pouchitis, with 50% of patients having sporadic bouts and 10–15% having more severe chronic inflammation in cohort studies [37]. Functional or technical failure necessitating excision of the pouch (pouch failure) still ranges around 5–15% in various series [38, 39]. Pelvic scarring and nerve damage is a risk with the surgery and sexual problems might occur [40]; dyspareunia and sexual uneasiness (fright of incontinence during intercourse) in women, whereas retrograde ejaculation and, more seldom, impotence may arise in men. A less-recognized problem with the pelvic pouch has been the diminished ability of operated women becoming pregnant. It has now has been convincingly demonstrated in cohort studies that female fecundity is reduced after IPAA, with a 3- to 5-fold longer time period needed for pregnancy and a lower number of children in total [40, 41].

In select cases, ileorectal anastomosis (IRA) can be an alternative [6, 20]. IRA is historically burdened with poor results because of persistent rectal inflammation and a high risk of later cancer [42]. More recent series have, however, shown better functional results and relatively low risks for cancer [43, 44], presumably due to better selection of patients and a consequent use of anti-inflammatory treatment. Moreover, because of no need for pelvic dissection during the operation, IRA seems to have less impact on sexual function and fertility than IPAA, as has been clearly shown in surgery for familial adenomatous polyposis [41, 45]. A modification in practice could therefore be considered, offering fertile female (and male) patients, not having had their children, an IRA as a temporary alternative (leaving the pelvis and pelvic nerves intact and with better anorectal function) with a view to later pouch surgery when the family is complete. To consider this option, however, at follow-up 3–6 months after colectomy the rectum should not be grossly inflamed and the proctitis must be easily kept in remission with basic medical treatment (e.g. mesalamine suppositories).

Permanent ileostomy is a valid option if the patient tolerates the stoma, particularly in elderly patients. In

Table 1. Summary of the pros and cons of the alternatives for reconstructive surgery after (procto)colectomy for UC

Technique	Pros	Cons
IPAA	Transanal defecation No follow-up needed	Pouchitis Risk for incontinence Fertility/fecundity Dyspareunia/sexual problems Impotence/retrograde ejaculation
Ileorectal anastomosis	Less effect sexual/fertility Good anorectal function	Medication needed Dysplasia/cancer risk Follow-up needed
Ileostomy	'Cured' from colitis No medication needed No follow-up needed Rectal stump issues	Ostomy problems Body image Sexual initiative
Kock pouch	Less ostomy problems No follow-up needed Improved body image	Multiple revision surgery Risk for pouchitis

It is pertinent to discuss these issues with the patient before a decision on restorative surgery is made.

case of intolerance to a regular ileostomy in the presence of contraindications to restorative surgery, for example severe proctitis with perianal fistulas or previous sphincter lesions due to childbirth, a continent ileostomy (Kock pouch) is an option. This is, however, demanding surgery not seldom requiring repeat revisions of the continent nipple [46]. Management of the rectal remnant in those cases where colectomy and ileostomy is considered as definitive surgery is an issue. If left in place, the rectal stump must be kept in surveillance as if the patient still was having an extensive colitis; if this is not possible or if there are severe symptoms with bleeding or anal discharge, the rectum should be removed. In this context it is important to remember that removal of the rectum in fertile women may lead to backward tilting of the vagina causing retention of vaginal discharge and sexual dysfunction [47].

The best choice for reconstruction is not always obvious and may differ depending on the circumstances of life, occupation, age, gender, etc. Therefore, the alternative options (table 1) with IPAA, IRA, Kock pouch or remaining ileostomy should always be thoroughly discussed with the patient, considering the pros and cons in each individual case over a lifetime perspective, before a final decision is made.

Medication and Surgery

While there is no doubt that corticosteroid use increases the risk for septic and anastomosis-related complications in elective UC surgery [16], there is less consensus regarding immunomodulators. It seems that purine analogues are safe to use perioperatively [6], whereas current studies on the effects of anti-TNF treatment (infliximab) on postoperative complications show contradictory results. Two recently presented series (n = 141 and 151, respectively) show no increase in complication risks with infliximab [48, 49], although the combination with cyclosporine did [49]. On the other hand, two large cohort studies (n = 301 and 523, respectively) [50, 51], where the outcome was adjusted for disease severity, showed increased risk of postoperative complications in pouch surgery for at least 4 months after i.v. therapy with infliximab. This is important to consider since many cases of severe acute colitis currently have been treated with high-dose steroids combined with rescue therapy with infliximab or cyclosporin. In addition, the experience from the Cleveland Clinic [52] showed an increased risk for intra-operative and postoperative complications if the restorative surgery was done within 6 months after acute colectomy. In our practice, reconstruction is done approximately 6 months from primary surgery, when the patient is back in a good general condition, medication has been discontinued or tapered to a minimum, and the rectal mucosa has been preoperatively assessed for the various surgical options.

Concluding Remarks

Surgery for UC should be seen as complementary to medical treatment and will, when used in the right situations, prevent complications, improve quality of life and occasionally even be life-saving. Correct diagnosis and assessment and optimized medical treatment are prerequisites for surgery on accurate indications and to achieve good surgical results. Therefore, close interactions between the gastroenterologist and the colorectal surgeon are needed for optimal patient outcome over a life-long perspective.

Disclosure Statement

The authors declare that no financial or other conflict of interest exists in relation to the content of the article.

References

1 Solberg IC, Lygren I, Jahnsen J, et al: Clinical course during the first 10 years of ulcerative colitis: results from a population-based inception cohort (IBSEN Study). Scand J Gastroenterol 2009;44:431–440.

2 Henriksen M, Jahnsen J, Lygren I, et al: Ulcerative colitis and clinical course: results of a 5-year population-based follow-up study (the IBSEN study). Inflamm Bowel Dis 2006; 12:543–550.

3 Langholz E, Munkholm P, Davidsen M, Binder V: Colorectal cancer risk and mortality in patients with ulcerative colitis. Gastroenterology 1992;103:1444–1451.

4 Leijonmarck CE, Persson PG, Hellers G: Factors affecting colectomy rate in ulcerative colitis: an epidemiologic study. Gut 1990;31: 329–333.

5 Cottone M, Scimeca D, Mocciaro F, Civitavecchia G, Perricone G, Orlando A: Clinical course of ulcerative colitis. Dig Liver Dis 2008;40(suppl 2):S247–S252.

6 Travis SP, Stange EF, Lemann M, et al: European evidence-based Consensus on the management of ulcerative colitis: current management. J Crohns Colitis 2008;2:24–62.

7 Travis SPL, Farrant JM, Ricketts C, et al: Predicting outcome in severe ulcerative colitis. Gut 1996;38:905–910.

8 Lindgren SC, Flood LM, Kilander AF, Lofberg R, Persson TB, Sjodahl RI: Early predictors of glucocorticosteroid treatment failure in severe and moderately severe attacks of ulcerative colitis. Eur J Gastroenterol Hepatol 1998;10:831–835.

9 Hancock L, Windsor AC, Mortensen NJ: Inflammatory bowel disease: the view of the surgeon. Colorectal Dis 2006;8(suppl 1):10–14.

10 Hyde GM, Jewell DP, Kettlewell MG, Mortensen NJ: Cyclosporin for severe ulcerative colitis does not increase the rate of perioperative complications. Dis Colon Rectum 2001;44:1436–1440.

11 Jarnerot G, Hertervig E, Friis-Liby I, et al: Infliximab as rescue therapy in severe to moderately severe ulcerative colitis: a randomized, placebo-controlled trial. Gastroenterology 2005;128:1805–1811.

12 Maser EA, Deconda D, Lichtiger S, Ullman T, Present DH, Kornbluth A: Cyclosporine and infliximab as rescue therapy for each other in patients with steroid-refractory ulcerative colitis. Clin Gastroenterol Hepatol 2008;6:1112–1116.

13 Hyman NH, Cataldo P, Osler T: Urgent subtotal colectomy for severe inflammatory bowel disease. Dis Colon Rectum 2005;48: 70–73.

14 Carter FM, McLeod RS, Cohen Z: Subtotal colectomy for ulcerative colitis: complications related to the rectal remnant. Dis Colon Rectum 1991;34:1005–1009.

15 McKee RF, Keenan RA, Munro A: Colectomy for acute colitis: is it safe to close the rectal stump? Int J Colorectal Dis 1995;10:222–224.

16 Aberra FN, Lewis JD, Hass D, Rombeau JL, Osborne B, Lichtenstein GR: Corticosteroids and immunomodulators: postoperative infectious complication risk in inflammatory bowel disease patients. Gastroenterology 2003;125:320–327.

17 Lake JP, Firoozmand E, Kang JC, et al: Effect of high-dose steroids on anastomotic complications after proctocolectomy with ileal pouch-anal anastomosis. J Gastrointest Surg 2004;8:547–551.

18 Thomas T, Abrams KA, Robinson RJ, Mayberry JF: Meta-analysis: cancer risk of low-grade dysplasia in chronic ulcerative colitis. Aliment Pharmacol Ther 2007;25:657–668.

19 Odze RD, Goldblum J, Noffsinger A, Alsaigh N, Rybicki LA, Fogt F: Interobserver variability in the diagnosis of ulcerative colitis-associated dysplasia by telepathology. Mod Pathol 2002;15:379–386.

20 Biancone L, Michetti P, Travis SP, et al: European evidence-based Consensus on the management of ulcerative colitis: special situations. J Crohns Colitis 2008;2: 63–92.

21 Befrits R, Ljung T, Jaramillo E, Rubio C: Low-grade dysplasia in extensive, long-standing inflammatory bowel disease: a follow-up study. Dis Colon Rectum 2002;45: 615–620.

22 Lim CH, Axon AT: Low-grade dysplasia: nonsurgical treatment. Inflamm Bowel Dis 2003;9:270–272.

23 Lovegrove RE, Tilney HS, Heriot AG, et al: A comparison of adverse events and functional outcomes after restorative proctocolectomy for familial adenomatous polyposis and ulcerative colitis. Dis Colon Rectum 2006;49: 1293–1306.

24 Silvestri MT, Hurst RD, Rubin MA, Michelassi F, Fichera A: Chronic inflammatory changes in the anal transition zone after stapled ileal pouch-anal anastomosis: is mucosectomy a superior alternative? Surgery 2008;144:533–537.

25 Remzi FH, Fazio VW, Delaney CP, et al: Dysplasia of the anal transitional zone after ileal pouch-anal anastomosis: results of prospective evaluation after a minimum of ten years. Dis Colon Rectum 2003;46:6–13.

26 Scarpa M, van Koperen PJ, Ubbink DT, Hommes DW, Ten Kate FJ, Bemelman WA: Systematic review of dysplasia after restorative proctocolectomy for ulcerative colitis. Br J Surg 2007;94:534–545.

27 Marcello PW, Milsom JW, Wong SK, et al: Laparoscopic restorative proctocolectomy: case-matched comparative study with open restorative proctocolectomy. Dis Colon Rectum 2000;43:604–608.

28 Dunker MS, Bemelman WA, Slors JF, van Duijvendijk P, Gouma DJ: Functional outcome, quality of life, body image, and cosmesis in patients after laparoscopic-assisted and conventional restorative proctocolectomy: a comparative study. Dis Colon Rectum 2001; 44:1800–1807.

29 Tan JJ, Tjandra JJ: Laparoscopic surgery for ulcerative colitis: a meta-analysis. Colorectal Dis 2006;8:626–636.

30 Maartense S, Dunker MS, Slors JF, Gouma DJ, Bemelman WA: Restorative proctectomy after emergency laparoscopic colectomy for ulcerative colitis: a case-matched study. Colorectal Dis 2004;6:254–257.

31 Ahmed AU, Keus F, Heikens JT, et al: Open versus laparoscopic (assisted) ileo pouch anal anastomosis for ulcerative colitis and familial adenomatous polyposis. Cochrane Database Syst Rev 2009;1:CD006267.

32 Wong KS, Remzi FH, Gorgun E, et al: Loop ileostomy closure after restorative proctocolectomy: outcome in 1,504 patients. Dis Colon Rectum 2005;48:243–250.

33 Williamson ME, Lewis WG, Sagar PM, Holdsworth PJ, Johnston D: One-stage restorative proctocolectomy without temporary ileostomy for ulcerative colitis: a note of caution. Dis Colon Rectum 1997;40:1019–1022.

34 Tjandra JJ, Fazio VW, Milsom JW, Lavery IC, Oakley JR, Fabre JM: Omission of temporary diversion in restorative proctocolectomy: is it safe? Dis Colon Rectum 1993;36: 1007–1014.

35 Matthiessen P, Hallbook O, Rutegard J, Simert G, Sjodahl R: Defunctioning stoma reduces symptomatic anastomotic leakage after low anterior resection of the rectum for cancer: a randomized multicenter trial. Ann Surg 2007;246:207–214.

36 Tjandra JJ, Fazio VW, Church JM, Oakley JR, Milsom JW, Lavery IC: Similar functional results after restorative proctocolectomy in patients with familial adenomatous polyposis and mucosal ulcerative colitis. Am J Surg 1993;165:322–325.

37 Stahlberg D, Gullberg K, Liljeqvist L, Hellers G, Lofberg R: Pouchitis following pelvic pouch operation for ulcerative colitis: incidence, cumulative risk, and risk factors. Dis Colon Rectum 1996;39:1012–1018.

38 Leowardi C, Hinz U, Tariverdian M, et al: Long-term outcome 10 years or more after restorative proctocolectomy and ileal pouch-anal anastomosis in patients with ulcerative colitis. Langenbecks Arch Surg 2009 DOI: 10.1007/s00423-009-0479-7.

39 Ferrante M, Declerck S, De Hertogh G, et al: Outcome after proctocolectomy with ileal pouch-anal anastomosis for ulcerative colitis. Inflamm Bowel Dis 2008;14:20–28.

40 Cornish JA, Tan E, Teare J, et al: The effect of restorative proctocolectomy on sexual function, urinary function, fertility, pregnancy and delivery: a systematic review. Dis Colon Rectum 2007;50:1128–1138.

41 Ording OK, Juul S, Berndtsson I, Oresland T, Laurberg S: Ulcerative colitis: female fecundity before diagnosis, during disease, and after surgery compared with a population sample. Gastroenterology 2002;122:15–19.

42 Aylett SO: Diffuse ulcerative colitis and its treatment by ileo-rectal anastomosis. Ann R Coll Surg Engl 1960;27:260–284.

43 Leijonmarck CE, Lofberg R, Ost A, Hellers G: Long-term results of ileorectal anastomosis in ulcerative colitis in Stockholm County. Dis Colon Rectum 1990;33:195–200.

44 Elton C, Makin G, Hitos K, Cohen CR: Mortality, morbidity and functional outcome after ileorectal anastomosis. Br J Surg 2003;90:59–65.

45 Olsen KO, Juul S, Bulow S, et al: Female fecundity before and after operation for familial adenomatous polyposis. Br J Surg 2003;90:227–231.

46 Nessar G, Fazio VW, Tekkis P, et al: Long-term outcome and quality of life after continent ileostomy. Dis Colon Rectum 2006;49:336–344.

47 Sjodahl R, Nystrom PO, Olaison G: Surgical treatment of dorsocaudal dislocation of the vagina after excision of the rectum. The Kylberg operation. Dis Colon Rectum 1990;33:762–764.

48 Ferrante M, D'Hoore A, Vermeire S, et al: Corticosteroids but not infliximab increase short-term postoperative infectious complications in patients with ulcerative colitis. Inflamm Bowel Dis 2009;15:1062–1070.

49 Schluender SJ, Ippoliti A, Dubinsky M, et al: Does infliximab influence surgical morbidity of ileal pouch-anal anastomosis in patients with ulcerative colitis? Dis Colon Rectum 2007;50:1747–1753.

50 Selvasekar CR, Cima RR, Larson DW, et al: Effect of infliximab on short-term complications in patients undergoing operation for chronic ulcerative colitis. J Am Coll Surg 2007;204:956–962.

51 Mor IJ, Vogel JD, da Luz MA, Shen B, Hammel J, Remzi FH: Infliximab in ulcerative colitis is associated with an increased risk of postoperative complications after restorative proctocolectomy. Dis Colon Rectum 2008;51:1202–1207.

52 Dinnewitzer AJ, Wexner SD, Baig MK, et al: Timing of restorative proctectomy following subtotal colectomy in patients with inflammatory bowel disease. Colorectal Dis 2006;8:278–282.

Dig Dis 2009;27:341–346
DOI: 10.1159/000228571

Management of Inflammatory Bowel Diseases during Pregnancy

Axel U. Dignass[a]   Franz Hartmann[b]   Andreas Sturm[c]   Jürgen Stein[d]

[a]Department of Medicine I – Gastroenterology, Hepatology, Oncology and Nutrition, Markus Hospital,
Goethe University, Frankfurt, [b]Department of Gastroenterology, Marien Hospital, Frankfurt,
[c]Department of Gastroenterology, Charité-Campus Virchow, Berlin, and [d]Department of Gastroenterology,
St. Elisabethen Krankenhaus, Frankfurt, Germany

Key Words

Azathioprine · 5-ASA · Anti-TNF · Methotrexate

Abstract

Inflammatory bowel diseases (IBD) have a high prevalence in younger patients with child-bearing potential. Usually, pregnancies in women with IBD will develop normally, if the patient is in remission or has minor disease activity at the time of conception. In contrast, the frequency of normal pregnancies is significantly reduced and the frequency of adverse outcomes like preterm birth or miscarriage is increased, when conception occurs in phases with active IBD. Therefore, it is generally recommended to women with IBD to conceive at a time with minor disease activity or in remission. IBD patients who plan to become pregnant or are pregnant should be treated adequately. Currently, it is widely accepted that the treatment of IBD with corticosteroids and 5-ASA derivatives does not increase the risk of malformations or adverse outcomes in pregnant IBD patients. However, a slight increase in the number of pre-term deliveries or reduced birth weight is observed. More recently, it has also been appreciated that azathioprine and 6-MP and presumably also infliximab and other TNF-α blockers can be safely used during pregnancy in IBD, as no significant increase of malformations, miscarriages or adverse pregnancy outcomes is observed. Information on cyclosporine and tacrolimus during pregnancy is scarcer, but it may be continued or started in some situations if clinically needed. Methotrexate is contraindicated, as this drug is known to sig-nificantly increase the risk of malformations and spontaneous abortion. Patients, who wish to nurse their babies, may be treated with steroids and 5-ASA derivatives without a significantly increased risk for the newborn.

Copyright © 2009 S. Karger AG, Basel

Introduction

The inflammatory bowel diseases (IBD) Crohn's disease (CD) and ulcerative colitis (UC) have a high prevalence in younger patients with child-bearing potential [1, 2]. Thus, uncertainties and a number of questions regarding medical treatment before and during pregnancy and the lactation period exist in IBD patients.

Several studies have demonstrated that most pregnancies in women with IBD will develop normal, if the patient is in remission or has only minor disease activity at the time of conception [3–5]. A meta-analysis by Miller [6] with more than 1,300 female patients with UC and over 700 patients with CD clearly demonstrated that normal pregnancies are observed in 83% of women with CD (71–93% in individual studies) and in 85% of women with UC (76–97% in individual studies) (table 1). Malformations were observed in about 1% of all pregnancies, and also the frequency of spontaneous abortions and still-births was in the same range as observed in the healthy normal population (table 1). In contrast, several studies [7–9] could demonstrate that the frequency of normal pregnancies is reduced and the frequency of adverse out-

Prof. Dr. med. Axel Dignass
Department of Medicine I, Markus-Krankenhaus
Wilhelm-Epstein-Strasse 4
DE–60431 Frankfurt/Main (Germany)
Tel. +49 69 9533 2201, Fax +49 69 9533 2291, E-Mail axel.dignass@fdk.info

Table 1. Outcome of pregnancy in IBD depends on disease activity

	Normal, % (range)	Malforma-tion, % (range)	Pre-term, %	Abortion, % (range)
Background population	83	2	6	9
Inactive CD	82 (71–93)	1 (0–6)	7	10 (3–27)
Active CD	54	1	25	20
Inactive UC	84 (76–97)	1 (0–3)	6	9 (1–16)
Active UC	65	2	12	21

Table 2. Mesalamine in pregnancy [14]

	Mesalamine (n = 165)	No mesalamine (n = 165)
Normal birth, %	88.5	89.7
Preterm (<37 PW)	13	4.7 (p < 0.02)
Spontaneous abortion, %	6.7	8.5
Induced abortion, %	4.2	1.8
Malformation, %	7.1	7.4
Birth weight, g	3,253 ± 546	3,461 ± 542 (p < 0.02)

comes of pregnancy is increased when pregnancies take place in phases with active IBD (table 1). In summary, these data indicate an uncomplicated outcome of pregnancies in IBD patients with inactive disease comparable to a pregnancy outcome in the general healthy population and an increased risk of adverse outcome in patients with active disease suggesting that inactive IBD generally do not affect the outcome of pregnancies. Therefore, it is generally recommended to women with IBD to conceive at a time with minor disease activity or in remission.

Conventional Medical Treatment of IBD during Pregnancy

The fact that adverse outcomes of pregnancy are observed more frequently in IBD patients with active disease indicates that IBD patients who plan to become pregnant or are pregnant should be treated adequately for active disease. Currently, it is widely accepted that the standard treatment of IBD with corticosteroids and 5-ASA derivatives is not significantly associated with malformations or adverse outcomes in pregnant IBD patients [10–12]. Therefore, corticosteroids and 5-ASA derivatives are used for the treatment of pregnant patients with active IBD and, when necessary, also to maintain remission during pregnancy. Treatment of active IBD with corticosteroids and 5-ASA derivatives during pregnancy does not significantly differ from treatment considerations in non-pregnant women, because these drugs can be used in almost usual dosage during pregnancy without any significantly increased adverse fetal outcomes. However, whenever possible, the lowest possible dosages should be used, especially for the new 5-ASA formulations, because limited information is available about adverse effects of high-dose 5-ASA treatment during pregnancy [13, 14]. It is generally accepted that the types and dosages of corti-costeroid preparations (prednisone, prednisolone, and hydrocortisone) usually prescribed for the treatment of IBD are not associated with an increased risk of miscarriage or fetal deformities. It is theoretically possible that very high doses of corticosteroids taken during the final phases of pregnancy might cause reduced corticosteroid production in the newborn's adrenal gland with resulting low levels of circulating cortisone after birth, together with apathy and reduced activity. Therefore, infants born to mothers taking large corticosteroid doses in late pregnancy should be closely followed by an experienced neonatologist. If necessary, the baby can receive cortisone substitution until the adrenal glands are able to produce sufficient cortisone.

Clinical experience with budesonide in pregnancy is more limited, but clinical experience and smaller studies indicate that also oral and rectal administration of budesonide can be used without any significantly increased risk [15, 16]. Our own experience with the use of budesonide in pregnancy has not shown any evidence for increased risk to mother or baby.

The use of 5-ASA derivatives has been demonstrated to be generally safe; however, a significant reduction of the birth weight and an increased frequency of premature births have been observed [14] (table 2).

Conventional therapy of IBD with pure 5-ASA or corticosteroids in fathers does not have any adverse effects on the progress of pregnancy. Sulfasalazine can cause temporary infertility in men, which normalizes about two months after discontinuing the drug or switching to pure mesalamine or 5-aminosalicylic acid (5-ASA) [17, 18]. The reasons for this temporary infertility include a decreased sperm count, a reduced amount of seminal fluid and abnormalities in the structure and motility of the sperm cells. These changes occur in about 80% of men treated with these drugs.

Table 3. 6-MP during pregnancy in female IBD patients [21]

	6-MP terminated before conception	Conception with 6-MP		No 6-MP
		terminated	continued	
Pregnancies	40	24	15	92
Normal	21	17	10	65
Preterm birth	3 (7.5%)	0 (0%)	4 (26.7%)	4 (4.3%)
Spontaneous abortion	15 (37.5%)	4 (16.6%)	1 (6.6%)	21 (22.8%)
Malformation	0 (0%)	0 (0%)	1 (6.6%)	4 (4.3%)
Infection	0	2	2	2
Neoplasia	0	0	0	0
Low birth weight	1	0	1 (6.7%)	5 (5.4%)

Immunosuppressive Therapy in Pregnant IBD Patients

In recent years, immunosuppressants play an increasingly important role in the medical management of patients with IBD. As a consequence the use of immunosuppressants in IBD patients with child-bearing potential has significantly increased and represents an important problem in the management of younger IBD patients requiring intensive counseling.

The use of immunosuppressive therapy during pregnancy in IBD patients is less clear because of limited clinical data about the use of these drugs in pregnant patients with IBD, which is limited to case reports and studies with limited numbers of patients [15, 19–24].

Early animal studies have demonstrated that very high doses of azathioprine/6-MP caused malformation of limbs, cleft palate and eye abnormalities in rat and rabbits [10, 15]. However, therapeutic doses have not been shown to cause an increase of malformation, but increased numbers of spontaneous abortions and growth retardation in animals. Significant clinical evidence regarding the use of immunosuppressants in pregnant women is provided by organ transplant patients and patients with rheumatoid arthritis, who became pregnant [22, 25–27]. The most extensive information is available regarding the use of azathioprine and 6-mercaptopurine in pregnant transplant patients. These studies clearly demonstrate that normal pregnancies are observed in the majority of women treated with azathioprine/6-MP and that no increased incidence of stillbirths, miscarriages and fetal abnormalities is observed in patients treated with usual doses of azathioprine and 6-MP [27, 28]. However, an increase of premature births and reduced weight at birth is frequent-

ly seen [25, 29]. Generally, no clinically relevant immunosuppression is observed in the newborn.

Although the existing data in IBD patients are less extensive, patients with IBD do not have an increased evidence of stillbirths, miscarriages and fetal abnormalities under therapy with azathioprine and 6-MP (table 3) [12, 19, 21, 30]. However, a tendency to more frequent premature births and reduced birth weight is also observed in IBD patients (table 3) [12, 21]. Despite the fact that the use of azathioprine during pregnancy seems to be safe, there are also small studies with limited numbers of patients showing that 6-MP or azathioprine may slightly increase the incidence of abortions, stillbirths or prematurity [31–33]. Currently, it is not clear if these observations are caused by the limited number of patient in these studies or if there is a real slightly increased risk of abortions, malformations and prematurity induced by azathioprine therapy during pregnancy. This information should be discussed carefully with the patient in order to obtain informed consent of both partners.

If treatment with azathioprine is necessary to maintain remission of IBD, it is currently accepted to continue treatment with azathioprine/6-MP following extensive counseling of the patient and spouse and getting informed consent for legal reasons. In patients who do not depend on treatment with azathioprine/6-MP, this therapy should be discontinued at least 3 months before a planned pregnancy. An involuntary pregnancy under treatment with azathioprine/6-MP does not represent a medical reason to terminate a pregnancy.

The effect of azathioprine/6-MP therapy in men who wish to conceive has recently been under discussion and the opinions are rather controversial. While the experience in the transplant population and in one study with

Table 4. Effect of 6-MP therapy in male IBD patients on pregnancy outcome [21]

	6-MP terminated before conception	Conception with 6-MP	No 6-MP
Pregnancies	44	37	73
Normal	32	27	59
Preterm birth	1 (2.2%)	3 (8.1%)	3 (4.1%)
Spontaneous abortion	4 (9.0%)	6 (16.2%)	11 (15.1%)
Malformation	2 (4.5%)	0 (0%)	2 (2.7%)
Infection	1	0	0
Neoplasia	0	1	0
Low birth weight	2 (4.5%)	2 (7.4%)	3 (4.1%)

Table 5. Therapy of IBD in pregnancy

Drug	Safety
5-ASA/SASP	safe
Olsalazine	caution
Corticosteroids	safe
Budesonide	probably safe
Azathioprine/6-MP	safe
Methotrexate	contraindicated
Thalidomide	contraindicated
Cyclosporine/tacrolimus	presumably safe
Infliximab/adalimumab	presumably safe
Loperamide	?, relatively safe
Metronidazole/ciprofloxacin	probably safe, 2nd line
Probiotics	safe

male IBD patients does not provide evidence for increased adverse effects with respect to the outcome of the pregnancy [21, 28] (table 4), a small study by Rajapakse et al. [33] reported a significantly increased incidence of pregnancy-related complications when the fathers used 6-MP within 3 months of conception. However, this study has some limitations and the results and conclusions are discussed controversially [34].

The use of methotrexate during pregnancy is not permitted because of well-characterized embryotoxicity and teratogenicity [10, 12]. Because of the ill-defined long-term effects of methotrexate on male and female reproductive organs, adequate contraception for at least 6 months following methotrexate therapy is recommended.

Experimental data in animals and clinical data regarding the use of infliximab in humans indicate that the use of this medication does not represent an increased risk for the pregnancy and the newborn. Animal studies provide no evidence for embryotoxicity and teratogenicity. Post-marketing data report a significant number of normal pregnancies; however, a few adverse outcomes have been observed as well [35, 36]. Because of limited data regarding the safety of infliximab, the manufacturer recommends adequate contraception. A recent study by Mahadevan et al. [37] reported no increased side effects when 10 patients with complicated IBD were intentionally treated with infliximab throughout their pregnancy. Elective termination of a pregnancy with infliximab medication is not necessary.

Post-marketing data also show no increased incidence of pregnancy complications with the use of adalimumab [38, 39]. Of note, both infliximab and adalimumab are IgG1 antibodies and may therefore allow placental transfer, especially in the last term of pregnancy, which may result in immunosuppression in the newborn following delivery [40]. As pointed out, no increased risk following the use of these antibodies during pregnancy has been observed in the newborn.

My personal recommendation for the use of immunosuppressive or biological therapy during pregnancy is to continue or even start these medications in those patients who need active treatment to control disease activity or maintain remission. My personal belief is that there is no indication for therapeutic abortions when pregnancy occurs following or in the course of treatment with azathioprine, infliximab, adalimumab, tacrolimus or cyclosporine. However, if the patient is worried or there is no definitive need for immunosuppressive therapy or biologicals, these medications should be terminated 3 months before planned conception and steroids should be started if needed.

Little information is available regarding the use of other immunosuppressants during pregnancy. A number of case reports describe normal pregnancies following treatment with cyclosporine A and tacrolimus [10, 12, 23, 24]. However, it seems to be inadequate to make general recommendations regarding the use of these immunosuppressants during pregnancy due to limited clinical evidence. Individual decisions based on the clinical situation of the individual patient are recommended. Again the transplant literature provides more encouraging data for the use of cyclosporine and tacrolimus [22, 41, 42].

Other Medications in Pregnant IBD Patients

Other medications that are occasionally used for the therapy of IBD like antibiotics, loperamide and probiotics are usually not used as first-line treatments and are only used in a subgroup of patients. Their use should be carefully evaluated. The short-term use of antibiotics such as metronidazole or ciprofloxacin during pregnancy requires a strict determination of indication; their long-term use is generally contraindicated. Table 5 provides a summary of some further IBD medications and their safety assessment during pregnancy [10, 15, 43].

Treatment of IBD in Nursing Women

Patients who wish to nurse their babies may be treated with steroids and 5-ASA derivatives without a significantly increased risk for the newborn [10, 15, 43].

The use of cortisone or 5-ASA preparations by the mother is not a problem during nursing since only negligible amounts of these drugs enter the child's organism through the milk and no permanent side effects for the baby are known. Since cortisone can pass through the milk into the baby, it is conceivable that an infant's cortisone intake during nursing could result in a depression of cortisone production in the baby's adrenal glands. If high doses of cortisone are required, careful follow-up of the infant by his pediatrician is important. The use of cortisone preparations should, however, be reduced as quickly as possible, both in pregnant and non-pregnant patients.

Immunosuppressants should be used with care in nursing women, as immunosuppressants are sometimes insufficiently metabolized in newborn with immature liver and may cause significant adverse events or unforeseeable long-term side effects [10, 15, 43].

Disclosure Statement

The authors declare that no financial or other conflict of interest exists in relation to the content of the article.

References

1 Timmer A, Goebell H: Incidence of ulcerative colitis, 1980–1995: a prospective study in an urban population in Germany. Z Gastroenterol 1999;37:1079–1084.
2 Timmer A, Breuer-Katschinski B, Goebell H: Time trends in the incidence and disease location of Crohn's disease 1980–1995: a prospective analysis in an urban population in Germany. Inflamm Bowel Dis 1999;5:79–84.
3 Hanan IM: Inflammatory bowel disease in the pregnant woman. Compr Ther 1998;24:409–414.
4 Nielsen OH, Andreasson B, Bondesen S, et al: Pregnancy in ulcerative colitis. Scand J Gastroenterol 1983;18:735–742.
5 Nielsen OH, Andreasson B, Bondesen S, et al: Pregnancy in Crohn's disease. Scand J Gastroenterol 1984;19:724–732.
6 Miller JP: Inflammatory bowel disease in pregnancy: a review. J R Soc Med 1986;79:221–225.
7 Khosla R, Willoughby CP, Jewell DP: Crohn's disease and pregnancy. Gut 1984;25:52–56.
8 Willoughby CP, Truelove SC: Ulcerative colitis and pregnancy. Gut 1980;21:469–474.
9 Woolfson K, Cohen Z, McLeod RS: Crohn's disease and pregnancy. Dis Colon Rectum 1990;33:869–873.

10 Connell WR: Safety of drug therapy for inflammatory bowel disease in pregnant and nursing women. Inflamm Bowel Dis 1996;2:33–47.
11 Alstead EM, Nelson-Piercy C: Inflammatory bowel disease in pregnancy. Gut 2003;52:159–161.
12 Subhani JM, Hamiliton MI: The management of inflammatory bowel disease during pregnancy. Aliment Pharmacol Ther 1998;12:1039–1053.
13 Habal FM, Hui G, Greenberg GR: Oral 5-aminosalicylic acid for inflammatory bowel disease in pregnancy: safety and clinical course. Gastroenterology 1993;105:1057–1060.
14 Diav-Citrin O, Park YH, Veerasuntharam G, et al: The safety of mesalamine in human pregnancy: a prospective controlled cohort study. Gastroenterology 1998;114:23–28.
15 Mottet C, Juillerat P, Pittet V, et al: Pregnancy and breastfeeding in patients with Crohn's disease. Digestion 2007;76:149–160.
16 Beaulieu DB, Ananthakrishnan AN, Issa M, et al: Budesonide induction and maintenance therapy for Crohn's disease during pregnancy. Inflamm Bowel Dis 2009;15:25–28.

17 O'Morain C, Smethurst P, Dore CJ, et al: Reversible male infertility due to sulphasalazine: studies in man and rat. Gut 1984;25:1078–1084.
18 Chatzinoff M, Guarino JM, Corson SL, et al: Sulfasalazine-induced abnormal sperm penetration assay reversed on changing to 5-aminosalicylic acid enemas. Dig Dis Sci 1988;33:108–110.
19 Alstead EM, Ritchie JK, Lennard-Jones JE, et al: Safety of azathioprine in pregnancy in inflammatory bowel disease. Gastroenterology 1990;99:443–446.
20 Rajapakse R, Korelitz BI: Inflammatory bowel disease during pregnancy. Curr Treat Options Gastroenterol 2001;4:245–251.
21 Francella A, Dyan A, Bodian C, et al: The safety of 6-mercaptopurine for childbearing patients with inflammatory bowel disease: a retrospective cohort study. Gastroenterology 2003;124:9–17.
22 Rayes N, Neuhaus R, David M, et al: Pregnancies following liver transplantation: how safe are they? A report of 19 cases under cyclosporine A and tacrolimus. Clin Transplant 1998;12:396–400.
23 Bertschinger P, Himmelmann A, Risti B, et al: Cyclosporine treatment of severe ulcerative colitis during pregnancy. Am J Gastroenterol 1995;90:330.

24 Baumgart DC, Sturm A, Wiedenmann B, et al: Uneventful pregnancy and neonatal outcome with tacrolimus in refractory ulcerative colitis. Gut 2005;54:1822–1823.

25 Marushak A, Weber T, Bock J, et al: Pregnancy following kidney transplantation. Acta Obstet Gynecol Scand 1986;65:557–559.

26 Huynh LA, Min DI: Outcomes of pregnancy and the management of immunosuppressive agents to minimize fetal risks in organ transplant patients. Ann Pharmacother 1994;28:1355–1357.

27 Roubenoff R, Hoyt J, Petri M, et al: Effects of anti-inflammatory and immunosuppressive drugs on pregnancy and fertility. Semin Arthritis Rheum 1988;18:88–110.

28 Penn I, Makowski EL, Harris P: Parenthood following renal transplantation. Kidney Int 1980;18:221–233.

29 Pirson Y, Van Lierde M, Ghysen J, et al: Retardation of fetal growth in patients receiving immunosuppressive therapy (letter). N Engl J Med 1985;313:328.

30 Dejaco C, Mittermaier C, Reinisch W, et al: Azathioprine treatment and male fertility in inflammatory bowel disease. Gastroenterology 2001;121:1048–1053.

31 Norgard B, Pedersen L, Fonager K, et al: Azathioprine, mercaptopurine and birth outcome: a population-based cohort study. Aliment Pharmacol Ther 2003;17:827–834.

32 Zlatanic J, Korelitz BI, Rajapakse R, et al: Complications of pregnancy and child development after cessation of treatment with 6-mercaptopurine for inflammatory bowel disease. J Clin Gastroenterol 2003;36:303–309.

33 Rajapakse RO, Korelitz BI, Zlatanic J, et al: Outcome of pregnancies when fathers are treated with 6-mercaptopurine for inflammatory bowel disease (see comments). Am J Gastroenterol 2000;95:684–688.

34 Kane SV: What's good for the goose should be good for the gander – 6-MP use in fathers with inflammatory bowel disease. Am J Gastroenterol 2000;95:581–582.

35 Katz JA, Antoni C, Keenan GF, et al: Outcome of pregnancy in women receiving infliximab for the treatment of Crohn's disease and rheumatoid arthritis. Am J Gastroenterol 2004;99:2385–2392.

36 O'Donnell S, O'Morain C: Review article: use of antitumour necrosis factor therapy in inflammatory bowel disease during pregnancy and conception. Aliment Pharmacol Ther 2008;27:885–894.

37 Mahadevan U, Kane S, Sandborn WJ, et al: Intentional infliximab use during pregnancy for induction or maintenance of remission in Crohn's disease. Aliment Pharmacol Ther 2005;21:733–738.

38 Vesga L, Terdiman JP, Mahadevan U: Adalimumab use in pregnancy. Gut 2005;54:890.

39 Coburn LA, Wise PE, Schwartz DA: The successful use of adalimumab to treat active Crohn's disease of an ileoanal pouch during pregnancy. Dig Dis Sci 2006;51:2045–2047.

40 Kane SV, Acquah LA: Placental transport of immunoglobulins: a clinical review for gastroenterologists who prescribe therapeutic monoclonal antibodies to women during conception and pregnancy. Am J Gastroenterol 2009;104:228–233.

41 Wu A, Nashan B, Messner U, et al: Outcome of 22 successful pregnancies after liver transplantation. Clin Transplant 1998;12:454–464.

42 Armenti VT, Moritz MJ, Davison JM: Drug safety issues in pregnancy following transplantation and immunosuppression: effects and outcomes. Drug Saf 1998;19:219–232.

43 Lamah M, Scott HJ: Inflammatory bowel disease and pregnancy. Int J Colorectal Dis 2002;17:216–222.

Dig Dis 2009;27:347–350
DOI: 10.1159/000228572

Mild to Moderate Crohn's Disease: Still Room for Step-Up Therapies?

Simon Bar-Meir

Sackler School of Medicine, Tel Aviv University, Tel Aviv, and Department of Gastroenterology, Chaim Sheba Medical Center, Tel Hashomer, Israel

Key Words

Immunosuppression · Crohn's disease · Infliximab · Step-up therapy · Top-down therapy

Abstract

Step-up therapy in Crohn's disease refers to the classic therapeutic approach resulting in progressive increase of therapies with the increasing severity of the disease. This approach has been recently challenged by the top-down strategy, where biologicals together with thiopurines were used as first-line therapy. Several arguments exist against the top-down therapy. The current ECCO recommendation is in favor of the step-up therapy. ECCO recommended budesonide 9 mg daily as the preferred treatment in mild to moderate Crohn's disease patients. The benefit of mesalazine in small bowel disease is limited and should be considered clinically no more effective than placebo. Antibiotics cannot be recommended unless septic complications are suspected. No treatment is an option for some patients with mild symptoms. Budesonide is preferred to prednisone for mild active Crohn's disease because it is associated with fewer side effects. Active mild colonic disease may be treated with sulfasalazine and when needed with systemic corticosteroids as well. Topical treatment should be considered for distal disease. The national cooperative Crohn's disease study and the European co-operative Crohn's disease study established corticosteroids as an effective therapy for inducing remission in Crohn's disease. Remission is achieved in 60–83% of the patients. A Cochrane review of the efficacy of azathioprine and 6-mercaptopurine for inducing remission in active Crohn's disease showed a benefit for thiopurine therapy compared with placebo. Methotrexate is another effective medication that has been confirmed in a systematic review. Once remission has been achieved with systemic corticosteroids, maintenance with azathioprine should be considered. For patients with extensive colitis, long-term treatment with mesalazine is an option as this may reduce the risk of colon cancer, although this is still unproved in Crohn's disease. In conclusion, the natural course of most patients with Crohn's disease is relatively mild and there is a room for step-up therapy. The efficacy of most medications is similar to the efficacy of infliximab but with less adverse effects. Infliximab should be reserved only for patients where other therapies failed.

Copyright © 2009 S. Karger AG, Basel

Step-up therapy in Crohn's disease refers to the classic therapeutic approach resulting in progressive increase of therapies with the increasing severity of the disease. This approach has been recently challenged by the top-down strategy, where biologicals and thiopurines are used as first-line therapy.

The author received research grants from the Falk Foundation for his research on the role of budesonide in Crohn's disease.

Prof. Simon Bar-Meir
Department of Gastroenterology, Chaim Sheba Medical Center
2 Sheba Road
IL–52621 Tel Hashomer (Israel)
E-Mail barmeirs@yahoo.com

It all started with studies like the one by Cosnes et al. [1] where despite earlier and widespread use of immunosuppressants in the last decade the cumulative need for intestinal resection has not been reduced. There is a stable percentage of 30% in the first 5 years after diagnosis. At the same time, in rheumatoid arthritis early introduction of anti- TNF therapy resulted in a modulation of the natural course [2]. Top-down therapy in rheumatoid arthritis was found to have a more rapid rate of improvement and less progression of joint damage compared to patients treated with methotrexate alone. The question is whether disease-modifying agents should be started first in Crohn's disease as well.

A recent paper by D'Haens et al. [3] seems to support this approach. In this study, patients with Crohn's disease were randomly assigned to either early combined immunosuppression or conventional treatment. The patients assigned to combined immunosuppression received 3 infusions of infliximab at weeks 0, 2 and 6, together with azathioprine. Additional treatment with infliximab and, if necessary, corticosteroids were administered to control disease activity. Azathioprine was administered during the entire study. Patients assigned to conventional management received corticosteroids, followed in sequence by azathioprine and infliximab. For those who responded to corticosteroid therapy the steroids were tapered to discontinuation. Patients were not given azathioprine unless they had relapsed. The primary outcome measures were remission without corticosteroids and without bowel resection at weeks 26 and 52. The investigators found that 60% of patients in the combined immunosuppression group were in remission compared with 35.9% in the conventional therapy. Corresponding rates at week 52 were 61.5 and 42.2%. Based on their results they concluded that combined immunosuppression was more effective than conventional management for induction of remission and reduction of corticosteroid use in patients recently diagnosed with Crohn's disease. They felt that initiation of more intensive treatment early in the course of the disease could result in better outcomes.

Several arguments exist against the top-down approach in Crohn's disease. First, data from a large population-based study performed in Copenhagen County showed that 80% of Crohn's disease patients maintain high disease activity only in the first year after diagnosis. This percentage decreases dramatically after the first year. At any given year after this, about 55% of Crohn's disease patients are in stable remission [4]. In addition, prospective studies from the GETAID included patients

in remission after corticosteroid treatment; the probability of remission off corticosteroid therapy was 60% at 12 months and 53% at 18 months. In addition, about half of the patients do have already a complication at the time of diagnosis [5]. Taken together, these data indicate that the indiscriminate use of infliximab as first-line therapy would represent an overtreatment for most of Crohn's disease patients.

Last but not least, in the study by D'Haens et al. [3], in the conventional arm no maintenance of azathioprine or methotrexate was given after the first course of corticosteroids. It has been already shown that in Crohn's disease the chance of relapse without maintenance over 1 year is 75%.

The lack of maintenance therefore may explain the high relapse rate. On the other hand, in the combined immunosuppression arm azathioprine was administered during the entire study, and this may play a major role in the higher remission rate in the combined immunosuppressant arm. It is of interest that in D'Haens study, at the end of 1 year, 76% of the patients in the conventional arm were on immunosuppressant drugs with disappearance of the difference in efficacy between the two therapeutic arms during the second year.

Infliximab is not an innocent medication, and the incidence of serious infections during infliximab therapy is increased compared to a control group (4–4.2 vs. 8.2–8.3%, respectively) [6], in particular the risk of active tuberculosis [7]. Hepatosplenic T cell lymphoma is another complication previously reported with infliximab [8]. In rheumatoid arthritis, infliximab was found to be associated with 3-fold increase in malignancy and 2-fold increase in serious infection [9]. In the study by D'Haens et al. [3], the top-down therapy was associated with a higher rate of serious adverse events than the conventional therapy – 31 vs. 25%, respectively.

Studies done separately on induction and maintenance of remission in Crohn's disease showed a similar efficacy for biological therapy and step-up therapy. In the ACCENT 1 study, 57% of Crohn's patients had an initial response and less than 20% of initial responders were in remission at the end of 1 year [10]. In the ACCENT 2 study, 58% showed an initial response and less than 20% of initial responders were healed at 1 year [11]. Conventional therapy with corticosteroids induced remission of 61% at 16 weeks [12], 83% at 6 weeks [13] and 92% at 7 weeks [14]. Azathioprine given for maintenance of remission was effective in two thirds of the patients [15]. Methotrexate given to Crohn's disease patients for 40 weeks maintained remission in 65% of the patients, which was significantly higher than the 39% in the placebo group. The prednisone requirement went down to 28 and 58%, respectively, in the methotrexate and placebo group, respectively [16]. Thus, conventional therapies do not seem to be less effective than biologicals.

Two important trials [12, 13] (The National Cooperative Crohn's Disease Study and the European Co-operative Crohn's Disease Study) established corticosteroids as an effective therapy for inducing remission in Crohn's disease. Remission was achieved in 60–83% of the patients.

ECCO statement therefore does not recommend starting with biological therapy in mild to moderate Crohn's disease [16]. Budesonide 9 mg daily is the preferred treatment in mild to moderate CD patients. The benefit of mesalazine is limited. At this stage, 5-ASA should be considered clinically no more effective than placebo for active ileal or colonic disease. Antibiotics cannot be recommended unless septic complications are suspected. No treatment is an option for some patients with mild symptoms. Budesonide 9 mg daily is favored because it is superior to both placebo (OR 2.85, 95% CI 1.67–4.87) and 5-ASA 4 g/day (OR 2.8, 95% CI 1.50–5.20) and achieves remission in 51–60% over 8–10 weeks. Budesonide is preferred to prednisolone for mild active Crohn's disease because it is associated with fewer side effects. Active mild colonic Crohn's disease may be treated with sulfasalazine and if needed with systemic corticosteroids as well. Topical treatment should be considered for distal disease. Any patient who has an early relapse is best started on an immunomodulator.

A Cochrane review found budesonide to be less effective than prednisone (RR = 0.87) for induction of remission in patients with Crohn's disease [17]. In our study which is part of this Cochrane review [18], 200 patients with mild to moderate Crohn's disease were randomized to receive either budesonide or prednisone. Both drugs turned out to be of similar efficacy. However, there were twice as many patients who responded without adverse effects in the budesonide group compared to the prednisone group. Budesonide had its maximal therapeutic effect in patients with disease of the terminal ileum. Once the colon became involved, the efficacy of budesonide decreased and it reached 20% only with left colonic involvement. The low efficacy of budesonide with colonic involvement is due to the location of budesonide absorption which is mainly in the distal small intestine. Only a small amount of budesonide is available for the right side of the colon and even less for the left colon.

For patients with Crohn's colitis sulfasalazine or corticosteroids are the treatment of choice. When the disease is in the distal colon, topical treatment should be considered. Infliximab should be considered if the disease is refractory to corticosteroids or immunomodulators.

There is inconsistent evidence for the efficacy of mesalazine in active Crohn's disease. A meta-analysis proved significant reduction of 18 points in CDAI in favor of mesalazine. However, from a clinical point of view this result is irrelevant.

Once medical induced remission has been achieved with systemic corticosteroids, thiopurine or methotrexate should be considered. Corticosteroids should not be used to maintain remission. Two meta-analyses failed to show any advantage of mesalamine over placebo in maintenance of remission of Crohn's disease [19, 20].

For patients with extensive colitis, long-term treatment with mesalamine is an option as this may reduce the risk of colon cancer, although this is still unproved in Crohn's disease.

A Cochrane review on the efficacy of azathioprine and 6-mercaptopurine for induction of remission in active CD showed a benefit for thiopurine therapy compared with placebo with an odds ratio of 2.36 (95% CI 1.57–3.53). This equates to an NNT of 5 and a number needed to harm (NNH) of 14 [21]. Methotrexate is another effective medication that has been confirmed in a systematic review [22]. In a controlled study, a larger number of the methotrexate-treated group was able to withdrawn from corticosteroids and also went into remission compared with placebo (39 vs. 19%; p = 0.025) [23].

ECCO recommends that if remission has been achieved with systemic corticosteroids, azathioprine should be considered. For patients with extensive colitis, long-term treatment with mesalamine is an option as this may reduce the risk of colon cancer, although this is still unproved in Crohn's disease. For patients in remission on azathioprine as maintenance treatment, cessation may be considered after 4 years of full remission, but a small treatment benefit persists even after 6 years.

Infliximab should be considered in addition to corticosteroids or immunomodulators in case the disease is refractory. It causes rapid mucosal healing while displaying steroid-sparing properties. It induces closure of perianal fistulas and fewer hospitalizations and operations related to Crohn's disease [24]. It is considered the last medical resort before handing over the patient to the surgeon.

In conclusion, the natural course of most patients with Crohn's disease is relatively mild and there is room for step-up therapy. The efficacy of most medications is similar to the efficacy of infliximab but with less adverse effects. Infliximab should be reserved only for patients where other therapies failed.

Disclosure Statement

The author declares that no financial or other conflict of interest exists in relation to the content of the article.

References

1 Cosnes J, Nion-Larmurier I, Beaugerie L, Afchain P, Tiret E, Gendre JP: Impact of the increasing use of immunosuppressants in Crohn's disease on the need for intestinal surgery. Gut 2005;54:237–241.
2 Goekoop-Ruiterman YP, de Vries-Bouwstra JK, Allaart CF, van Zeben D, Kerstens PJ, Hazes JM, Zwinderman AH, Ronday HK, Han KH, Westedt ML, Gerards AH, van Groenendael JH, Lems WF, van Krugten MV, Breedveld FC, Dijkmans BA: Clinical and radiographic outcomes of four different treatment strategies in patients with early rheumatoid arthritis (the BeSt study): a randomized, controlled trial. Arthritis Rheum 2005;52:3381–3390.
3 D'Haens G, Baert F, van Assche G, Caenepeel P, Vergauwe P, Tuynman H, De Vos M, van Deventer S, Stitt L, Donner A, Vermeire S, Van de Mierop FJ, Coche JC, van der Woude J, Ochsenkühn T, van Bodegraven AA, Van Hootegem PP, Lambrecht GL, Mana F, Rutgeerts P, Feagan BG, Hommes D: Early combined immunosuppression or conventional management in patients with newly diagnosed Crohn's disease: an open randomised trial. Lancet 2008;371:660–667.
4 Munkholm P, Langholz E, Davidsen M, Binder V: Disease activity courses in a regional cohort of Crohn's disease patients. Scand J Gastroenterol 1995;30:699–706.
5 Papi C, Festa V, Fagnani C, Stazi A, Antonelli G, Moretti A, Koch M, Capurso L: Evolution of clinical behaviour in Crohn's disease: predictive factors of penetrating complications. Dig Liver Dis 2005;37:247–253.
6 Sandborn WJ, Loftus EV: Balancing the risks and benefits of infliximab in the treatment of inflammatory bowel disease. Gut 2004;53: 780–782.
7 Keane J, Gershon S, Wise RP, Mirabile-Levens E, Kasznica J, Schwieterman WD, Siegel JN, Braun MM: Tuberculosis associated with infliximab, a tumor necrosis factor alpha-neutralizing agent. N Engl J Med 2001;345:1098–1104.

8 Thayu M, Markowitz JE, Mamula P, Russo PA, Muinos WI, Baldassano RN: Hepatosplenic T-cell lymphoma in an adolescent patient after immunomodulator and biologic therapy for Crohn disease. J Pediatr Gastroenterol Nutr 2005;40:220–222.
9 Bongartz T, Sutton AJ, Sweeting MJ, Buchan I, Matteson EL, Montori V: Anti-TNF antibody therapy in rheumatoid arthritis and the risk of serious infections and malignancies: systematic review and meta-analysis of rare harmful effects in randomized controlled trials. JAMA 2006;295:2275–2285.
10 Hanauer SB, Feagan BG, Lichtenstein GR, Mayer LF, Schreiber S, Colombel JF, Rachmilewitz D, Wolf DC, Olson A, Bao W, Rutgeerts P: Maintenance infliximab for Crohn's disease: the ACCENT I randomised trial. Lancet 2002;359:1541–1549.
11 Present DH, Rutgeerts P, Targan S, Hanauer SB, Mayer L, van Hogezand RA, Podolsky DK, Sands BE, Braakman T, DeWoody KL, Schaible TF, van Deventer SJ: Infliximab for the treatment of fistulas in patients with Crohn's disease. N Engl J Med 1999;340:1398–1405.
12 Summers RW, Switz DM, Sessions JT Jr, Becktel JM, Best WR, Kern F Jr, Singleton JW: National Cooperative Crohn's Disease Study: results of drug treatment. Gastroenterology 1979;77:847–869.
13 Malchow H, Ewe K, Brandes JW, Goebell H, Ehms H, Sommer H, Jesdinsky H: European Cooperative Crohn's Disease Study (ECCDS): results of drug treatment. Gastroenterology 1984;86:249–266.
14 Modigliani R, Mary JY, Simon JF, Cortot A, Soule JC, Gendre JP, Rene E: Clinical, biological, and endoscopic picture of attacks of Crohn's disease: evolution on prednisolone. Gastroenterology 1990;98:811–818.
15 Pearson DC, May GR, Fick G, Sutherland LR: Azathioprine for maintaining remission of Crohn's disease. Cochrane Database Syst Rev 2009;1:CD000067.
16 Travis SP, Stange EF, Lémann M, Oresland T, Chowers Y, Forbes A, D'Haens G, Kitis G, Cortot A, Prantera C, Marteau P, Colombel JF, Gionchetti P, Bouhnik Y, Tiret E, Kroesen J, Starlinger M, Mortensen NJ; European Crohn's and Colitis Organisation: European evidence based consensus on the diagnosis and management of Crohn's disease: current management. Gut 2006;55(suppl 1):i16–i35.

17 Otley A, Steinhart AH: Budesonide for induction of remission in Crohn's disease. Cochrane Database Syst Rev 2008;3: CD000296.
18 Bar-Meir S, Chowers Y, Lavy A, Abramovitch D, Sternberg A, Leichtmann G, Reshef R, Odes S, Moshkovitz M, Bruck R, Eliakim R, Maoz E, Mittmann U: Budesonide versus prednisone in the treatment of active Crohn's disease. The Israeli Budesonide Study Group. Gastroenterology 1998;115:835–840.
19 Cammà C, Giunta M, Rosselli M, Cottone M: Mesalamine in the maintenance treatment of Crohn's disease: a meta-analysis adjusted for confounding variables. Gastroenterology 1997;113:1465–1473.
20 Akobeng AK, Gardener E: Oral 5-aminosalicylic acid for maintenance of medically induced remission in Crohn's disease. Cochrane Database Syst Rev 2005;1: CD003715.
21 Sandborn W, Sutherland L, Pearson D, May G, Modigliani R, Prantera C: Azathioprine or 6-mercaptopurine for inducing remission of Crohn's disease. Cochrane Database Syst Rev 2000;2:CD000545.
22 Alfadhli AA, McDonland JW, Feagan BG: Methotrexate for induction of remission in refractory Crohn's disease. Cochrane Database Syst Rev 2005;1:CD003459.
23 Feagan BG, Fedorak RN, Irvine EJ, Wild G, Sutherland L, Steinhart AH, Greenberg GR, Koval J, Wong CJ, Hopkins M, Hanauer SB, McDonald JW: A comparison of methotrexate with placebo for the maintenance of remission in Crohn's disease. North American Crohn's Study Group Investigators. N Engl J Med 2000;342:1627–1632.
24 Lichtenstein GR, Yan S, Bala M, Blank M, Sands BE: Infliximab maintenance treatment reduces hospitalizations, surgeries, and procedures in fistulizing Crohn's disease. Gastroenterology 2005;128:862–869.

Dig Dis 2009;27:351–357
DOI: 10.1159/000228573

Anti-Tumor Necrosis Factor Nonresponders in Crohn's Disease: Therapeutic Strategies

E. Louis   J. Belaiche   C. Reenaers

Department of Gastroenterology, CHU of Liège, and GIGA Research, University of Liège, Liège, Belgium

Key Words
Anti-TNF · Crohn's disease · Nonresponders

Abstract

Anti-TNF antibodies have revolutionized the treatment of Crohn's disease. In pivotal trials, however, the frequencies of primary and secondary nonresponders appeared rather high with, by the end of 1 year of scheduled treatment, only one fifth of the patients initially treated still in sustained remission. Other studies and monocentric experiences have indicated that these seemingly disappointing results were partly due to suboptimal selection of the patients and absence of treatment optimization. Optimal selection of the patient includes proving active intestinal lesions and systemic inflammation as well as excluding stricturing or infectious complications. Treatment optimization includes potential immunosuppressive co-treatment and dose or administration interval adjustment of the anti-TNF. When a failure is confirmed with an anti-TNF despite such optimization, second- or third-line anti-TNFs have proved useful. Beyond that, a transient steroid course and surgical procedures still represent rescue option, waiting for new promising biologics in development.   Copyright © 2009 S. Karger AG, Basel

Introduction

Anti-TNF treatments have dramatically changed the disease outcome in Crohn's disease (CD). Infliximab and then adalimumab and certolizumab pegol have shown a significant efficacy in severe CD refractory to conventional treatments, including immunosuppressive drugs [1–3]. A significant efficacy has also been proven for fistulizing CD, in a specific placebo-controlled trial with infliximab and in a post hoc analysis of a general pivotal trial with adalimumab [2, 4]. This clinical efficacy has been associated with mucosal healing and improvement of quality of life. The clinical efficacy of anti-TNF has also a major impact on important disease outcomes, with a reduction of hospitalization and surgeries [5, 6]. However, some patients do not respond to anti-TNF treatments and a significant proportion of responders may lose response over time. After the hope for the patients generated by the advent of anti-TNF, it is now time to try and optimize our strategies to prevent non-response or loss of response as well as develop new treatment options for these patients.

Primary Nonresponse

The frequency of primary nonresponse with anti-TNF varies according to the treatment strategies that have been used, the definition of nonresponse and the popula-

Prof. Edouard Louis
Service de Gastroentérologie
CHU de Liège, Domaine du Sart Tilman
BE–4000 Liège (Belgium)
Tel. +32 4366 7256, Fax +32 4366 7889, E-Mail edouard.louis@ulg.ac.be

tion studied. The variation is huge as it goes from 10% for nonresponse in monocentric uncontrolled experiences [7, 8] to 75% for the absence of remission in pivotal placebo-controlled clinical trials [9–11]. Placebo-controlled trials with infliximab, adalimumab and certolizumab pegol of course give the most robust data. However, the analysis of remission and response rates in these different trials gives us some insight into the mechanisms of primary nonresponse.

Magnitude and Mechanisms of Primary Nonresponse
In the placebo-controlled trials, the percentages of response and remission after induction ranged from 58–64% and from 18–36%, respectively [9–11]. These trials have also shown the crucial importance of an induction regimen. Particularly with adalimumab, only the induction with 160 mg followed 2 weeks later by 80 mg gave a remission rate greater than placebo at 4 weeks [10]. However, response rates were higher than with placebo also with lower-dosage induction regimens. With certolizumab pegol, only one induction scheme was tested with 400 mg at weeks 0, 2 and 4. This scheme failed to show any significant difference in remission rate as compared to placebo at week 6, while there was a significant difference in response rate [11]. With infliximab, an induction with an infusion of 5 mg/kg at weeks 0, 2 and 6 was superior to only one infusion at week zero for the response rate at week 10 [1]. However, a single infusion at week 0 was already superior to placebo when assessing remission rate at week 4 [9].

Post hoc analysis of the trials with these three anti-TNFs has also shown that the response and remission rates were higher in patients with a shorter duration of the disease [2, 3]. Particularly with certolizumab pegol, the response rates were 90% and 57% for disease duration shorter than 1 year and longer than 5 years, respectively, while it was 37 and 33%, respectively, for the placebo with the same disease durations [3]. This difference may indicate either a change in the immunoinflammatory process over the course of the disease [12] or the development of fibrotic lesions and after-effects that are less responsive to anti-TNF [13].

Various types of cotreatment have been tested across the controlled trials with anti-TNF. Even if post hoc analyses of pivotal placebo-controlled trials failed to show in the majority of cases a significant difference in response or remission rates according to the concomitant use of steroids or immunosuppressive treatments [1–3], other trials, including some specifically designed to answer this question, have indicated significant differences. In the

GETAID so-called 'bridge' study, steroid-dependent patients were put or kept under purine analogues and received either a placebo or infliximab 3-dose induction [14]. The remission rate without steroid at 12 weeks in the arm receiving an infliximab induction on the top of purine analogues and, at the beginning steroid treatment, was historically high at 75%. Likewise, in the COMMIT study comparing a treatment with infliximab and methotrexate to a treatment with infliximab and placebo, all the patients received an induction regimen with 3 weeks of steroids [15]. While in this study there was no difference between the placebo and methotrexate groups, the remission rate without steroids at 14 weeks was above 75% in both groups. These two studies, albeit not specifically designed to answer this question, indicate the potential added value of a course of steroids during induction with anti-TNF. More recently, the SONIC study has clearly shown the benefit of a co-treatment with immunosuppressive drug (at least purine analogues) during infliximab induction [16]. In this study specifically designed to compare azathioprine monotherapy, infliximab monotherapy and infliximab + azathioprine combined therapy in patients naïve from immunosuppressive drugs, the steroid-free remission at 26 weeks was 30.6, 44.4 and 56.8%, respectively. Although the remission rate with an anti-TNF monotherapy is already reasonably high and significantly superior to placebo, the results also indicate that more than 10% of nonresponse could be avoided by a concomitant immunosuppressive treatment. However, the benefit of such combined treatment is still not proven in patients who are not naïve from immunosuppressive drugs. Furthermore, in immunosuppressive-naïve patients, owing to the potential increase in the risk of lymphoma [17] and opportunistic infections [18] with combined treatment, the benefit/risk ratio of such combined therapy should be discussed on a case-by-case basis.

Another aspect that has been clearly confirmed by the SONIC study, but that had already been shown in previous studies [19], is the suboptimal response in patients having no increase in C-reactive protein (CRP). Although there is no significant correlation between the magnitude of the response to anti-TNF and the blood concentration of CRP, the patients who have a normal CRP, indicating the absence of significant systemic inflammation, have a significantly lower response rate. In this group of patients, the response to combined therapy was not superior to the one to anti-TNF or azathioprine alone. The same holds true for the group of patients without endoscopic evidence of active disease. A way to significantly reduce anti-TNF nonresponse is thus to avoid treating patients with normal CRP or at least to check for signs of active disease in these patients at endoscopy or imaging, although the criteria for definition of active disease at imaging are less clearly defined than at endoscopy. Other particular clinical situations are also associated with suboptimal response to anti-TNF: fibrotic strictures and insufficiently drained perianal lesions. In a monocentric series analyzing nonresponse or loss of response to infliximab in CD, 2/3 of these nonresponders had a luminal stricture, mainly in the small bowel [13]. However, clinical experience shows that some active inflammatory stricturing CD can improve with anti-TNF [20]. Important ongoing studies are aiming at precisely defining the type of stricturing disease that could still respond to infliximab, particularly using imaging techniques such as magnetic resonance imaging. As far as perianal disease is concerned, a perianal abscess not properly drained is a contraindication to anti-TNF treatment. Uncontrolled studies have also indicated an optimization of the response to anti-TNF treatment with strategy combining exploration under anesthesia (possibly preceded by MRI or ultrasound endoscopy), full drainage of the lesion and sometimes antibiotics [21].

Other features that have been associated with lower response rates to infliximab are older age, small bowel location and smoking [22]. Smoking is particularly relevant since the start of an anti-TNF treatment as it is for surgery can be a good occasion to try and motivate the patient to stop smoking.

Since the beginning of the use of anti-TNF in CD, hope has existed that one could predict response and select appropriate patients by using biomarkers. Hence, a large number of studies have evaluated serological markers [23], pharmacogenetics [24–27], proteomics [28] and tissue micro-array [29] searching for the Holy Grail. However, until now these studies have been disappointing, either finding markers that have not been replicated and representing probably false-positive results, or confirming markers which have such a weak impact that they are not useful in clinical practice.

Therapeutic Strategy in Primary Nonresponders
Published results from the experience of referral centers in routine practice have shown that appropriate patient selection and induction strategy could lead to response rates higher than in controlled trials reaching 60–90%. However, even in routine practice, there is still a proportion of patients not responding to an appropriate induction to anti-TNF. There are very little data in the literature on such patients. Infliximab primary nonresponders have usually been excluded from controlled clinical trials with new anti-TNF including adalimumab and certolizumab pegol, and phase-3 controlled trials with new biologics such as anti-IL-12/anti-IL-23 or anti-alpha4-beta7, that will include anti-TNF primary nonresponders, are only currently starting. However, these infliximab primary nonresponders could be included in the CARE trial, an open label trial with adalimumab having included more than 900 patients in Europe. The remission rate at week 20 in this subgroup of patients was not significantly different from the one of secondary loss of response and reached 36%, indicating a relevant benefit also in this category of patients [30].

Secondary Nonresponse (Loss of Response)

The secondary nonresponse to anti-TNF treatment is defined by a loss of response in a patient having primarily responded to the drug. As for primary nonresponse, the frequency varies according to the definition used to determine loss of response. In the literature, its frequency ranges from 50% over 1 year in the placebo-controlled phase 3 trials [1–3] to 35% over 5 years in large monocentric experience [7]. The main difference between clinical trials and routine practice is the possibility of optimizing treatment. Any relapse with the need of optimizing treatment has been considered as a failure in clinical trials, while in routine practice, the drug is still used and still benefits the patient.

Magnitude and Mechanisms of Secondary Nonresponse
In the pivotal placebo-controlled trials with infliximab, adalimumab or certolizumab pegol, the loss of response rate was approximately 50% over 1 year. The loss of response has usually been described as an increase of 70 points in CDAI and 25% judged in comparison to the CDAI reached at the time of assessment of response to the induction treatment.

When anti-TNFs were used episodically, essentially infliximab, the main mechanism of loss of response was the development of anti-therapeutic antibody antibodies [31]. This mechanism has been well described as a cause of not only loss of response or shortening of the response but also infusion reactions. It was clearly associated with episodic infliximab monotherapy and was much less frequent when using immunosuppressive cotreatment [31–33]. When using systematic scheduled maintenance treatment, as in the phase 3 pivotal trials with infliximab, adalimumab and certolizumab pegol, the influence of immunosuppressive cotreatment was much weaker and no longer statistically significant [1–3]. When comparing controlled trials with scheduled anti-TNF maintenance, there was no relevant difference between infliximab, adalimumab and certolizumab pegol, indicating that the humanization of the antibody had no strong influence on immunization when the drug was used on a scheduled basis. In a controlled trial specifically designed to determine whether the prolongation of immunosuppressive drug was useful beyond 6 months after the induction, no clear clinical benefit was found in the group of patients in whom the immunosuppressive drug was maintained over a 2-year period, indicating that after a 6-month induction with combined therapy, an anti-TNF monotherapy was probably sufficient [34]. However, when analysing more profoundly their data, the authors found both lower CRP and higher infliximab trough levels in patients maintained on the combined therapy with immunosuppressive drug. This may indicate a relevant difference with potential clinical impact over a longer period of time. Indeed, in other studies both with infliximab and adalimumab, the trough levels of the therapeutic antibody have been associated with the clinical efficacy [33, 35].

Although one of the reasons for low therapeutic antibody trough level is the development of antitherapeutic antibody antibodies, this is not the only mechanism since up to 25% of the patients with such low levels have no antibodies [33]. The clearance of the therapeutic antibodies considerably varies among patients and antitherapeutic antibodies development is only one of the reasons. Cotreatment with immunosuppressive drug, particularly methotrexate in patients with rheumatoid arthritis, has been shown to significantly delay the clearance of infliximab independently from antibody formation [36]. The mechanism by which immunosuppressive treatment could influence the clearance of therapeutic antibodies remains unclear. When the loss of response is due to an increased clearance of the anti-TNF, optimization of the treatment is required. This can be achieved either by increasing the dosage of the anti-TNF or by reducing the interval between administrations. According to pharmacokinetic modeling, this second option appears more effective and should be preferred unless the response after an injection is completely absent [37]. In this particular case, a transient increase in dosage is certainly to be tested. According to large monocentric experiences, such anti-TNF optimization allows a sus-

tained benefit over 5 years in approximately two thirds of the patients [7].

Beside the disappearance of the therapeutic antibody from the organism, mainly two other reasons may explain loss of response to anti-TNF: first, the escape of the immuno-inflammatory process with the development of a TNF-independent inflammation, and second, the development of complications. The first reason is theoretically plausible but has never really been proven: it remains a working hypothesis. The second reason has clearly been shown in routine practice and published trials and series. The three main complications that may induce a loss of response are concurrent gastrointestinal tract infection, the development of a fibrotic stricture and intra-abdominal or perianal abscess. A flare between two anti-TNF injections should always prompt the search for an infectious complication. Particularly, *Clostridium difficile* infection is not a rare finding in CD patients and is more frequent than in the general population [38]. While some case reports of intestinal strictures developing under anti-TNF treatment have been reported, a post-hoc analysis of the ACCENT 1 trial did not show an increase in the development of symptomatic strictures in patients treated with infliximab as compared to placebo [39]. Over 10 years after the diagnosis of CD, up to one third of the patient develop stricturing disease and a fibrotic stricture is probably part of healing inflammation in some patients. The development of a perianal abscess may be the consequence of an inappropriate drainage before starting anti-TNF treatment but can also develop during the scheduled maintenance treatment in an appropriately drained patient. A full drainage of the lesions, possibly leaving in place a loose seton and in association with a short course of antibiotics, usually solves the problem and often even does not require to stop or change anti-TNF. A short interruption to allow full healing of the infection is sometimes necessary. In more severe cases of relapsing abscesses despite apparently optimal drainage, usually linked to complex multiple fistulas, a protection stoma is required to allow the action of anti-TNF.

Therapeutic Strategy in Loss of Response to Anti-TNF
The first anti-TNF used in CD has been infliximab. Therefore, the data available for second-line anti-TNF essentially concerns treatment of infliximab failure with adalimumab or certolizumab pegol. For adalimumab, both uncontrolled trials and the placebo-controlled GAIN trial have shown good efficacy [40–41]. Although slightly lower than for anti-TNF-naïve patients, the re-

sponse and remission rates were superior to placebo and indicate a relevant benefit for the patients with a remission and a response at 4 weeks in one quarter and one half of the patients, respectively [41]. For certolizumab pegol, only an uncontrolled trial was performed [42]. This trial indicates a response rate similar to the one observed with adalimumab, i.e. slightly above half of the patients. Recently, a multicentric retrospective study also analyzed the response rate in patients treated with a third-line anti-TNF [43]. These patients had in the vast majority first failed infliximab and were secondarily treated with either adalimumab or certolizumab pegol. The third-line anti-TNF was thus either adalimumab or certolizumab pegol. While the remission and response rates were quantitatively close to the one observed in the second-line GAIN trial, the loss of response to this third-line anti-TNF was rather sharp with approximately 2/3 of the responders stopping the treatment over 1 year due to loss of benefit or intolerance.

The patients who failed a third-line anti-TNF have usually already failed purine analogues and methotrexate and have got a high cumulated dose of steroids. Even if steroids very often remain transiently efficacious in these situations, they do not represent a good long-term option. Alternative options are surgery or inclusion in trials with new promising drugs. Surgery remains acceptable when the resection is limited and does not affect a critical part of the gastrointestinal tract. In other situations, new medical treatment is certainly preferable. Among the new promising treatments, natalizumab is already available in the United States as a rescue treatment after anti-TNF failure. This antibody interacts with the alpha-4 integrin, which is part of several dimeric integrins involved in lymphocyte homing and costimulatory signals. Its efficacy, particularly as a maintenance treatment, has been well demonstrated in placebo-controlled trials [44, 45]. Globally, the tolerance was excellent and this drug was considered as having a top profile as a maintenance drug, until progressive multifocal leukoencephalopathy appeared to affect 1/1,000 patients treated [46]. This pathology, usually fatal, is due to the reactivation of the ubiquitous JC virus and can currently not be prevented. That is the reason why this drug has not been introduced on the European market for CD yet, while, due to an estimation of a favorable benefit/risk profile, it is available for multiple sclerosis. Beyond this, a more specific inhibitor of lymphocyte homing is currently entering phase 3 trials in CD: MLN-0002, interacting with alpha 4-beta 7 integrin, which binds to Mad-cam 1, mainly expressed in intestinal endothelium and involved in gut lymphocyte homing. Another promising track for the treatment of CD is IL-23/IL-12 inhibition. Two antibodies directed towards the common p40 subunit are currently entering phase 3 trials.

Conclusions

Anti-TNF has revolutionized the treatment of severe CD. A good pretreatment workup allows to select optimal indication for such treatment and to reduce the rate of nonresponse below one quarter of the patients. The use of an optimal induction scheme together with immunosuppressive and/or steroid cotreatment leads to an even higher response rate. However, the benefit/risk ratio of such combined treatment should be discussed on a case-by-case basis. Secondary loss of response is mainly due to rapid clearance of the anti-TNF from the organism and is associated with low trough levels of these drugs. This rapid clearance is partly linked to the development of antitherapeutic antibody formation, but other mechanisms are also involved. The problem may be solved in approximately half of the cases by either increasing the dosage or decreasing the interval between anti-TNF administrations. In case of loss of response to an anti-TNF, stricturing complication, abdominal and perianal abscesses as well as superinfection must always be excluded. In case of failure to an anti-TNF despite optimization and absence of complication, a second or even a third anti-TNF may reveal effective. Surgery or temporary steroid treatment are rescue options.

Disclosure Statement

The authors declare that no financial or other conflict of interest exists in relation to the content of the article.

References

1 Hanauer S, Feagan B, Lichtenstein G, et al: Maintenance infliximab for Crohn's disease: the ACCENT I randomised trial. Lancet 2002;359:1541–1549.

2 Colombel J, Sandborn W, Rutgeerts P, et al: Adalimumab for maintenance of clinical response and remission in patients with Crohn's disease: the CHARM trial. Gastroenterology 2007;132:52–65.

3 Schreiber S, Khaliq-Kareemi, Lauwrance I, et al: Maintenance therapy with certolizumab pegol for Crohn's disease. N Engl J Med 2007;357:239–250.

4 Present DH, Rutgeerts P, Targan S, Hanauer SB, Mayer L, van Hogezand RA, Podolsky DK, Sands BE, Braakman T, DeWoody KL, Schaible TF, van Deventer SJ: Infliximab for the treatment of fistulas in patients with Crohn's disease. N Engl J Med 1999;340: 1398–1405.

5 Lichtenstein GR, Yan S, Bala M, Blank M, Sands BE: Infliximab maintenance treatment reduces hospitalizations, surgeries, and procedures in fistulizing Crohn's disease. Gastroenterology 2005;128:862–869.

6 Feagan BG, Panaccione R, Sandborn WJ, D'Haens GR, Schreiber S, Rutgeerts PJ, Loftus EV Jr, Lomax KG, Yu AP, Wu EQ, Chao J, Mulani P: Effects of adalimumab therapy on incidence of hospitalization and surgery in Crohn's disease: results from the CHARM study. Gastroenterology 2008;135:1493–1499.

7 Schnitzler F, Fidder H, Ferrante M, Noman M, Arijs I, Van Assche G, Hoffman I, Van Steen K, Vermeire S, Rutgeerts P: Long-term outcome of treatment with infliximab in 614 patients with Crohn's disease: results from a single-centre cohort. Gut 2009;58:492–500.

8 Marting A, Belaiche J, Louis E: Long term safety and efficacy of infliximab in routine practice. Acta Gastroenterol Belg 2007;10: D45.

9 Targan SR, Hanauer SB, van Deventer SJ, Mayer L, Present DH, Braakman T, DeWoody KL, Schaible TF, Rutgeerts PJ: A short-term study of chimeric monoclonal antibody cA2 to tumor necrosis factor alpha for Crohn's disease. Crohn's Disease cA2 Study Group. N Engl J Med 1997;337:1029–1035.

10 Hanauer SB, Sandborn WJ, Rutgeerts P, Fedorak RN, Lukas M, MacIntosh D, Panaccione R, Wolf D, Pollack P: Human anti-tumor necrosis factor monoclonal antibody (adalimumab) in Crohn's disease: the CLASSIC-I trial. Gastroenterology 2006;130:323–333.

11 Sandborn WJ, Feagan BG, Stoinov S, Honiball PJ, Rutgeerts P, Mason D, Bloomfield R, Schreiber S, PRECISE 1 Study Investigators: Certolizumab pegol for the treatment of Crohn's disease. N Engl J Med 2007;357:228–238.

12 Kugathasan S, Saubermann L, Smith L, et al: Mucosal T-cell immunoregulation varies in early and late inflammatory bowel disease. Gut 2007;56:1696–1705.

13 Prajapati D, et al: Symptomatic luminal stricture underlies infliximab non-response in Crohn's disease. Gastroenterology 2002; 122:A777.

14 Lémann M, Mary JY, Duclos B, Veyrac M, Dupas JL, Delchier JC, Laharie D, Moreau J, Cadiot G, Picon L, Bourreille A, Sobahni I, Colombel JF, Groupe d'Etude Therapeutique des Affections Inflammatoires du Tube Digestif (GETAID): Infliximab plus azathioprine for steroid-dependent Crohn's disease patients: a randomized placebo-controlled trial. Gastroenterology 2006;130:1054–1061.

15 Feagan BG, McDonald J, Panaccione, et al: A randomized trial of methotrexate in combination with infliximab for the treatment of Crohn's disease. Gut 2008;57(suppl 2):A66.

16 Colombel JF, Rutgeerts P, Reinisch W, et al: A randomized, double-blind, controlled trial comparing infliximab and infliximab plus azathioprine to azathioprine in patients with Crohn's disease naive to immunomodulators and biologic therapy. Gut 2008; 57(suppl 2):A1.

17 Mackey A, Green L, Liang L, Dinndorf P, Avigan M: Hepatosplenic T cell lymphoma associated with infliximab use in young patients treated for inflammatory bowel disease. J Pediatr Gastroenterol Nutr 2007;44: 265–267.

18 Toruner M, Loftus E, Harmsen W, et al: Risk factors for opportunistic infections in patients with inflammatory bowel disease. Gastroenterology 2008;134:929–936.

19 Louis E, Vermeire S, Rutgeerts P, et al: A positive response to infliximab in Crohn's disease is associated with a higher systemic inflammation before treatment but not with -308 TNF gene polymorphism. Scand J Gastroenterol 2002;37:818–824.

20 Louis E, Boverie J, Dewit O, Baert F, De Vos M, D'Haens G: Treatment of small bowel subocclusive Crohn's disease with infliximab: an open pilot study. Acta Gastroenterol Belg 2007;70:15–19.

21 Hyder S, Travis S, Jewell D, Mortensen N, Georges B: Fistulating anal Crohn's disease: results of combined surgical and infliximab treatment. Dis Colon Rectum 2006;49:1837–1841.

22 Vermeire S, Louis E, Carbonez A, et al: Demographic and clinical parameters influencing the short-term outcome of anti-tumor necrosis factor (infliximab) treatment in Crohn's disease. Am J Gastroenterol 2002; 97:2357–2363.

23 Esters N, Vermeire S, Joossens S, et al: Serological markers for prediction of response to anti-tumor necrosis factor treatment in Crohn's disease. Am J Gastroenterol 2002; 97:1458–1462.

24 Vermeire S, Louis E, Rutgeerts, et al: NOD2/CARD15 does not influence response to infliximab in Crohn's disease. Gastroenterology 2002;103:106–111.

25 Hlavaty T, Ferrante M, Henckaerts L, Pierik M, Rutgeerts P, Vermeire S: Predictive model for the outcome of infliximab therapy in Crohn's disease based on apoptotic pharmacogenetic index and clinical predictors. Inflamm Bowel Dis 2007;13:372–379.

26 Dideberg V, Théâtre E, Farnir F, Vermeire S, Rutgeerts P, Vos MD, Belaiche J, Franchimont D, Gossum AV, Louis E, Bours V: The TNF/ADAM 17 system: implication of an ADAM 17 haplotype in the clinical response to infliximab in Crohn's disease. Pharmacogenet Genomics 2006;16:727–734.

27 Louis EJ, Watier HE, Schreiber S, Hampe J, Taillard F, Olson A, Thorne N, Zhang H, Colombel JF: Polymorphism in IgG Fc receptor gene FCGR3A and response to infliximab in Crohn's disease: a subanalysis of the ACCENT I study. Pharmacogenet Genomics 2006;16:911–914.

28 Meuwis MA, Fillet M, Lutteri L, Marée R, Geurts P, de Seny D, Malaise M, Chapelle JP, Wehenkel L, Belaiche J, Merville MP, Louis E: Proteomics for prediction and characterization of response to infliximab in Crohn's disease: a pilot study. Clin Biochem 2008;41: 960–967.

29 Arijs I, Quintens R, Van Lommel L, et al: Effect of infliximab treatment on colonic mucosal gene expression profiles in patients with inflammatory bowel disease. Gut 2008; 57(suppl 2):A39.

30 Löfberg R, Louis E, Reinisch W, et al: Response to adalimumab in bionaive and anti-TNF exposed patients with Crohn's disease: results of a phase IIIb clinical trial. Gut 2008; 57(suppl 2):A248.

31 Baert F, Noman M, Vermeire S, Van Assche G, D'Haens G, Carbonez A, Rutgeerts P: Influence of immunogenicity on the long-term efficacy of infliximab in Crohn's disease. N Engl J Med 2003;348:601–608.

32 Hanauer SB, Wagner CL, Bala M, Mayer L, Travers S, Diamond RH, Olson A, Bao W, Rutgeerts P: Incidence and importance of antibody responses to infliximab after maintenance or episodic treatment in Crohn's disease. Clin Gastroenterol Hepatol 2004;2: 542–553.

33 Maser EA, Villela R, Silverberg MS, Greenberg GR: Association of trough serum infliximab to clinical outcome after scheduled maintenance treatment for Crohn's disease. Clin Gastroenterol Hepatol 2008;6:1112–1116.

34 Van Assche G, Magdelaine-Beuzelin C, D'Haens G, Baert F, Noman M, Vermeire S, Ternant D, Watier H, Paintaud G, Rutgeerts P: Withdrawal of immunosuppression in Crohn's disease treated with scheduled infliximab maintenance: a randomized trial. Gastroenterology 2008;134:1861–1868.

35 Karmiris K, Paintaud G, Degenne D, et al: Antibodies against adalimumab in Crohn's disease patients who failed infliximab treatment: correlation with clinical response and trough levels. Gut 2008;57(suppl 2):A67.

36 Maini RN, Breedveld FC, Kalden JR, Smolen JS, Davis D, Macfarlane JD, Antoni C, Leeb B, Elliott MJ, Woody JN, Schaible TF, Feldmann M: Therapeutic efficacy of multiple intravenous infusions of anti-tumor necrosis factor alpha monoclonal antibody combined with low-dose weekly methotrexate in rheumatoid arthritis. Arthritis Rheum 1998;41:1552–1563.

37 St Clair EW, Wagner CL, Fasanmade AA, Wang B, Schaible T, Kavanaugh A, Keystone EC: The relationship of serum infliximab concentrations to clinical improvement in rheumatoid arthritis: results from ATTRACT, a multicenter, randomized, double-blind, placebo-controlled trial. Arthritis Rheum 2002;46:1451–1459.

38 Nguyen GC, Kaplan GG, Harris ML, Brant SR: A national survey of the prevalence and impact of *Clostridium difficile* infection among hospitalized inflammatory bowel disease patients. Am J Gastroenterol 2008;103:1443–1450.

39 Lichtenstein GR, Olson A, Travers S, Diamond RH, Chen DM, Pritchard ML, Feagan BG, Cohen RD, Salzberg BA, Hanauer SB, Sandborn WJ: Factors associated with the development of intestinal strictures or obstructions in patients with Crohn's disease. Am J Gastroenterol 2006;101:1030–1038.

40 Sandborn WJ, Hanauer S, Loftus EV Jr, Tremaine WJ, Kane S, Cohen R, Hanson K, Johnson T, Schmitt D, Jeche R: An open-label study of the human anti-TNF monoclonal antibody adalimumab in subjects with prior loss of response or intolerance to infliximab for Crohn's disease. Am J Gastroenterol 2004;99:1984–1989.

41 Sandborn WJ, Rutgeerts P, Enns R, Hanauer SB, Colombel JF, Panaccione R, D'Haens G, Li J, Rosenfeld MR, Kent JD, Pollack PF: Adalimumab induction therapy for Crohn disease previously treated with infliximab: a randomized trial. Ann Intern Med 2007;146:829–838.

42 Vermeire S, Abreu M, D'Haens G, et al: Efficacy and safety of certolizumab pegol in patients with active Crohn's disease who previously lost response or were intolerant to infliximab: open-label induction preliminary results of the welcome study. Gastroenterology 2008;134(suppl 1):A-67.

43 Mozziconacci N, Vermeire S, Laharie D, et al: Efficacy of a third anti-TNF monoclonal antibody in Crohn's disease after failure of two other anti-TNF. Gastroenterology 2008;34(suppl 1):A-663.

44 Targan SR, Feagan BG, Fedorak RN, Lashner BA, Panaccione R, Present DH, Spehlmann ME, Rutgeerts PJ, Tulassay Z, Volfova M, Wolf DC, Hernandez C, Bornstein J, Sandborn WJ, International Efficacy of Natalizumab in Crohn's Disease Response and Remission (ENCORE) Trial Group: Natalizumab for the treatment of active Crohn's disease: results of the ENCORE Trial. Gastroenterology 2007;132:1672–1683.

45 Sandborn WJ, Colombel JF, Enns R, Feagan BG, Hanauer SB, Lawrance IC, Panaccione R, Sanders M, Schreiber S, Targan S, van Deventer S, Goldblum R, Despain D, Hogge GS, Rutgeerts P, International Efficacy of Natalizumab as Active Crohn's Therapy (ENACT-1) Trial Group; Evaluation of Natalizumab as Continuous Therapy (ENACT-2) Trial Group: Natalizumab induction and maintenance therapy for Crohn's disease. N Engl J Med 2005;353:1912–1925.

46 Yousry TA, Major EO, Ryschkewitsch C, Fahle G, Fischer S, Hou J, Curfman B, Miszkiel K, Mueller-Lenke N, Sanchez E, Barkhof F, Radue EW, Jäger HR, Clifford DB: Evaluation of patients treated with natalizumab for progressive multifocal leukoencephalopathy. N Engl J Med 2006;354:924–933.

Dig Dis 2009;27:358–365
DOI: 10.1159/000228574

Early Inflammatory Bowel Disease: Different Treatment Response to Specific or All Medications?

James Markowitz

Division of Pediatric Gastroenterology and Nutrition, Schneider Children's Hospital, North Shore – LIJ Health System, New Hyde Park, N.Y., USA

Key Words
Crohn's disease, children · Crohn's disease, adults · Therapeutic response

Abstract
Background: The literature suggests that medications prescribed for the treatment of inflammatory bowel disease may be more efficacious in children than adults. Care must be exercised in comparing these data, however, as significant differences in disease duration and concomitant therapy are present among studies. **Methods:** Review of key clinical trials, meta-analyses and observational registries for which there are treatment response data from both pediatric and adult Crohn's disease (CD) populations. **Results:** Acute response to corticosteroids is similar in children (84–89%) and adults (80–84%), but prolonged response may be better in children (50–61 vs. 32–44%). Differences in duration of CD among the various studies' subjects and the proportion of subjects receiving concomitant immunomodulators probably explain much of these differences. CD remission rates with thiopurines appear higher in children at both 6 months (85 vs. 31%) and 15–18 months (81 vs. 42%), but the reported outcomes are likely influenced by very short duration of CD in the pediatric populations studied. Similarly, remission of CD 1 year following initiation of infliximab also appears higher in children (56%) than adults (28%), but again differences in study populations' durations of CD and use of concomitant immunomodulators likely are responsible for the observed differences. **Conclusion:** Differences between pediatric and adult responses to a variety of IBD treatments appear to be due more to study design than the age of the subjects evaluated. As published pediatric trials have generally evaluated subjects with potent treatments at or shortly after diagnosis, the consistently higher rates of responses seen in children lend weight to the argument that some form of 'top-down' therapy offers the best option to maximize remission rates in all patients with IBD.

Copyright © 2009 S. Karger AG, Basel

Introduction

Children who develop inflammatory bowel disease (IBD) represent an important clinical model of 'early IBD'. Many clinical researchers have postulated that children with IBD represent a population with disease in its purest and most inflammatory stage. Aggravating environmental factors such as cigarette smoking are commonly absent, suggesting that genetic factors may be more likely to play a role in disease pathogenesis than in adult populations.

However, observations drawn from longitudinal follow-up of well-defined populations suggest that children and adults with Crohn's disease (CD) do not appear to have significantly different CD behavior, either at the

James Markowitz, MD
Division of Pediatric Gastroenterology and Nutrition, Schneider Children's Hospital
269-01 76 Avenue
New Hyde Park, NY 11040 (USA)
Tel. +1 718 470 3430, Fax +1 718 962 2908, E-Mail jmarkowi2@nshs.edu

time of diagnosis or over time. Cosnes et al. [1] in France have described the change in CD phenotype over time in a large cohort of adults followed over 20 years. While the great majority have an inflammatory phenotype in the first few years of disease, as many as 20% present with penetrating or stricturing disease at the time of diagnosis. Over time, an increasing proportion develops these complications, such that the 20-year actuarial rate for persistent inflammatory phenotype is only 12% [1]. Similar long-term longitudinal data in children with CD are sparse, but disease phenotype during the first few years after diagnosis has been reported from a prospectively followed pediatric inception cohort derived from the combined databases of three North American observational registries, the Pediatric IBD Collaborative Research Group, the Western Regional Pediatric IBD Research Alliance and the Wisconsin Pediatric IBD Alliance [2]. Among 796 children with CD, 88% present with an inflammatory phenotype and only 12% had penetrating or stricturing disease at diagnosis. However, another 20% developed these complications during a median follow-up of 32 months. Recent data from New Zealand support the observations that high proportions of both children (76%) and adults (73%) have uncomplicated inflammatory CD when they are diagnosed [3]. However, the data also reveal that adults older than 40 years of age at diagnosis are more likely to already have a stricturing phenotype at diagnosis than children (20 vs. 11%, p = 0.044). Importantly, however, age at diagnosis did not predict the rate of progression from inflammatory to either stricturing or penetrating complications in this population [3].

Published data suggest that the medications prescribed for the treatment of IBD may be more efficacious in children than adults. If the evolution of CD phenotype over time is not significantly different in pediatric and adult populations, why do children appear to have a better response to treatment? The answer may lie in the demographics of the specific study populations being compared, or in factors hidden in study design. In addition, extreme care must be exercised when evaluating the available data, especially when comparing rates of response among different trials, as there are significant differences among studies in factors beyond the age of the subjects such as disease duration, drug doses evaluated and concomitant therapy. Given the observed evolution of CD phenotype over time, it appears likely that a study population's duration of disease at the onset of a clinical trial might be a critical factor in interpreting the response to any treatment. Increasing disease duration potentially increases the inclusion of subjects with fibrotic rather than inflammatory CD, thereby decreasing the likelihood of therapeutic response to any anti-inflammatory intervention.

This review will summarize observations from a number of different medication classes and highlight the similarities and differences in responses between pediatric and adult populations. In doing so, it will attempt to focus on the factors that could be affecting the results of the various trials. Unfortunately, no study has directly evaluated pediatric versus adult population cohorts in direct, head-to-head comparisons of treatment response. This review will therefore focus on pertinent data from key clinical trials, meta-analyses and observational registries for which there are data from both pediatric and adult populations. As there are very few large clinical trials in children with ulcerative colitis, this review will focus on treatments for CD.

Corticosteroids

Acute Response

Few prospective trials specifically designed to assess the response of patients with active CD to a course of corticosteroids have been published. In 1979, Summers et al. [4] reported data from the National Cooperative Crohn's Disease Study (NCCDS). In addition, there are 2 clinical trials, one adult and one pediatric, in which the control arms of the studies utilized a corticosteroid as the only active therapy [5, 6]. In the NCCDS study, about 30% of adults with active CD responded to prednisone within 30 days of initiating treatment, and 47% responded by 3 months. Somewhat better results were seen in the clinical trial by Candy et al. [5], in which 63% of adults treated solely with prednisolone were in remission by 12 weeks. Acute response rates in children appear to be even better, however, as 79% of newly diagnosed children with moderately to severely active CD who were treated only with prednisone in the control arm of a multicenter trial had inactive CD by 30 days, and 89% were in remission by 3 months [6].

Despite the relatively large differences seen among these clinical trials, in routine clinical practice acute corticosteroid responsiveness appears to be similar between age groups. Munkholm et al. [7] described outcomes following a course of corticosteroids in a population-based adult CD population in Denmark. Thirty days after starting corticosteroids, 48% were in remission, 32% had a partial response, and 20% no response [7]. Similar find-

Table 1. Demographic characteristics of study populations from selected publications: corticosteroids

	Number	Age, years	Duration of CD	Corticosteroid-naïve, %
Controlled trials				
Summers, 1979 [4]	85	mean: 31.8; SD: 11.7	mean: 3.4 years; SD: 4.3 years	–
Candy, 1995 [5]	30	median: 31.8; range: 21–62	median: 3.7 years; range: 0.1–18.7 years	7
Markowitz, 2000 [6]	28	mean: 13.4; SD: 2.5	89% at diagnosis; 11% by 4 weeks after diagnosis	100
Clinical experience				
Munkholm, 1994 [7]	109	median: 28.6; range: 14–84	84% within 1 year of diagnosis	100
Faubion, 2001 [8]	74	median: 27.6	median: 1.0 years; range: 0–18.4 years	100
Tung, 2006 [9]	26	median: 15.2; range: 8.4–18.8	median: 0.02 years; range: 0–2.1 years	100
Markowitz, 2006 [10]	109	mean: 11.8; SD: 2.8	100% by 1 month after diagnosis	100

ings were described by Faubion et al. [8] using the Olmstead County, Minnesota nonreferral CD population followed at the Mayo Clinic. In this population, 58% had a complete remission at 30 days, 26% had a 'partial remission' and 16% did not respond. In a subsequent publication evaluating children diagnosed in the same Olmstead County population, acute outcomes 30 days after starting corticosteroids included complete remission in 62%, partial remission in 27% and no response/surgery in 12% [9]. These rates appear virtually identical to those described in a large North American pediatric multicenter observational registry, in which 60% had a complete response, 24% a partial response, and 17% no response to a course of corticosteroid [10].

Prolonged Response

Prolonged responsiveness to a course of corticosteroid appears more common in children than in adults. In the pediatric multicenter trial described above [6], about 50% of children who entered remission following a course of corticosteroids remained in remission at 18 months despite weaning off prednisone and receiving no additional maintenance therapy. This prolonged responsiveness was not seen in adults in clinical trials, as only 7% of the prednisolone-treated subjects in the Candy trial remained in remission at 15 months [5].

Interestingly, this tendency towards more prolonged corticosteroid responsiveness in children also appears to be evident in clinical practice settings. The North American pediatric registry cohort found 61% of children remaining in remission 1 year after a course of corticosteroids [10]. By contrast, only 32% of the Mayo Clinic adult cohort, and 48% of the Danish cohort were in remission after 1 year [7, 8].

Overall Assessment

Clinical trial data suggest that children are more sensitive to corticosteroid treatment than adults, as evidenced by both their acute (30-day to 3-month) and long-term (1-year) outcomes. The data may well be affected, however, by the characteristics of the specific study populations studied (table 1). All children enrolled in the prospective multicenter clinical trial were newly diagnosed, with 89% of them receiving corticosteroid therapy as their initial treatment, and the other 11% starting within 4 weeks of diagnosis [6]. All were corticosteroid-naïve prior to study inclusion. By contrast, the mean time following diagnosis of CD to study treatment was 41 months in the NCCDS trial [4]. Similarly, the median time from diagnosis to study inclusion in the Candy study was 3.7 years and only 7% were corticosteroid-naïve [5].

By contrast, demographic differences between studies in the published clinical practice populations are much less apparent (table 1). All four studies cited in table 1 evaluated subjects receiving their first course of corticosteroid. However, the North American pediatric registry population included only children receiving corticosteroid within 30 days of diagnosis [10], and the median duration of CD in the Mayo pediatric cohort was also very short [9]. While the adult populations evaluated had somewhat longer duration of disease, 84% of the Danish cohort received treatment within the first year after diagnosis [7], and the median duration of CD in the adult Mayo Clinic population was 1 year (range 0–18.4 years) [8].

Bottom Line

Children with CD appear to be more responsive to corticosteroids than adults.

Thiopurines

Acute Response

Multicenter, placebo-controlled trials exploring the efficacy of thiopurine treatment in both adult and pediatric populations with CD have been published. Overall, the data appear to demonstrate that a greater proportion of children than adults benefit from maintenance thiopurine treatment, although the reverse might be true for induction of remission.

In an early seminal paper, Present et al. [11] reported that 67–79% of adults with active CD improved after starting 6-MP, compared to only 8–29% of those receiving placebo. Eighty-one percent of responders did so by 4 months after initiating treatment. A somewhat lower rate of response (54%; CI 47–61%) was identified in a subsequent Cochrane meta-analysis of thiopurine therapy for induction of remission in adults, with the likelihood of response increasing with duration of therapy ≥17 weeks [12]. More recently, the ongoing SONIC trial [13] has provided additional data regarding the short-term response to azathioprine in an adult CD population. SONIC is a study designed to provide data regarding the differences in outcome between adults treated with azathioprine, infliximab, or infliximab plus azathioprine. In the azathioprine only treatment arm, corticosteroid-free remission following initiation of azathioprine for active CD was only 24.1% at 10 weeks and 25.9% at 18 weeks (data reported at the 2008 national meeting of the American College of Gastroenterology, Orlando, Fla., USA).

In children, acute CD response to a thiopurine has never been prospectively assessed in a clinical trial. Small retrospective case series of children with CD who were corticosteroid dependent or corticosteroid resistant have described response rates of 33% at 3 months and 50–67% at 6 months after starting azathioprine or 6-MP [14, 15]. While corticosteroid use was markedly diminished in these children, the rates of corticosteroid-free remission were not specifically described. The only controlled trial to assess thiopurine response in a pediatric population evaluated newly diagnosed children with moderate-severe CD [6]. Subjects were randomized to treatment with either prednisone + placebo, or prednisone + 6-mercaptopurine, and no differences between groups were seen in response at 30 days or 3 months [6]. However, this study mandated a protocolized corticosteroid-tapering schedule over at least 17 weeks, making it impossible to determine whether there was significant induction effect from 6-MP therapy.

Prolonged Response

By contrast, observations in children appear to demonstrate better long-term responses to thiopurine treatment than that seen in adults. In the multicenter, placebo-controlled 6-MP trial described above, 91% of the children who entered remission and were treated with 6-MP maintained remission over 18 months of follow-up [6], compared to only 50% of those entering remission after treatment with only prednisone. By contrast, the study by Candy et al. [5], incorporating a similar study design to the pediatric trial, reported remission at 15 months in only 42% in the thiopurine treated subjects, compared to 7% in those treated with corticosteroid. Interestingly, however, in routine clinical practice only 60% of children treated with a thiopurine are maintained in remission 1 year after starting therapy [16], irrespective of whether the thiopurine is started within the first 3 months after diagnosis, or 4–12 months after diagnosis. This appears roughly comparable to the overall maintenance rate in adults of 67% (CI 59–75%) reported in a Cochrane meta-analysis of maintenance thiopurine therapy in adults with CD [17].

Study Assessments

The meta-analyses of thiopurine effect in the treatment of CD identified no significant demographic differences among the different studies. Representative demographic data from the larger trials are summarized in table 2, and compared to the pediatric controlled trial. Apart from the age of the subjects, the primary difference between the pediatric and adult trials is the duration of CD at the time thiopurine therapy was started. The pediatric study included only newly diagnosed children, 89% of whom started 6-MP as initial therapy and the other 11% within 30 days of diagnosis. By contrast, the adult subjects in the various trials generally started thiopurine therapy 2–5 years or more after CD diagnosis.

Bottom Line

Study populations with significantly different durations of disease confound comparisons of thiopurine response rates between adults and children. In contrast to the adults enrolled in published controlled trials, children in the pediatric clinical trial were not only treated with a thiopurine very early in their disease course, but they also were naïve to all other treatments except concomitant corticosteroids. Study design and population demographics appear to bias the results in favor of the pediatric study.

Table 2. Demographic characteristics of study populations from selected publications: thiopurines

	Number	Age, years	Duration of CD, years	Medication
Controlled trials				
Summers, 1979 [4]	59	mean: 29.8; SD: 11.0	mean: 3.3; SD: 5.1	AZA
Present, 1980 [11]	83	mean: 31; range: 15–70	mean: 8.3; range: 0.75–35	6-MP
Ewe, 1994 [18]	21	mean: 27.3; range: 18–43	mean 4.6 years	AZA
Candy, 1995 [5]	33	median: 33.9; range: 15–60	median: 2.6; range: 0.1–19.0	AZA
Markowitz, 2000 [6]	27	mean:13.0; SD: 2.3	newly diagnosed	6-MP
Sandborn, 2008 [13]; AZA + placebo arm	107	median: 35; IQR: 26, 43	median: 2.4; IQR: 1, 8	AZA
Clinical experience				
O'Brien, 1991 [19]	78	median: 29; range: 14–70	–	6-MP/AZA
Punati, 2008 [16]	199	mean: 12.0; SD: 2.4	75% ≤3 months from Dx 25% 4–12 months from Dx	6-MP/AZA

Dx = Diagnosis; AZA = azathioprine; 6-MP = 6-mercaptopurine.

Infliximab

Comparisons between age groups regarding response to infliximab are facilitated by the completion of a controlled pediatric clinical trial that was designed to mirror the study design in the adult ACCENT I trial. In one of the 3 treatment arms evaluated in ACCENT I, adults with moderate-severe CD received a 3-dose induction of 5 mg/kg infliximab at 0, 2 and 6 weeks, followed by 5 mg/kg maintenance infusions every 8 weeks [20]. In the comparable arm of the pediatric REACH trial, children with moderate-severe CD were induced with the identical 3-dose 5 mg/kg regimen, and responders at 10 weeks were then randomized to 5 mg/kg maintenance infusions every 8 weeks [21]. Clinical remission at week 30 in the ACCENT I subjects treated with 5 mg/kg infusions every 8 weeks was 39%, compared to 60% in the children treated with the same therapy in REACH. Remission rates at 54 weeks were also markedly better in the children (28% in ACCENT, 56% in REACH).

By contrast, comparison of the REACH data to those recently reported in the SONIC trial reveal less clear-cut differences. In SONIC, adult subjects with moderate-severe CD were treated with infliximab alone or infliximab plus azathioprine [13], utilizing the same 5-mg/kg 3-dose induction and every-8-weeks' maintenance schedule for infliximab used in REACH. At week 26, remission was seen in 44% of those treated with infliximab only and in 57% of those treated with both infliximab and azathioprine (data reported at the 2008 national meeting of the American College of Gastroenterology,

Orlando, Fla., USA). These rates approach the 60% remission rate seen in the children of the REACH trial at 30 weeks [21].

Study Assessments

Despite the comparable treatment arms in ACCENT I and REACH, significant differences in study methods and study populations are present (table 3). To be included in REACH, all children were required to be on a concomitant immunomodulator, an inclusion criterion not present in ACCENT I. The result was that the entire REACH cohort was on an immunomodulator at the onset of infliximab treatment, compared to only 29% of the ACCENT cohort. Disease duration was also considerably longer in the ACCENT population. By contrast, the adult cohort enrolled in the combined treatment arm of the SONIC trial appears to be much more comparable to the REACH population than that enrolled in ACCENT I (table 3). In SONIC, all of the subjects in the combined treatment arm received both infliximab and azathioprine. Duration of disease was also much shorter in SONIC than ACCENT I, and quite comparable to the duration of disease in the pediatric study.

Bottom Line

Response to infliximab appears similar in children and adults, when concomitant immunomodulator therapy and duration of disease are comparable.

Table 3. Demographic characteristics of study populations from selected publications: infliximab

	Number	Age, years	Duration of CD, years	Concomitant immuno-modulators	Concomitant cortico-steroids
ACCENT I 2002 [20] Total study population	573	median: 35; IQR: 28, 46	median: 7.9; IQR: 3.9, 14.7	29%	51%
REACH 2007 [21] Total study population	112	mean: 13.7; SD: 3.3	mean: 2.4; SD: 1.6	100%	33.3%
SONIC 2008 [13] Azathioprine + infliximab group	169	median: 34; IQR: 26, 45	median: 2.2; IQR: 1, 9	100%	41.8%

Adalimumab/Certolizumab

Data allowing comparison between pediatric and adult responses to other biologics are more limited. No pediatric data have been reported with the use of certolizumab pegol. Similarly, no prospective clinical trial data evaluating pediatric response to adalimumab exist, although a multicenter trial is currently underway. The largest pediatric experience, published only in abstract form to date, comes from a multicenter retrospective evaluation of 115 children who had initially responded to and then failed or been intolerant of infliximab [22]. In this group, steroid-free remission at 3, 6 and 12 months after starting adalimumab was 30, 41 and 52%, respectively. Two smaller open label pediatric series have described somewhat similar responses. An Italian study of 23 children noted remission of symptoms in 60.8% at 4 weeks, 30.5% at 3 months, and 50% at 12 months [Cucchiara, pers. commun., 2008]. A smaller (n = 15) open-label pediatric study observed a steroid-free remission at 3 months in 50% [23]. These data can be compared to the adult GAIN trial that evaluated adults who had initial infliximab response and then became resistant or intolerant. Among these subjects, a remission rate of 21% at 4 weeks was seen [24]. The CLASSIC I and II trials [25, 26] recruited only infliximab-naïve subjects. Remission at 4 weeks was noted in up to 36% of subjects in the highest dosage studied [25]. Among subjects initially responding to adalimumab therapy, remission rates of 79–83% were seen at 1 year [26]. Among those not in remission at 4 weeks but subsequently treated with open-label adalimumab, 46% were in remission by 1 year [26].

Study Assessments

Comparisons among the pediatric and adult trials of adalimumab are particularly difficult, as the available studies are significantly different (table 4). No blinded prospective clinical trials have been completed in children, nor are there any pediatric trials that control the use of concomitant therapy. Compared to the adult populations studied, children receiving adalimumab were more likely to have shorter duration of disease, and been previously treated with immunomodulators and infliximab.

Bottom Line

While preliminary data suggest that remission rates may be higher in children than in adults, disease duration, concomitant therapies and associated factors such as smoking likely reduce the response rates seen in the adult populations compared to children.

Natalizumab

Responses to natalizumab have been investigated in adolescents with moderate-to-severe CD in a single, small, open-label clinical trial [27]. All received 3 mg/kg infusions of natalizumab at 0, 4 and 8 weeks. About 40% of subjects demonstrated a clinical response and about 10% were in remission 4 weeks following the first natalizumab infusion. By comparison, pooled data from 2 adult trials suggest that 4 weeks following a single 300-mg infusion of natalizumab 51% of subjects were in response and 24% in remission [28]. At 10 weeks after starting natalizumab given as 3 monthly infusions, 55% of the pediatric population was in response and 29% in remission [27]. These results are quite comparable to the 48–56% response and 26–37% remission rates described in adults at 8–12 weeks [29, 30].

Table 4. Demographic characteristics of study populations from selected publications: adalimumab

	Number	Mean age ± SD, years	Duration of CD, years	Infliximab-naïve	Concomitant immunosuppressant	Smoker
Controlled trials						
CLASSIC I 2006 [25]						
160/80 mg arm	76	39 ± 11	–	100%	29%	42%
CLASSIC II 2007 [26]						
40 mg q2 weeks	19	34 ± 12	7.7 ± 6.5	100%	21%	68%
40 mg q1 week	18	38 ± 10	9.1 ± 9.8	100%	28%	56%
Open label	204	40 ± 12	9.6 ± 8.8	100%	33%	59%
GAIN 2007 [24]	159	39 ± 12	–	0%	46%	35%
Clinical experience						
Rosh, 2008 [22]	115	11 ± 3	4.7 ± 2.8	5%	63%	–
Wyneski, 2008 [23]	15	16.6 ± 3.1	5.7 ± 4.7	0%	87%	–

Study Assessments

Data from subanalyses of a number of adult trials suggest that natalizumab is most efficacious in patients with objective evidence of active inflammatory disease, as demonstrated by elevated CRP or failure to respond to immunosuppressive or other biologic treatment. In the open-label pediatric trial, 74% of the subjects had an elevated CRP [27] compared to 73% in ENACT-I [29], and 100% of the subjects in ENCORE [30]. The 3 study populations had similar proportions of subjects on corticosteroids (37–42%). By contrast, a greater proportion of children (76%) than adults (34–37%) had failed immunosuppressive therapy prior to receiving natalizumab. Duration of CD at entry into the natalizumab studies was also markedly different (children: 35 ± 24 months; ENACT-I: 121 ± 92 months; ENCORE: 121.4 months).

Bottom Line

Children and adults appear to have similar short-term rates of response and remission to natalizumab.

Conclusions

Published data suggest that children with CD are more likely than adults to respond to treatment with corticosteroids, thiopurines and infliximab. By and large, however, the pediatric clinical trials and data arising from pediatric observational registries have focused on evaluating treatment response in children within the first 1–2 years after diagnosis. In some cases, the pediatric trials also include a much greater proportion of patients on potent concomitant therapies than do the comparable adult trials. These differences likely bias comparisons of response rates in favor of the pediatric trials. When clinical trials allow comparison of pediatric and adult study populations with similar durations of CD and similar rates of concomitant therapies, apparent differences in response rates between the two age groups tend to disappear. This effect can be seen most clearly in the comparison of the infliximab trials.

These observations appear to have particular relevance as future therapeutic paradigms for the treatment of CD are developed. As a much higher proportion of children than adults receive potent immunomodulators early in their course, the pediatric experience lends weight to the argument that some form of 'top-down' therapy offers the best option to maximize remission rates in all patients with IBD.

Disclosure Statement

Centocor (consultant, research support), Abbott Labs (research support), UCB (consultant), and Prometheus (consultant, research support).

References

1 Cosnes J, Cattan S, Blaine A, Beaugerie L, Carbonnel F, Parc R, Gendre JP: Long-term evolution of disease behavior of Crohn's disease. Inflamm Bowel Dis 2002;8:244–250.

2 Dubinsky M, Kugathasan S, Mei L, et al: Increased immune reactivity predicts aggressive complicating Crohn's disease in children. Clin Gastroenterol Hepatol 2008;6:1105–1111.

3 Tarrant KM, Barclay ML, Frampton CMA, Gearry RB: Perianal disease predicts changes in Crohn's disease phenotype: results of a population-based study of inflammatory bowel disease phenotype. Am J Gastroenterol 2008;103:3082–3093.

4 Summers RW, Switz DM, Sessions JT Jr, Becktel JM, Best WR, Kern F Jr, Singleton JW: National cooperative Crohn's disease study: results of drug treatment. Gastroenterology 1979;77:847–869.

5 Candy S, Wright J, Gerber M, Adams G, Gerig M, Goodman R: A controlled double blind study of azathioprine in the management of Crohn's disease. Gut 1995;37:674–678.

6 Markowitz J, Grancher K, Kohn N, Lesser M, Daum F: A multicenter trial of 6-mercaptopurine and prednisone in children with newly diagnosed Crohn's disease. Gastroenterology 2000;119:985–902.

7 Munkholm P, Langholz E, Davidsen M, Binder V: Frequency of glucocorticoid resistance and dependency in Crohn's disease. Gut 1994;35:360–362.

8 Faubion WA Jr, Loftus EV Jr, Harmsen WS, Zinsmeister AR, Sandborn WJ: The natural history of corticosteroid therapy for inflammatory bowel disease: a population-based study. Gastroenterology 2001;121:255–260.

9 Tung J, Loftus EV Jr, Freese DK, El-Youssef M, Zinsmeister AR, Melton LJ 3rd, Harmsen WS, Sandborn WJ, Faubion WA Jr: A population-based study of the frequency of corticosteroid resistance and dependence in pediatric patients with Crohn's disease and ulcerative colitis. Inflamm Bowel Dis 2006;12:1093–1100.

10 Markowitz J, Hyams J, Mack D, et al: Corticosteroid therapy in the age of infliximab: acute and 1-year outcomes in newly diagnosed children with Crohn's disease. Clin Gastroenterol Hepatol 2006;4:1124–1129.

11 Present DH, Korelitz BI, Wisch N, Glass JL, Sachar DB, Pasternack BS: Treatment of Crohn's disease with 6-mercaptopurine: a long-term, randomized, double-blind study. N Engl J Med 1980;302:981–987.

12 Sandborn W, Sutherland L, Pearson D, May G, Modigliani R, Prantera C: Azathioprine or 6-mercaptopurine for inducing remission of Crohn's disease. Cochrane Database Syst Rev 2000;2:CD000545.

13 Sandborn W, Rutgeerts P, Reinsch W, Kornbluth A, Lichtiger S, D'Haens G, van der Woude C, Diamond R, Broussard D, Colombel J: Sonic: a randomized, double-blind, controlled trial comparing infliximab and infliximab plus azathioprine to azathioprine in patients with Crohn's disease naïve to immunomodulators and biologic therapy (abstract). Am J Gastroenterol 2008;103(suppl 1):S436.

14 Verhave M, Winter HS, Grand RJ: Azathioprine in the treatment of children with inflammatory bowel disease. J Pediatr 1990;117:809–814.

15 Markowitz J, Rosa J, Grancher K, Aiges H, Daum F: Long term 6-mercaptopurine treatment in adolescents with Crohn's disease. Gastroenterology 1990;99:1347–1355.

16 Punati J, Markowitz J, Lerer T, et al: Effect of early immunomodulator use in moderate to severe pediatric Crohn disease. Inflamm Bowel Dis 2008;14:949–954.

17 Pearson DC, May GR, Fick G, Sutherland LR: Azathioprine for maintenance of remission in Crohn's disease. Cochrane Database Syst Rev 1998;4:CD000067.

18 Ewe K, Press AG, Singe CC, Stufler M, Ueberschaer B, Hommel G, Meyer zum Büschenfelde KH: Azathioprine combined with prednisolone or monotherapy with prednisolone in active Crohn's disease. Gastroenterology 1993;105:367–372.

19 O'Brien JJ, Bayless TM, Bayless JA: Use of azathioprine or 6-mercaptopurine in the treatment of Crohn's disease. Gastroenterology 1991;101:39–46.

20 Hanauer SB, Feagan BG, Lichtenstein GR, Mayer LF, Schreiber S, Colombel JF, Rachmilewitz D, Wolf DC, Olson A, Bao W, Rutgeerts P, ACCENT I Study Group: Maintenance infliximab for Crohn's disease: the ACCENT I randomised trial. Lancet 2002;359:1541–1549.

21 Hyams J, Crandall W, Kugathasan S, et al: Induction and maintenance infliximab therapy for the treatment of moderate-to-severe Crohn's disease in children. Gastroenterology 2007;132:863–873.

22 Rosh JR, Lerer T, Markowitz J, Goli SR, Mamula P, Noe JD, Pfefferkorn MD, Kelleher KT, Griffiths AM, Kugathasan S, Keljo D, Oliva-Hemker M, Crandall W, Carvalho R, Mack DR, Hyams JS: Retrospective evaluation of the safety and effect of adalimumab therapy (Reseat) on pediatric Crohn's disease (abstract). Gastroenterology 2008;134(suppl 1):A-657.

23 Wyneski MJ, Green A, Kay M, Wyllie R, Mahajan L: Safety and efficacy of adalimumab in pediatric patients with Crohn disease. J Pediatr Gastroenterol Nutr 2008;47:19–25.

24 Sandborn WJ, Rutgeerts P, Enns R, Hanauer SB, Colombel JF, Panaccione R, D'Haens G, Li J, Rosenfeld MR, Kent JD, Pollack PF: Adalimumab induction therapy for Crohn disease previously treated with infliximab: a randomized trial. Ann Intern Med 2007;146:829–838.

25 Hanauer SB, Sandborn WJ, Rutgeerts P, Fedorak RN, Lukas M, MacIntosh D, Panaccione R, Wolf D, Pollack P: Human anti-tumor necrosis factor monoclonal antibody (adalimumab) in Crohn's disease: the CLASSIC-I trial. Gastroenterology 2006;130:323–333.

26 Sandborn WJ, Hanauer SB, Rutgeerts PJ, Fedorak RN, Lukas M, MacIntosh DG, Panaccione R, Wolf D, Kent JD, Bittle B, Li J, Pollack PF: Adalimumab for maintenance treatment of Crohn's disease: results of the CLASSIC II trial. Gut 2007;56:1232–1239.

27 Hyams JS, Wilson DC, Thomas A, Heuschkel R, Mitton S, Mitchell B, Daniels R, Libonati MA, Zanker S, Kugathasan S, International Natalizumab CD305 Trial Group: Natalizumab therapy for moderate to severe Crohn disease in adolescents. J Pediatr Gastroenterol Nutr 2007;44:185–191.

28 MacDonald JK, McDonald JW: Natalizumab for induction of remission in Crohn's disease. Cochrane Database Syst Rev 2007;1:CD006097.

29 Sandborn WJ, Colombel JF, Enns R, et al: Natalizumab induction and maintenance therapy for Crohn's disease. N Engl J Med 2005;353:1912–1925.

30 Targan SR, Feagan BG, Fedorek RN, et al: Natalizumab for the treatment of active Crohn's disease: results of the ENCORE trial. Gastroenterology 2007;132:1672–1683.

Dig Dis 2009;27:366–369
DOI: 10.1159/000228575

Beyond Tumor Necrosis Factor: Next-Generation Biologic Therapy for Inflammatory Bowel Disease

Daniel K. Podolsky

University of Texas Southwestern Medical Center, Dallas, Tex., USA

Key Words

Crohn's disease · Ulcerative colitis · Biologics

Abstract

Even as further refinements of anti-TNF continue to emerge, new biologics targeting alternative mechanisms are progressing through clinical development programs and offer the opportunity for categorically new therapeutics in the years ahead. Several of these target regulatory cytokines occupy important nodal positions in the intricate pathways mediating immune and inflammatory injury. A number of agents which antagonize the IL-12/IL-23 axis appear to offer promise. The apparent efficacy of these anti-cytokine agents has served as a stimulus for development of therapeutics that inhibits the signaling pathway common to their action. In addition to the focus of new biologic development on additional components of the cytokine network, other biologics target mechanisms of recruitment of various key cell populations to mucosa involved in inflammatory bowel disease. Natalizumab is already approved for clinical use and targets $\alpha4$ with proven efficacy in Crohn's disease. A more specific antibody designated finds $\alpha4\beta7$ (also known as MAdCAM) trials has had efficacy in ulcerative colitis and probable efficacy in Crohn's disease. Efforts continue to exploit increasing understanding of the mechanisms necessary for T cell activation, and most especially co-stimulatory molecules to intervene in immune-related injury. A chimeric protein encompassing CTLA4 and an immunoglobulin tail (abatacept) has yielded promising results. Another mechanistic strategy to intervene with recruitment of key leukocytes to sites of disease activity has focused on members of the chemokine family that appear to be especially critical to the intestinal mucosa. In summary, the expanding knowledge of mechanisms that contribute to the pathogenesis of inflammatory bowel diseases has yielded a wealth of new potential targets and the results of the variety of agents currently being developed offer promise for a rich mix of next-generation biologics.

Copyright © 2009 S. Karger AG, Basel

Recent progress in the understanding of key elements in the pathogenesis of the major forms of inflammatory bowel disease promises the potential for more effective mechanism-based therapy. Given that many of these involve regulation of dynamic biological processes, it is likely that many of the most effective agents will fall within the broad rubric of biologic therapy. The current working model of inflammatory bowel disease highlights the dynamic interaction between luminal flora and their products and the mucosal surface which is influenced by the integrity of the epithelial barrier and homeostasis controlled by innate immune responses. In part, as a result of inherited variants of various genes which influence the mucosal integrity and state of immune activa-

Daniel K. Podolsky
University of Texas Southwestern Medical Center
5323 Harry Hines Blvd.
Dallas, TX 75390-9046 (USA)
E-Mail daniel.podolsky@utsouthwestern.edu

tion, there is inappropriate regulation of the steady-state balance between flora and immune response which eventuates in the downstream activation of adaptive immune pathways that are ultimately deleterious in driving perpetuation of immune activation and actual tissue destruction responsible for the clinical manifestations of these disorders.

Genome-wide association studies have proven a major catalyst in understanding host susceptibility, but even more importantly in pointing to key dimensions of the pathogenesis of inflammatory bowel disease which offer new therapeutic targets for future therapy. Beyond these broad components that are integral to the pathogenesis of inflammatory bowel disease, many details of the 'software' that mediate the interactions between various key cell populations have been delineated. These include intracellular signaling of pathways through which regulatory proteins stimulate cell responses as well as the wide variety of regulatory peptides and other mediators that serve as wiring between the different cell populations that ultimately are involved in inflammatory bowel disease.

The prototypic example of the ability of a biologic agent to effectively recast the therapeutic landscape is provided by anti-TNF, first demonstrated through clinical validation of the prototypic agent infliximab. It is both notable and humbling that a decade after approval of this agent for the treatment of subsets of patients with inflammatory bowel disease, understanding of the mechanisms through which it achieves that therapeutic benefit beyond the obvious targeting of anti-TNF remains, at best, uncertain. Nevertheless, moving forward, considering the fundamentally different target for future biological therapies it is reasonable to speculate that continued refinement of anti-TNF cells will eventually lead to even more effective agents pivoting off the role of TNF, whether through the expanding menu of new anti-TNF agents, per se, or targeting some of the downstream effects and signaling pathways normally activated by TNF.

Looking beyond TNF, it is clear that an important opportunity has emerged from the identification of the key role that the IL-12/IL-23 family of cytokines plays in driving differentiation of key effector T-cell populations. The evolution of the development of biologics targeting this family of cytokines is a cautionary tale. Initially, it focused on the important role of IL-12 in driving Th1-mediated responses which have been well known to be associated with active Crohn's disease. It was therefore both satisfying and important that early phase-2 trials suggested a therapeutic benefit to an anti-IL-12. We now appreciate that this antibody directed against the p40 subunit of the IL-12 heterodimeric cytokine was also targeting IL-23, which shares the p40 subunit.

It is now clear that IL-23 is also likely a critical regulator, most notably in driving differentiation of Th17 cells, a subset not known at the time anti-p40 was being developed initially, but yet, appears to be directly involved in generating products that eventuate in tissue injury as well as sustaining overall inflammatory activity. The particular importance of IL-23 is also underscored by identification of the gene encoding the receptor for this cytokine as modifying host susceptibility (ironically a variant of the receptor confers relative resistance to Crohn's disease). It is equally plausible as a hypothesis that the beneficial effects from anti-p40 might be attributed to its blockade of IL-12, blockade of IL-23 or both.

In any case, the recent trials of the prototypic anti-p40 ustekinumab as well as ABT-874 human monoclonal antibodies have therapeutic benefit. Both prevent IL-12 and IL-23 from binding the IL-12-R1 receptor and normalize IL-12- and IL-23-mediated signaling. ABT-874 has a particularly high affinity and is very potent in neutralizing p40 in vitro as well as neutralizing IL-12-induced responses in vivo in animal models. In a phase-2 trial involving two different cohorts of approximately 40 patients, in which those receiving an active agent received seven weekly injections, there was a significant benefit as judged by clinical response through week 8, and it is especially notable that this was even more accentuated when analysis focused on patients with active Crohn's disease who had prior infliximab experience.

Other biologics will likely emerge from focus on the molecular machinery involved in T cell activation. Among these is the humanized non-FCR-binding anti-CD3 visilizumab. This antibody targets CD3 variant in part of the T cell receptor complex, and in phase-1 and early phase-2 trials among patients with either moderate-to-severe refractory Crohn's disease or ulcerative colitis demonstrated some evidence of clinical activity. Perhaps, and most importantly, within these relatively small trials this anti-CD3 agent appeared to be relatively safe despite the potential for profound and broad immunosuppression.

An alternative approach to abrogating effective T cell activation focuses on the requirement for effective costimulation in the presence of a MHC presentation of antigen. Thus, abatacept, a fusion protein as an immunoglobulin backbone fused to a fragment of the co-stimulatory molecule CTLA4 effectively competes with cell surface CTLA4 presumably preventing effective costimulation – and in theory, should be at least as effective and perhaps more selective than a strategy focused on CD3. Other biologic strategies aimed at minimizing T cell activation have focused not on the primary activation, but on the self-reinforcing cytokines necessary to sustain that activation. Two antibodies, dacilizumab and basiliximab, target IL-2 or its receptor which abrogate the otherwise reinforcing production of IL-2 that follows T cell activation.

It is noteworthy that each of these potential new classes of biologics progressing through the clinical development reflects the former focus on the key role of adaptive immune responses. The evolving model summarized above which has focused attention increasingly on innate immune response is now leading to the development of strategies focused on that facet of inflammatory bowel disease pathogenesis as a lagging indicator of the processes recognized to be important in the pathogenesis of IBD.

One intriguing approach has been the use of GM-CSF (sargramostin) which has been evaluated in phase-2 trials of patients with moderate to severe Crohn's disease. Ironically, this is an agent known to stimulate many dimensions of innate immune responses. This may be consistent with the counteractive, but nonetheless increasingly plausible notion that inflammatory bowel disease may be more reflective of relatively inadequate rather than excessive innate immune activation. While the early experience with sargramostin was suggestive, evaluation of otherwise unstratified patients in a larger phase-2 trial was not able to document significant effect. However, re-evaluation in a subsequent trial with the primary endpoint of clinical steroid-free remission showed significant difference to suggest that this may yet be a viable approach.

Other strategies to capitalize on the insight into the importance of regulating innate immune responses have focused less on biologics, per se, than on small molecules which can modulate pathways mediated by pattern recognition receptors. Of interest, the therapeutic effect may depend on both which members of the key families of pattern recognition receptors are targeted and the situational context of that modulation. Thus, in some settings agonists of members of the toll-like receptor family appear to be protective, while in others antagonists have effected therapeutic benefits in pre-clinical models. At the very least, this points to the potential complexities and caution will need to be exercised in strategies which target the modulation of innate immune pathways mediated through pattern recognition receptors.

In parallel with the increasing sophistication in targeting the pathways of immune activation and tissue injury, the potential benefits for biologics which focus on a categorically distinct mechanism, the process of recruitment of lymphocyte and other key populations to sites affected by inflammatory bowel disease are now well demonstrated. The prototypic agent natalizumab targets the α4 subunit which is present as a component of two distinct integrin, α4β1 and α4β7, that likely each contribute to processes leading to inflammatory bowel disease. Controlled trials have demonstrated the therapeutic benefit to this agent in patients with moderate to severe active Crohn's disease. Although enthusiasm for this use must be tempered by the rare, but nonetheless dread, complication of progressive multifocal leukoencephalopathy (PML), this agent appears effective even in those who have either failed to respond to anti-TNF or have lost that initial response, so that it represents a valuable addition to our armamentarium. Clearly, further clinical experience will help determine how best to calibrate the risk/benefit ratio for optimal clinical decision making.

A number of additional agents which focus on the mechanics of cell recruitment also appear promising. Among these, vedolizumab may be most promising therapeutically and also provide additional insights into the mechanism in which natalizumab achieves its benefit. As noted, the latter monoclonal antibody targets an α4 chain which is a partner to both β1 and β7 subunits. In contrast, vedolizumab is specific to α4β7 which is known to be essential for homing of lymphocytes to intestinal mucosa. Preliminary studies have demonstrated clinical benefits for patients with moderate to severe ulcerative colitis. More recently, a phase-2 study of patients with Crohn's disease suggests equal benefit consistent with the premise that this agent is targeting a process important in sustaining inflammatory activity in both major forms of inflammatory bowel disease.

Thus, in looking beyond TNF, one can reasonably anticipate that the biologic agents targeting disruption of the cell recruitment may fill an important, complementary role in the therapeutic armamentarium. It is worth noting that in parallel to the development of these biologics, a number of alternative strategies which use small molecules to target other dimensions of the overall process of cell recruitment are advancing in their clinical development and may prove equally therapeutically useful. These include antagonists for a member of the cytokine receptor family which are critical to initiating cell recruitment and migration, while other nonbiologic approaches may directly target some other members of the integrin family known to be involved in cell-cell recognition that leads to cell migration. The latter is exemplified by the use of antisense agents to drive downregulation of the integrin ICAM-1. Potential therapeutic efficacy has been suggested by trials with alicaforsen administered as enemas in patients with active distal ulcerative colitis. Thus, the landscape for development of agents that modulate cell adhesion and migration will likely be dynamic and complex.

At this time, there is remarkable vitality in the variety and intensity of biological therapeutic strategies currently being developed. Beyond those described here, these include such diverse and innovative approaches as the administration of genetically engineered probiotics which secrete therapeutically active biologic compounds once resident in the GI tract and a variety of cell-based therapies including bone marrow transplantation. Which of these may truly transform clinical care of patients with inflammatory bowel disease remains to be determined through careful clinical investigation.

One can note that in general, the explosion of new therapeutic strategies relying on biological agents has proceeded in parallel with a better understanding of mechanism, and in a complementary fashion demonstration of efficacy has helped provide new insights into pathophysiology. In defining the potential therapeutic benefit of each new biologic treatment, it will be important to further delineate risk profiles so that the benefits can be fairly weighed against the potential unwanted effects. Undoubtedly, the number of new strategies will continue to expand driven by recent recognition of the remarkable number of genes that confer some risk of inflammatory bowel disease and the new insights that they are providing in suggesting previously unappreciated mechanisms that might be relevant to the pathogenesis of these disorders. Without doubt, the years ahead will be both exciting for investigators and enormously promising for patients.

Disclosure Statement

The author declares that no financial or other conflict of interest exists in relation to the content of the article.

Dig Dis 2009;27:370–374
DOI: 10.1159/000228576

How Do We Manage Vaccinations in Patients with Inflammatory Bowel Disease?

Maria Esteve Comas   Carme Loras Alastruey   Fernando Fernandez-Bañares

Department of Gastroenterology, Hospital Universitari Mútua de Terrassa, University of Barcelona, Barcelona, Spain

Key Words

Vaccination · Inflammatory bowel disease · Opportunistic infections · Immunosuppression

Abstract

The mortality in inflammatory bowel disease (IBD) has been reported similar or slightly increased as compared to that of the general population. However, deaths related to infectious and parasitic diseases have been repeatedly reported in clinical trials, open series and registries. The IBD patients are exposed to the same infections affecting the community, added to opportunistic infectious related to the immunosuppression. Some of these infectious diseases may be prevented by the appropriate use of a vaccination program. Thus, vaccination status should be assessed at IBD diagnosis, and from time to time, and vaccination should be updated to every patient as soon as possible, since deaths due to preventable diseases should never occur. Present recommendations include vaccination for influenza (annually), for pneumococcal disease with the 23-valent strain (every 5 years), for hepatitis B virus (in patients with no detectable hepatitis B surface antibodies), combined vaccination against tetanus, diphtheria and inactivated poliomyelitis (every 10 years). The role of human papillomavirus vaccine preventing cervical dysplasia and neoplasia in IBD women taking immunosuppressive are at present unknown. In patients lacking varicella immunization, specific vaccination should be considered. Nevertheless, it should be taken into account that varicella vaccine contains live attenuated virus that cannot be administered in patients taking immunosuppressive. The same consideration should be kept in mind for patients travelling to endemic areas for yellow fever. Finally, IBD patients on immunosuppressive may have an altered response to vaccine immunization. Decreased response has been reported for hepatitis B and pneumoccocal vaccination. In those cases, testing for serological responses to vaccine should be performed and booster doses may be required.

Copyright © 2009 S. Karger AG, Basel

The mortality in inflammatory bowel disease patients (IBD) was reported to be similar or slightly higher when compared to that of the general population. In the most recently published population-based study, a higher mortality was reported in Crohn's disease (CD) but not in ulcerative colitis (UC) patients. However, in both diseases, a large proportion of deaths was related to infectious diseases [1]. The IBD patients are exposed to the same infections affecting the community plus to opportunistic infections related to the immunosuppression.

The number of potential opportunistic infections that may affect patients with IBD is very large. The true prevalence of specific infections is not known and may vary from country to country. Therefore, reactivation of some infections such as tuberculosis, histoplasmosis or hepati-

KARGER

Fax +41 61 306 12 34
E-Mail karger@karger.ch
www.karger.com

© 2009 S. Karger AG, Basel
0257–2753/09/0273–0370$26.00/0

Accessible online at:
www.karger.com/ddi

Maria Esteve, MD
Department of Gastroenterology, Hospital Universitari Mútua de Terrassa
University of Barcelona, Plaça Dr Robert n° 5, ES–08221 Terrassa, Barcelona (Spain)
Tel. +34 93 736 5050 ext. 1215, Fax +34 93 736 5043
E-Mail mestevecomas@telefonica.net

Table 1. Current recommended vaccination program for adult IBD patients [2, 13]

Illness	Vaccine	Recommendation	Schedule
Tetanus, diphtheria	purified anatoxin	recommended	every 10 years
Poliomyelitis	injectable:inactivated	recommended	every 10 years
Pertussis	acellular antigen	authorized	every 10 years
Hepatitis B	recombinant peptide	recommended	single/double doses? booster?
Pneumococcal disease	23-valent purified antigen	recommended	every 5 years
Influenza	inactivated virus	recommended	annually
Human papillomavirus infection	recombinant L1 protein	authorized	??
Measles, mumps, rubella	live attenuated	contraindicated during immunosuppression	??
Varicella	live attenuated	contraindicated during immunosuppression	double dose (4 weeks' interval)
Haemophilus influenzae B disease	conjugated capsular polyosidique antigen	authorized	single dose

tis B will be much more frequent in endemic areas of these infections than in others [2]. So, this aspect should be taken into account when specific preventive measures are applied in a particular country.

The majority of opportunistic infections reported in our hospital in anti-TNF-treated patients appeared in previous years before a systematic work-up assessment for detection of latent or active infections was implemented. Nine infections were reported in 94 infliximab-treated patients for both rheumatologic diseases and Crohn's disease. A clear predominance of *Mycobacterium tuberculosis* was observed, followed by visceral leishmaniasis, pyogenic muscular abscess (one *Salmonella* spp. and one *Streptococcus pneumoniae*), and two viral infections due to hepatitis B virus reactivation and zoster ophthalmicus. The risk of opportunistic infection was significantly higher in the first year of treatment, probably due to the lack of a specific policy for opportunistic infection detection at that moment. This fact illustrates the 'learning curve' inherent in new drug use. The only factor related to such infections was the simultaneous use of more than 2 immunosuppressors (OR 8.6; 95% CI 1.8–39.9) [3]. This relation of opportunistic infections with the number of simultaneous immunosuppressors administered was stressed in another study performed at the Mayo Clinic including 100 IBD patients in the same period of 6 years from January 1, 1998, to December 31, 2003. No patient died due to these opportunistic infections. Corticosteroids (OR 3.4; 95% CI 1.8–6.2), azathioprine/6-mercaptopurine (OR 3.1; 95% CI 1.7–5.5), and infliximab (OR 4.4; 95% CI 1.2–17.1) were independently associated with in-

creased risk of opportunistic infections. Immunosuppressors, especially when used in combination, increased this risk 4-fold with an OR of 14.5 (95% CI 4.9–43). At an age over 50 there was a significantly higher risk of opportunistic infections than in patients younger than 24. Consequently, combined immunosuppression should be avoided when possible, particularly in patients older than 50. In contrast, when compared to our more limited series, no cases of tuberculosis were found, emphasizing the importance of local environment in the incidence of specific infections [4].

Therefore, preventive measures are warranted to minimize the risk. This includes: (1) A good control of the environmental exposure, which is particularly important in the hospital setting to avoid a nosocomial transmission of infections. (2) To be aware of factors related to opportunistic infections as previously mentioned. (3) Chemoprophylaxis and when indicated a control of underlying chronic viral infections. (4) Use of a vaccination program.

Current recommendation for adult IBD patients vaccination (table 1) [2] includes vaccination against tetanus, diphtheria and inactivated poliomyelitis administered every ten years. There is no universal recommendation regarding vaccination against pertussis. However, due to the resurgence of the infection in some countries its administration in combination with tetanus, poliomyelitis and diphtheria is advisable.

Influenza vaccine should be administered annually, and vaccine for pneumococcal disease with the 23-valent strain should be administered every 5 years.

Antibodies against hepatitis B and against varicella should be tested and vaccination considered for those who are not immunized. However, it is important to keep in mind that varicella vaccine is a live attenuated vaccine and cannot be administered if the patient is undergoing immunosuppressive treatment. Immunosuppressors can be safely administered 3 months after the last dose of vaccine dose and can be initiated 3 months after removing the immunosuppressor.

Regarding human papillomavirus infection, there is a growing concern about this infection and its relation with cervical displasia and cancer in IBD patients taking immunosuppressors. However, available data for immune response to such a vaccination of the general population is limited and there is not enough information about the efficacy in immunosuppressed patients, including IBD patients.

Immunization against rubella, measles and mumps should be checked if there is no certainty that they were administered. However, in the majority of industrialized countries the general population is universally vaccinated against these viral infections, making the risk of acquisition very low. A population-based study performed using the Manitoba Health Population Registry demonstrated that the majority of individuals, both patients and controls, were immunized against these viral infections [5]. In addition, as it occurs with the varicella vaccine, they are live attenuated vaccines, making their administration in immunosuppressed patients difficult.

The established general recommendations of vaccination for IBD should be adapted, from time to time, to the specific public health reality of any particular country. In this sense, an epidemiological study assessing the prevalence of viral markers for hepatitis B and C of more than 2,000 IBD patients in Spain found that the global percentage of effective B virus immunization was very low. However, the progressive implementation of B virus vaccine to preadolescents at school or in children at birth since 1983 has increased the number of vaccinated IBD patients younger than 27 to around 60% as compared to 10% in the older patients, and this figure will probably increase in the future [6].

In order to know if we are managing our IBD patients well, the following questions should be answered concerning vaccine administration: Firstly, at what point in time should patients be immunized? Secondly, are vaccines systematically utilized in IBD patients? Thirdly, are patients properly immunized if the current recommended schedule is applied?

The answer to the first question is as soon as possible after diagnosis. However, a checkup from time to time should be performed following the schedule shown in table 1, as well as before treatment starting with immunomodulators or biologics.

A study performed in the Cedars-Sinai Inflammatory Bowel Disease Center in Los Angeles showed that vaccines are underutilized in patients with IBD. Thus, this study emphasizes the need for a specific control of the vaccination program in the IBD units apart from the general recommendations for the community in any given country [7].

Finally, another important issue is to be aware if patients are well immunized when current recommended schedule is applied. The information in this field is very limited. Three studies regarding the immune response to influenza vaccine are available, 2 of them performed in children with IBD [8, 9] and 1 in an adult population [10] treated with anti-TNF.

In the pediatric population, a variable percentage of serologic conversion ranging from 33 to 85% was observed [8]. In one study from the Children' Hospital in Boston, the response to influenza vaccine was not related to the administration of immunosuppressors, except for a lower serologic conversion for the influenza B strain in infliximab-treated patients [9]. However, in another study of the Children's Hospital of Philadelphia, a decreased response was observed related to immunomodulators and infliximab for strains influenza B and A/H1N1 [8].

In the adult population receiving anti-TNF for rheumatic diseases and Crohn's disease, a high proportion ranging from 80 to 94% of both patients and controls had protective titers ≥40 irrespective of whether they were or were not under anti-TNF therapy. However, as expected, post-vaccination geometric mean antibody titers of 2 strains of influenza (A/H3N3 and B) were lower in patients receiving anti-TNF as compared with patients not receiving anti-TNF and controls [10]. Thus, the conclusion is that IBD patients receiving standard trivalent influenza vaccine are, in general, reasonably protected, mainly in the adulthood.

It is also unknown whether pneumoccocal vaccination in adults with IBD induces measurable immunity in immunosuppressed patients. In a study presented at the last DDW in San Diego [11], 64 subjects were included: 20 in the group immunosuppressors plus biologics, 25 in the group of IBD not receiving immunosuppressors and 19 healthy controls. All subjects received a single dose of 23-valent pneumococcal polysaccharide vaccine (PPV).

Esteve Comas/Loras Alastruey/
Fernandez-Bañares

Table 2. Current recommended vaccination program for adult IBD patients to prevent travel-related illnesses [2, 13]

Illness	Vaccine	Recommendation
Hepatitis A	inactivated virus	authorized
Yellow fever	live attenuated	contraindicated
Cholera	oral killed	use with caution
	oral live	contraindicated
Meningoccocal disease	conjugate polysaccharide C	authorized
	polysaccharide combined A+C	authorized
	polysaccharide combined A+C+W+Y	authorized
Typhoid	i.v. capsular polysaccharide	authorized
Rabies	cell culture-derived vaccine	authorized
Japanese encephalitis	inactivated virus	authorized
Tick-borne encephalitis	inactivated virus	use with caution

Blood was collected prior to vaccination and one month later and antibody titers to 5 antigens were measured (6B, 9V, 14, 19F, 23F). The response was defined as >2-fold rise in geometric mean antibody and absolute geometric mean antibody >1 μg/ml. There were no differences between the non-immunosuppressed group of IBD and controls, but immunosuppressed patients showed a slightly impaired response to pneumococcal vaccination. Therefore, these patients should be vaccinated as soon as possible to optimize the response to vaccination.

A more marked impairment of the immune response to hepatitis B vaccine has been described in a study performed in Spain and including 129 IBD patients negative for hepatitis B surface antibodies, who were given the 3 standard doses at 1, 2 and 6 months [12]. Detectable antibodies higher than 10 IU were found in only 34% of the patients. The youngest patients had the highest response rate and a non-significant trend for a worse response was observed in those patients treated with steroids and immunosuppressors. These results emphasize the need for the use of higher doses in IBD patients than those recommended for the general population.

Finally, those patients traveling abroad should adhere to a specific vaccination program depending on the country they are traveling to. Specific advice by specialists in tropical medicine may be required. Again, it should be kept in mind that live attenuated vaccines, such as those for yellow fever, cannot be administered to immunosuppressed patients (table 2).

To summarize, a vaccination program should be applied in all IBD units, since deaths due to preventable diseases should never occur. Patients should be vaccinated as soon as possible after diagnosis and be checked up periodically.

The immunosuppression status of IBD patients may impair the immune response to some vaccines making the administration of booster doses necessary in some cases.

Disclosure Statement

The authors declare that no financial or other conflict of interest exists in relation to the content of the article.

References

1 Hutfless SM, Weng X, Liu L, Allison J, Herrinton LJ: Mortality by medication use among patients with inflammatory bowel disease, 1996–2003. Gastroenterology 2007; 133:1779–1786.
2 Viget N, Vernier-Massouille G, Salmon-Ceron D, Yazdanpanah Y, Colombel JF: Opportunistic infections in patients with inflammatory bowel disease: prevention and diagnosis. Gut 2008;57:549–558.
3 Garcia-Vidal C, Rodríguez-Fernández S, Teijón S, Esteve M, Rodríguez-Carballeira M, Lacasa JM, Salvador G, Garau J: Risk factors for opportunistic infections in infliximab-treated patients: the importance of screening in prevention. Eur J Clin Microbiol Infect Dis 2009;28:331–337.
4 Toruner M, Loftus EV Jr, Harmsen WS, Zinsmeister AR, Orenstein R, Sandborn WJ, Colombel JF, Egan LJ: Risk factors for opportunistic infections in patients with inflammatory bowel disease. Gastroenterology 2008;134:929–936.

5 Bernstein CN, Rawsthorne P, Blanchard JF: Population-based case-control study of measles, mumps, and rubella and inflammatory bowel disease. Inflamm Bowel Dis 2007;13: 759–762.

6 Loras C, Saro C, Gonzalez-Huix F, Mínguez M, Merino O, Gisbert JP, Barrio J, Bernal A, Gutiérrez A, Piqueras M, Calvet X, Andreu M, Abad A, Ginard D, Bujanda L, Panés J, Torres M, Fernández-Bañares F, Viver JM, Esteve M; REPENTINA study, Grupo Español de Enfermedades de Crohn y Colitis Ulcerosa: Prevalence and factors related to hepatitis B and C in inflammatory bowel disease patients in Spain: a nationwide, multicenter study. Am J Gastroenterol 2009;104:57–63.

7 Melmed GY, Ippoliti AF, Papadakis KA, Tran TT, Birt JL, Lee SK, Frenck RW, Targan SR, Vasiliauskas EA: Patients with inflammatory bowel disease are at risk for vaccine-preventable illnesses. Am J Gastroenterol 2006;101:1834–1840.

8 Mamula P, Markowitz JE, Piccoli DA, Klimov A, Cohen L, Baldassano RN: Immune response to influenza vaccine in pediatric patients with inflammatory bowel disease. Clin Gastroenterol Hepatol 2007;5:851–856.

9 Lu Y, Jacobson DL, Ashworth LA, Grand RJ, Meyer AL, McNeal MM, Gregas MC, Burchett SK, Bousvaros A: Immune response to influenza vaccine in children with inflammatory bowel disease. Am J Gastroenterol 2009;104:444–453.

10 Gelinck LB, van der Bijl AE, Beyer WE, Visser LG, Huizinga TW, van Hogezand RA, Rimmelzwaan GF, Kroon FP: The effect of anti-tumour necrosis factor alpha treatment on the antibody response to influenza vaccination. Ann Rheum Dis 2008;67:713–716.

11 Melmed GY, Frenck R, Barolet-Garcia C, Ibanez P, Simpson P, Papadakis KA, Ward J, Ippoliti A, Targan SR, Vasiliauskas EA: TNF blockers and immunomodulators impair antibody response to pneumococcal polysaccharide vaccine (PPV) in patients with inflammatory bowel disease. Gastroenterology 2008;134:A68.

12 Vida Pérez L, Gómez Camacho F, García Sánchez V, Iglesias Flores EM, Castillo Molina L, Cerezo Ruiz A, Casáis Juanena L, De Dios Vega JF: Adequate rate of response to hepatitis B virus vaccination in patients with inflammatory bowel disease. Med Clin (Barc) 2009;132:331–335.

13 Sands BE, Cuffari C, Katz J, Kugathasan S, Onken J, Vitek C, Orenstein W: Guidelines for immunizations in patients with inflammatory bowel disease. Inflamm Bowel Dis 2004;10:677–692.

Esteve Comas/Loras Alastruey/
Fernandez-Bañares

Dig Dis 2009;27:375–381
DOI: 10.1159/000228577

Noncolorectal Malignancies in Inflammatory Bowel Disease: More than Meets the Eye

Laurent Beaugerie   Harry Sokol   Philippe Seksik

Department of Gastroenterology, Saint-Antoine Hospital, and Pierre et Marie Curie University (UPMC), Paris, France

Key Words

Inflammatory bowel disease · Cancer risks · Small bowel adenocarcinoma · Lymphoma · Immunosuppressive therapy

Abstract

In patients with Crohn's disease, the risk of small bowel adenocarcinoma is 20–40 times higher than the low background risk of the general population. In the subset of patients with longstanding small bowel lesions, the absolute risk of small bowel adenocarcinoma exceeds 1 per 100 patient-years after 25 years of follow-up and becomes equivalent to the risk of colorectal cancer. Growing evidence suggests that the pathogenesis of small bowel adenocarcinoma arising in inflammatory lesions of Crohn's disease is similar to that of colorectal cancer complicating chronic colonic inflammation (inflammation-dysplasia-cancer sequence). However, contrasting with the established endoscopic detection of colonic advanced neoplasias in patients with longstanding extensive colitis, there is no consensus at this time how to face the excess-risk of small bowel adenocarcinoma in patients at high risk. There are no specific clinical or imaging alert signs and endoscopic surveillance of the totality of the inflamed small bowel mucosa would suppose to perform repeated enteroscopies, with the potential limiting factor of stenosis. Very preliminary data suggest that chemoprevention with salicylates could be an alternative way for reducing the risk. Data from referral centers and from the CESAME cohort suggest that intestinal lymphomas may arise in the chronically inflamed segments in patients with inflammatory bowel disease (IBD). Regarding nonintestinal lymphomas, it is now established that IBD patients treated with thiopurines have an excess risk of lymphomas, exhibiting in most cases pathological features of lymphomas associated with immunosuppression, including the frequent presence of EBV in neoplastic tissues. There is growing evidence that treatment with thiopurines is responsible by itself for this excess risk. IBD patients receiving immunomodulators, especially young men, are also at risk (0.4 for 10,000 patient-years in the CESAME study) for developing fatal early post-mononucleosis lymphomas, like in Purtilo's syndrome, maybe in association with a background genetic susceptibility. Finally, patients receiving thiopurines and/or TNF-inhibitors are at risk for developing fatal hepatosplenic T cell lymphomas, but this risk is low (no case in the CESAME study). Whether patients receiving a monotherapy with methotrexate and/or TNF inhibitors are at increased risk of lymphomas is not known. Concordant data suggest that women receiving immunosuppressive therapy are at increased risk for developing uterine cervix dysplasia and require closer surveillance. But it is not established whether the risk of uterine cervix cancer and basal and squamous cell skin cancers (that may be associated with chronic human papillomavirus infection) is increased in patients receiving immunomodulators.

Copyright © 2009 S. Karger AG, Basel

Prof. Laurent Beaugerie
Service de Gastroentérologie et Nutrition, Hôpital Saint-Antoine
184, rue du faubourg Saint-Antoine
FR–75571 Paris Cedex 12 (France)
Tel. +33 1 49 28 31 71, Fax +33 1 49 28 31 88, E-Mail laurent.beaugerie@sat.aphp.fr

Population Background

In industrialized countries, cancer has become a considerable concern of public health. Taking the example of France, cancer was the second cause of mortality in 2000 (www.e-cancer.fr). Among incident cancers, sporadic colorectal cancer had the third and second highest annual rate in men and women, respectively. 27 and 11% of the incident cancers were attributable to smoking and alcohol abuse, respectively. In the general French population, it is estimated that almost one individual out of two is prone to develop a cancer during his/her life, in 40% of the cases before the age of 65.

Mortality, Inflammatory Bowel Disease (IBD) and Cancers

Data from the most recent population-based studies suggest that life expectancy is similar to that of the general population in ulcerative colitis [1] but slightly reduced in Crohn's disease [2]. The overall incidence and mortality from cancer are similar to those of the general population [3], both in Crohn's disease [4] and ulcerative colitis [1].

IBD-Related Cancers

The specificities of cancers occurring in patients with IBD may be related to a genetic background or environmental factors shared by cancers and IBD. Cancers occurring in IBD patients may also be due to chronic biliary or intestinal inflammation or to drug-induced immunosuppression.

Common Genes

There are no data suggesting that susceptibility genes to IBD may promote the development of cancers.

Common Environment: Smoking

Smoking is a major risk factor for ear-nose-throat, esophagus and lung cancer. Compared with the general population, smokers are over-represented in Crohn's disease and under-represented in ulcerative colitis. As an illustration, in the early 2000s in France, the prevalence

of smokers was 30, 55 and 15% in the general population, Crohn's disease and ulcerative colitis population, respectively. This distribution of smokers according the type of IBD probably explains why a decreased incidence of lung cancer has been reported in ulcerative colitis [1] while a trend towards the opposite figure has been reported in Crohn's disease [3].

Cancers Associated with Chronic Tissue Inflammation

Cholangiocarcinoma Complicating Primary Sclerosing Cholangitis

The excess risk of IBD-related cholangiocarcinoma is restricted to IBD patients with concurrent primary sclerosing cholangitis who represent less than 5% of the total IBD population. In those patients, the crude incidence rate of cholangiocarcinoma is approximately 1% per year [5]. This excess risk is present from the diagnosis, as the associated excess risk of colorectal cancer [6]. Some data suggest that a prolonged treatment with ursodeoxycholic acid could reduce theses risks [5, 7].

Anal Squamous Cell Carcinoma Complicating Chronic Anal Crohn's Disease

There are numerous case reports of anal squamous cell carcinomas occurring in patients with longstanding anal lesions (including fistulas [8] and tags) in the literature [9]. The reality and the extent of this putative excess risk are not established in the absence of reference incidence rates in the general population discriminating between perianal and anal carcinomas. If this excess risk exists, the respective roles of chronic inflammation, human papillomavirus (HPV) infection [10] and drug-induced immunosuppression (when patients receive immunosuppressants) are unknown.

Small Bowel Adenocarcinoma Complicating Small Bowel Inflammation in Crohn's Disease

In the general population, small bowel adenocarcinoma is rare (60-fold less frequent than colorectal cancer, with a lifelong cumulative risk of <1/1,000) and affects the jenunum and the ileum in similar proportions. In patients with Crohn's disease, the risk of small bowel adenocarcinoma is 20–50 times higher than the low background risk of the general population [2, 11]. In the subset of patients with longstanding small bowel lesions, the absolute risk of small bowel adenocarcinoma exceeds 1 per 100 patient-years after 25 years of follow-up and becomes equivalent to the risk of sporadic colorectal cancer [12]. Small bowel adenocarcinomas occurring in patients with Crohn's disease usually arise in the intestinal segments chronically affected by the IBD, thus in most cases in the ileum. The median time between the diagnosis of Crohn's disease and the diagnosis of small bowel adenocarcinoma is 15 years, but in some instances symptoms of small bowel adenocarcinoma may reveal a longstanding undiagnosed paucisymptomatic Crohn's disease. Given the usual absence of clinical symptoms or imaging features discriminating between inflammatory intestinal lesions of Crohn's disease and intestinal cancer, the diagnosis of small bowel adenocarcinoma is rarely made preoperatively [12]. In most cases, the diagnosis is made either intra-operatively in case of advanced neoplasia or, as a bad surprise, after the microscopic examination of the resected specimens, often under the form of a small cancer surrounded by usual inflammatory lesions of Crohn's disease. Signet ring cells are found in up to one third of the histological specimens of adenocarcinomas arising in patients with Crohn's disease while this feature is usually absent in de novo adenocarcinomas [12].

Despite surgical treatment, when feasible, the 5-year survival rate of patients with Crohn's disease developing small bowel adenocarcinomas is <50%. Growing evidence suggests that pathogenesis of small bowel adenocarcinoma arising in inflammatory lesions of Crohn's disease is similar to that of colorectal cancer complicating chronic colonic inflammation (inflammation-dysplasia-cancer sequence). As described for adenocarcinomas complicating IBD colitis, some adjacent or distant foci of dysplasia may be evidenced around small bowel adenocarcinomas occurring in inflamed intestinal segments of patients with Crohn's disease affecting the small bowel [13]. In addition, individual accounts of small bowel adenocarcinoma with pre-existing dysplasia have been reported [14]. However, contrasting with the established endoscopic detection of colonic advanced neoplasias in patients with longstanding extensive colitis, there is no consensus at this time how to face the excess risk of small bowel adenocarcinoma in patients at high risk. There are no specific clinical or imaging alert signs, irrespective of the imaging technique used (CT scan, MRI, PET scan) discriminating between inflammatory and neoplastic lesions. The endoscopic surveillance of the totality of the inflamed small bowel mucosa would suppose to perform in most of the patients at risk repeated enteroscopies, with the potential limiting factor of stenosis. Preliminary data suggest that chemoprevention with salicylates could be an alternative way for reducing the risk [15, 16].

Cancers and Drug-Induced Immunosuppression

Lymphoproliferative Disorders (LD)

LD are clonal B or T cell proliferative diseases. The incidence of LD has risen markedly in developed countries since the 1970s. Several causes of immunosuppression (primary immune deficiency, HIV infection, post-transplant immunosuppression) are responsible for an excess risk of LD that often involve diffuse large B cells and arise in extranodal sites (especially the gastrointestinal tract and central nervous system). Some of these LD are due to defective immune surveillance of Epstein-Barr virus (EBV); in these cases, signs of EBV replication can be evidenced in the neoplastic lymphocytes. Other infections and genetic factors may be involved, as many cases of LD in the context of immunosuppression are EBV-negative.

In IBD population-based studies [3, 17–25], there is no background excess risk of LD (table 1). However, among the patients with IBD developing LD, a significantly high proportion of LD affecting the gastrointestinal tract, ranging from 27% in population-based studies [20] to 65% in a tertiary care medical center-based study [26], has been reported. This subset of LD observed in patients with IBD could be partly related to chronic inflammatory intestinal lesions, since in other contexts, chronic localized tissue inflammation may lead to an in situ genesis of LD [27].

Thiopurines have a cytotoxic effect on activated T cells and NK cells [28] that are involved in the control of EBV-induced lymphocyte proliferation [29]. This is one possible explanation for the excess incidence of EBV-associated LD reported in patients with IBD receiving thiopurines [26, 30]. This epidemiological feature was precised in the specifically designed CESAME cohort that included prospectively almost 20,000 IBD patients. In this cohort, about one third of the patients were receiving thiopurines at entry into the study, in most cases as a monotherapy [25]. This large study (49,713 patient-years of follow-up) confirmed an independent association between ongoing thiopurine therapy and the risk of LD. Most cases of LD observed in IBD patients treated with thiopurines were associated with EBV and belonged histologically to the post-transplant type. Extrapolating the results of the CESAME cohort, the absolute cumulative risk of LD in young patients receiving a 10-year course of thiopurines remains low (below 1%) and does not significantly undermine the positive risk-benefit ratio of these drugs [31]. In addition, it may become possible in the future to better manage this risk with innovative biological

Table 1. Risk of lymphoproliferative disorders in patients with IBD: population-based studies

Authors	Year of publication	Setting	Patients	SIR (95% CI)
Ekbom et al.	1991	Uppsala, Sweden	CD: 1,665 UC: 3,121 IBD: 4,786	0.4 (0.0–2.4) 1.2 (0.5–2.4) 1.0 (0.5–1.9)
Persson et al.	1994	Stockholm, Sweden	CD: 1,251	1.4 (0.4–3.5)
Karlen et al.	1999	Stockholm, Sweden	UC: 1,547	1.2 (0.3–3.5)
Loftus et al.	2000	Olmsted County, USA	CD: 216 UC: 238 IBD: 454	2.4 (0.1–13.1) 0.0 (0.0–6.4) 1.0 (0.03–5.6)
Palli et al.	2000	Florence, Italy	CD: 231 UC: 689 IBD: 920	NA HD: 9.3 (2.5–23.8) NHL: 1.8 (0.2–6.5) HD: 8.6 (2.8–20.1) NHL: 1.4 (0.2–5.2)
Bernstein et al.	2001	Manitoba, Canada	CD: 2,857 UC: 2,672 IBD: 5,529	2.4 (1.2–5.0)* 1.03 (0.5–2.2)* 1.52 (0.9–2.6)*
Lewis et al.	2001	United Kingdom	CD: 6,605 UC: 10,391 IBD: 16,996	1.59 (0.6–3.3) 1.2 (0.6–2.2) 1.32 (0.8–2.1)
Winther et al.	2004	Copenhagen County, Denmark	UC: 1,160	0.5 (0.1–1.8)
Jess et al.	2004	Copenhagen County, Denmark	CD: 374	none observed
Askling et al.	2005	multiple Swedish cohorts	CD: 20,120 UC: 27,759 IBD: 47,679	1.3 (1.0–1.6) 1.0 (0.8–1.3) NA
Beaugerie et al.	2008	CESAME French nationwide cohort	CD: 11,759 UC: 7,727 IBD: 19,486	1.86 (1.1–3.0)

* Incidence rate ratio (IRR). CESAME is very similar to a population-based study, as it involved a well-balanced proportion of patients from hospitals and private practices. In addition, each consecutive patient from each investigator was enrolled in the study.

SIR = Standardized incidence ratio; UC = ulcerative colitis; CD = Crohn's disease; IBD = inflammatory bowel disease; HD = Hodgkin's disease; NHL = non-Hodgkin lymphoma; NA = not applicable.

tools such as the monitoring of systemic or tissue EBV viral load or the ex vivo assessment of EBV-directed cytotoxic activity of patient lymphocytes. The benefit ratio could be less favorable, however, for elderly patients and unlimited treatment periods.

Beside PTLD-like B cell LD, 2 cases of early fatal post-mononucleosis LD were observed in the CESAME cohort in young men receiving thiopurines, previously reported as sporadic cases [32]. These cases were reminiscent of LD observed in the X-linked lymphoproliferative syndrome [33], further pointing to a combined effect of genetic predisposition and thiopurine treatment. This specific risk, although very rare, should be kept in mind before initiating thiopurine treatment in young EBV-negative males.

Recently, concerns were expressed regarding the risk of hepatosplenic T cell lymphoma in IBD patients receiving anti-TNF-α therapy [34]. In 2007, 8 cases of this rare and rapidly fatal lymphoproliferative disorder were reported in young IBD patients treated with a combination of infliximab and thiopurines. The general incidence of hepatosplenic T cell lymphoma is not known, but fewer than 200 cases have been reported in the literature. Some of these cases involved post-transplant immunosuppression, and 6 cases have also been reported in IBD patients receiving thiopurines alone [35]. Among the 8 cases reported in 2007, 7 involved young males and 7 occurred in CD patients (the 8th patient had UC), leading to concerns regarding anti-TNF-α and thiopurine co-prescription. Since this first publication, 9 other cases have been reported, 3 of which involved adalimumab and 1 an RA patient. Interestingly, while the first 8 cases were described over an 8-year period, the following 9 cases were reported in a period of only 15 months, suggesting that the incidence of this type of LD might have been underestimated in IBD patients. Nevertheless, the true incidence of hepatosplenic T cell lymphoma is probably low, as no cases were recorded in the CESAME study [25].

Whether monotherapy with methotrexate and TNF inhibitors in IBD patients is associated with an overall excess risk of LD has not been properly assessed yet, since few patients worldwide are receiving methotrexate and most of the patients receiving TNF inhibitors have been co-treated up to now with immunomodulators, making it impossible to determine the proper role of TNF inhibitors.

Thiopurine Use and HPV-Related Tumors

Chronic infection with various subtypes of HPV is the cause of benign skin and genital warts and is involved in the pathogenesis of some of the cancers affecting skin, anus and uterine cervix. Because patients receiving thiopurines may have an impaired T lymphocyte-related control of chronic viral infections (see above), we should address the question whether patients receiving thiopurines have a specific thiopurine-related increase in the risk of HPV-related cancers.

IBD outpatients with controlled intestinal disease receiving thiopurines have a slightly increased risk for developing benign skin warts [36]. Regarding nonmelanoma skin cancers, it is now established that thiopurine metabolites both increase photosensitivity of human skin to UVA radiations [37] and UVA-induced mutagenesis of human epithelial cells [38]. These proper effects of thiopurines on skin epithelial cells are sufficient per se for recommending a strict skin protection against UVA radiation in IBD patients. The direct effects of thiopurine metabolites on skin cells could also come in addition to the putative thiopurine-induced promotion of skin HPV infection for increasing the individual risk of nonmelanoma skin cancers in IBD patients receiving thiopurines. However, while it is established that post-transplant patients receiving immunosuppressants have a markedly increased risk of nonmelanoma skin cancer [39], there are no data at this time in the literature supporting the fact that IBD patients receiving thiopurines or another immunosuppressive therapy are at risk of developing nonmelanoma skin cancers.

Concordant recent data suggest that women with IBD have an increased risk of abnormal Pap smears with an over-representation of higher-grade lesions [40–42]. The specific role of thiopurines or other immunosuppressants, via the promotion of HPV infection, in the increased risk for abnormal Pap smears, is not yet quantified among the other established risk factors (smoking, contraceptive pill, etc.). From a practical point of view, strict surveillance of the cervix should be recommended to all women with IBD, with special attention given to those who smoke or are receiving immunosuppressants.

Overall Risk of Cancers in IBD Patients Receiving Methotrexate or Anti-TNF

The proportion of IBD patients receiving methotrexate worldwide has been up to now too small for adequately assessing a putative overall increased risk of cancer due to methotrexate. In the population of patients with rheumatoid arthritis receiving methotrexate as an immunosuppressive monotherapy, sporadic cases of reversible early lymphomas have been reported [43], but no overt excess risk of cancers has been demonstrated [44].

Regarding a potential specific role of anti-TNF in the overall risk of cancers occurring in IBD patients, no conclusion can be made because most of the patients are co-treated with immunomodulators (mainly thiopurines), making it impossible to discriminate between the respective roles of anti-TNF and immunomodulators. In huge cohorts of patients with rheumatoid arthritis receiving TNF antagonists, often as an immunosuppressive monotherapy, no overt excess risk of cancer has been evidenced [45, 46].

Practical Recommendations

In order to limit the risks of noncolorectal cancers and given the epidemiological features detailed here, we are able at this time to recommend smoking cessation in all

IBD patients, strict protection against UV radiations and periodical skin examination in IBD patients receiving immunosuppressants, and strict Pap smear screening protocols in female IBD patients, especially those who are smoking or receiving immunosuppressants.

Disclosure Statement

The authors declare that no financial or other conflict of interest exists in relation to the content of the article.

References

1 Jess T, Gamborg M, Munkholm P, Sorensen TI: Overall and cause-specific mortality in ulcerative colitis: meta-analysis of population-based inception cohort studies. Am J Gastroenterol 2007;102:609–617.

2 Canavan C, Abrams KR, Mayberry JF: Meta-analysis: mortality in Crohn's disease. Aliment Pharmacol Ther 2007;25:861–870.

3 Bernstein CN, Blanchard JF, Kliewer E, Wajda A: Cancer risk in patients with inflammatory bowel disease: a population-based study. Cancer 2001;91:854–862.

4 Persson PG, Bernell O, Leijonmarck CE, Farahmand BY, Hellers G, Ahlbom A: Survival and cause-specific mortality in inflammatory bowel disease: a population-based cohort study. Gastroenterology 1996;110:1339–1345.

5 Talwalkar JA, Lindor KD: Primary sclerosing cholangitis. Inflamm Bowel Dis 2005;11:62–72.

6 Sokol H, Cosnes J, Chazouilleres O, et al: Disease activity and cancer risk in inflammatory bowel disease associated with primary sclerosing cholangitis. World J Gastroenterol 2008;14:3497–3503.

7 Pardi DS, Loftus EV, Jr, Kremers WK, Keach J, Lindor KD: Ursodeoxycholic acid as a chemopreventive agent in patients with ulcerative colitis and primary sclerosing cholangitis. Gastroenterology 2003;124:889–893.

8 Ky A, Sohn N, Weinstein MA, Korelitz BI: Carcinoma arising in anorectal fistulas of Crohn's disease. Dis Colon Rectum 1998;41:992–996.

9 Connell WR, Sheffield JP, Kamm MA, Ritchie JK, Hawley PR, Lennard-Jones JE: Lower gastrointestinal malignancy in Crohn's disease. Gut 1994;35:347–352.

10 Kuhlgatz J, Golas MM, Sander B, Fuzesi L, Hermann RM, Miericke B: Human papilloma virus infection in a recurrent squamous cell carcinoma associated with severe Crohn's disease. Inflamm Bowel Dis 2005;11:84–86.

11 Jess T, Gamborg M, Matzen P, Munkholm P, Sorensen TI: Increased risk of intestinal cancer in Crohn's disease: a meta-analysis of population-based cohort studies. Am J Gastroenterol 2005;100:2724–2729.

12 Palascak-Juif V, Bouvier AM, Cosnes J, et al: Small bowel adenocarcinoma in patients with Crohn's disease compared with small bowel adenocarcinoma de novo. Inflamm Bowel Dis 2005;11:828–832.

13 Sigel JE, Petras RE, Lashner BA, Fazio VW, Goldblum JR: Intestinal adenocarcinoma in Crohn's disease: a report of 30 cases with a focus on coexisting dysplasia. Am J Surg Pathol 1999;23:651–655.

14 Watermeyer G, Locketz M, Govender D, Mall A: Crohn's disease-associated small bowel adenocarcinoma with pre-existing low-grade dysplasia: a case report. Am J Gastroenterol 2007;102:1545–1546.

15 Piton G, Cosnes J, Monnet E, et al: Risk factors associated with small bowel adenocarcinoma in Crohn's disease: a case-control study. Am J Gastroenterol 2008;103:1730–1736.

16 Solem CA, Harmsen WS, Zinsmeister AR, Loftus EV, Jr: Small intestinal adenocarcinoma in Crohn's disease: a case-control study. Inflamm Bowel Dis 2004;10:32–35.

17 Ekbom A, Helmick C, Zack M, Adami HO: Extracolonic malignancies in inflammatory bowel disease. Cancer 1991;67:2015–2019.

18 Persson PG, Karlen P, Bernell O, et al: Crohn's disease and cancer: a population-based cohort study. Gastroenterology 1994;107:1675–1679.

19 Karlen P, Lofberg R, Brostrom O, Leijonmarck CE, Hellers G, Persson PG: Increased risk of cancer in ulcerative colitis: a population-based cohort study. Am J Gastroenterol 1999;94:1047–1052.

20 Loftus EV Jr, Tremaine WJ, Habermann TM, Harmsen WS, Zinsmeister AR, Sandborn WJ: Risk of lymphoma in inflammatory bowel disease. Am J Gastroenterol 2000;95:2308–2312.

21 Lewis JD, Bilker WB, Brensinger C, Deren JJ, Vaughn DJ, Strom BL: Inflammatory bowel disease is not associated with an increased risk of lymphoma. Gastroenterology 2001;121:1080–1087.

22 Winther KV, Jess T, Langholz E, Munkholm P, Binder V: Long-term risk of cancer in ulcerative colitis: a population-based cohort study from Copenhagen County. Clin Gastroenterol Hepatol 2004;2:1088–1095.

23 Jess T, Winther KV, Munkholm P, Langholz E, Binder V: Intestinal and extra-intestinal cancer in Crohn's disease: follow-up of a population-based cohort in Copenhagen County, Denmark. Aliment Pharmacol Ther 2004;19:287–293.

24 Askling J, Brandt L, Lapidus A, et al: Risk of haematopoietic cancer in patients with inflammatory bowel disease. Gut 2005;54:617–622.

25 Beaugerie L, Carrat F, Bouvier AM, et al: Excess risk of lymphoproliferative disorders (LPD) in inflammatory bowel diseases (IBD): interim results of the CESAME cohort. Gastroenterology 2008;134:A116.

26 Dayharsh GA, Loftus EV Jr, Sandborn WJ, et al: Epstein-Barr virus-positive lymphoma in patients with inflammatory bowel disease treated with azathioprine or 6-mercaptopurine. Gastroenterology 2002;122:72–77.

27 Takakuwa T, Tresnasari K, Rahadiani N, Miwa H, Daibata M, Aozasa K: Cell origin of pyothorax-associated lymphoma: a lymphoma strongly associated with Epstein-Barr virus infection. Leukemia 2008;22:620–627.

28 Taylor M, Ajayi F, Almond M: Enterocolitis caused by methicillin-resistant *Staphylococcus aureus*. Lancet 1993;342:804.

29 Rezk SA, Weiss LM: Epstein-Barr virus-associated lymphoproliferative disorders. Hum Pathol 2007;38:1293–1304.

30 Kandiel A, Fraser AG, Korelitz BI, Brensinger C, Lewis JD: Increased risk of lymphoma among inflammatory bowel disease patients treated with azathioprine and 6-mercaptopurine. Gut 2005;54:1121–1125.

31 Lewis JD, Schwartz JS, Lichtenstein GR: Azathioprine for maintenance of remission in Crohn's disease: benefits outweigh the risk of lymphoma. Gastroenterology 2000;118:1018–1024.

32 Posthuma EF, Westendorp RG, van der Sluys Veer A, Kluin-Nelemans JC, Kluin PM, Lamers CB: Fatal infectious mononucleosis: a severe complication in the treatment of Crohn's disease with azathioprine. Gut 1995;36:311–313.

33 Engel P, Eck MJ, Terhorst C: The SAP and SLAM families in immune responses and X-linked lymphoproliferative disease. Nat Rev Immunol 2003;3:813–821.

34 Mackey AC, Green L, Liang LC, Dinndorf P, Avigan M: Hepatosplenic T cell lymphoma associated with infliximab use in young patients treated for inflammatory bowel disease. J Pediatr Gastroenterol Nutr 2007;44:265–267.

35 Shale M, Kanfer E, Panaccione R, Ghosh S: Hepatosplenic T cell lymphoma in inflammatory bowel disease. Gut 2008;57:1639–1641.

36 Seksik P, Cosnes J, Sokol H, Nion-Larmurier I, Gendre JP, Beaugerie L: Incidence of benign upper respiratory tract infections, HSV and HPV cutaneous infections in inflammatory bowel disease patients treated with azathioprine. Aliment Pharmacol Ther 2009;29: 1106–1113.

37 Perrett CM, Walker SL, O'Donovan P, et al: Azathioprine treatment photosensitizes human skin to ultraviolet A radiation. Br J Dermatol 2008;159:198–204.

38 O'Donovan P, Perrett CM, Zhang X, et al: Azathioprine and UVA light generate mutagenic oxidative DNA damage. Science 2005; 309:1871–1874.

39 Euvrard S, Kanitakis J, Claudy A: Skin cancers after organ transplantation. N Engl J Med 2003;348:1681–1691.

40 Kane S: Abnormal Pap smears in inflammatory bowel disease. Inflamm Bowel Dis 2008; 14:1158–1160.

41 Kane S, Khatibi B, Reddy D: Higher incidence of abnormal Pap smears in women with inflammatory bowel disease. Am J Gastroenterol 2008;103:631–636.

42 Bhatia J, Bratcher J, Korelitz B, et al: Abnormalities of uterine cervix in women with inflammatory bowel disease. World J Gastroenterol 2006;12:6167–6171.

43 Kamel OW, van de Rijn M, Weiss LM, et al: Brief report: reversible lymphomas associated with Epstein-Barr virus occurring during methotrexate therapy for rheumatoid arthritis and dermatomyositis. N Engl J Med 1993;328:1317–1321.

44 Buchbinder R, Barber M, Heuzenroeder L, et al: Incidence of melanoma and other malignancies among rheumatoid arthritis patients treated with methotrexate. Arthritis Rheum 2008;59:794–799.

45 Wolfe F, Michaud K: Biologic treatment of rheumatoid arthritis and the risk of malignancy: analyses from a large US observational study. Arthritis Rheum 2007;56:2886–2895.

46 Askling J, Fored CM, Brandt L, et al: Risks of solid cancers in patients with rheumatoid arthritis and after treatment with tumour necrosis factor antagonists. Ann Rheum Dis 2005;64:1421–1426.

Specific Management Issues

Dig Dis 2009;27:382–386
DOI: 10.1159/000228578

Transition from Pediatric to Adult Health Care in Inflammatory Bowel Disease

Johanna C. Escher

Department of Pediatric Gastroenterology, Erasmus MC-Sophia Children's Hospital, University Medical Center, Rotterdam, The Netherlands

Key Words

Transition · Inflammatory bowel disease · Adolescents

Abstract

Inflammatory bowel disease (IBD) is a lifelong disease that has great psychosocial impact on the adolescent patient and his/her family. Starting around age 12–14 years, many changes take place related to school, work, and sexual development. At some point, usually around the age of 16–18 years, these patients need to move from the pediatric clinic to the adult caregivers. A stepwise program for transition of care, aimed at coaching the adolescent patient into self-management will benefit patients, parents, and the 'adult gastroenterologist' who will take over the care from the pediatric gastroenterologist. Differences in pediatric and adult health care, transition goals, tips and tools for successful transition will be discussed.

Copyright © 2009 S. Karger AG, Basel

Definitions

Transition is a process that may take some years, ideally starting at age 14. During this process, patients and parents will be prepared for the transfer to an adult gastroenterologist (fig. 1). The actual transfer takes place somewhere between age 16 and 18, depending on the lo-cal regulation. The timing of this transfer should be carefully planned together with the patient and parents. Preferably, it should be planned in a period of quiescent disease. In addition, study or work plans and concomitant move from the family home need to be taken into account before identifying the adult gastroenterologist. This new doctor should be apprehensive of the specific psychosocial issues that adolescents and young adults with IBD may have. Patients with early onset IBD tend to have a more severe course of disease, longer duration of exposure to immunomodulators and biologics, and a high lifetime risk of malignancy. Therefore, most adolescent patients will be transferred to an IBD-dedicated gastroenterologist in an academic setting. A transitional clinic, where IBD outpatients are seen (either simultaneously or alternating) by the pediatric and adult gastroenterologist, and a transition nurse seem essential for a well-coordinated transition process.

Why Do We Need Transition?

Transition is needed to bridge the differences between pediatric and adult health care in IBD (table 1). Successful transition will guarantee continuity of care and is aimed at better adherence, a higher level of self-management and hopefully effective disease control in young adult patients.

Johanna C. Escher, MD, PhD
Department of Pediatric Gastroenterology, Erasmus MC-Sophia Children's Hospital
University Medical Center, Dr. Molewaterplein 60
NL–3015 GJ Rotterdam (The Netherlands)
Tel. +31 10 703 6049, Fax +31 10 703 6811, E-Mail j.escher@erasmusmc.nl

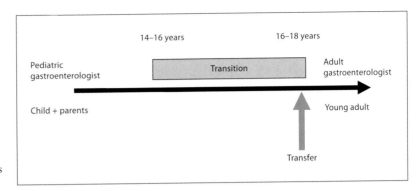

Fig. 1. Transition is a process that takes place between ages 14 and 18 years.

In our experience, abrupt transfer at the age of 18 years (as we used to do before we started our transitional clinic in 2006) may cause unnecessary harm in patients, insufficient confidence in parents, and frustration in the adult gastroenterologist.

We can define three goals in transition:
– to get the patient ready for transfer, having attained specific skills and knowledge;
– to get the parents ready for transfer;
– to get the adult gastroenterologist ready and well-informed at the time of transfer.

Table 1. Differences in pediatric and adult health care in IBD

Pediatric IBD care	Adult IBD care
Focus on: growth, puberty, nutrition	Focus on: malignancy, surveillance, new drugs
Endoscopy: general anesthesia	Endoscopy: conscious sedation or no anesthesia
Family oriented	Parents not appreciated
Child is a special patient – child-friendly approach	Patient is one of many – neutral approach
Pediatricians: nice, take more time	Adult gastroenterologists: business-like approach, less time

The Adolescent IBD Patient

Adolescence is a time of growth and change that causes frustration about the present and anxiety about the future, and the adolescent must shed the sheltered environment of childhood and achieve self-reliance and self-dependent living [1]. Adolescents with IBD should in addition to all this come to terms with a life-long disease, and meanwhile get ready to self-manage their illness. Hait et al. [2] give practical recommendations for a stepwise transition protocol with age-appropriate checklists of tasks for the patient and medical team. For example, at age 14–16 years, the patient is able to identify the medical team, knows names and purposes of procedures and tests done on him or her, knows his or her medical history, knows about the IBD patient organization, understands the medical risk of non-adherence and the impact of drugs and alcohol on their illness. Next, beyond the age of 16, a patient knows how to gather information about IBD, is able to book his or her own appointments, fill prescriptions and contact the medical team if needed.

In parallel, the medical team should direct all questions and explanations to the patient, determine when the parents can be in and out of the room at the outpatient clinic, and instruct the patient how to acquire the specific skills.

It is important for the pediatric gastroenterologist to discuss the high life-time cancer risk that young patients have, as this will have direct implications for endoscopic surveillance. As yearly surveillance is advised after a disease duration of 8 years, patients with a diagnosis in their teens may be faced with screening colonoscopy directly after transfer. Patients and parents need to understand about the risks and anticipate to concomitant surveillance.

The Parents

For parents, transfer to a new doctor is often accompanied by fear and a sense of loss. After having been involved in all treatment decisions, they are now faced with a new situation where that need to let go and gain trust as the adolescent will become more self-dependent.

It is therefore important for the medical team to also coach the parents in order for them to have faith in their child's newly achieved self-management as well as to trust the new doctor. In other words, transition is a family matter.

The Adult Gastroenterologist

The adult gastroenterologist needs to be provided with a written, detailed history of the patient's disease, past and present medications, initial and most recent investigations, and surgery. It is important for the adult gastroenterologist to understand and know about growth failure, residual growth potential and target height of the individual patient. In addition, specific information on childhood diseases and vaccinations have to be provided.

In the ideal setting of a transitional clinic, the adult gastroenterologist will already be involved in the care of the patient before transfer. This will enable useful discussions between the pediatric and adult caregivers, who may have a different treatment approach. In a survey by Hait et al. [3], adult gastroenterologists reported that young IBD patients often demonstrated deficits in knowledge about their medical history (55% of respondents) and medical regimens (69%). In addition, 51% reported to have received inadequate information from the pediatric gastroenterologists at transfer.

Interestingly, adult gastroenterologists were less concerned about the ability of patients to attend office visits by themselves (15%) or to undergo endoscopic procedures under conscious sedation (13%).

As for understanding growth and mental development in adolescence, 89% thought this was important, while only 46% felt competent in these issues.

The Transition Protocol

Transition is more successful if it is well-coordinated. A hospital-based or national protocol provides guidance in the individual transition plan. A protocol can be disease-specific, but general protocols for transition of adolescents with chronic disease may also be helpful. Depending on the local situation and the availability of the adult gastroenterologist, a transition strategy will be chosen, as exemplified in figure 2a–c. Figure 2a shows major involvement of the adult gastroenterologist as each patient is seen 3–5 times at yearly combined visits with both doctors present in the room. The situation in figure 2b shows the strategy of several alternating visits, and in figure 2c only one combined visit, just prior to transfer is organized.

It is unknown which strategy is most effective, but when asked, most adolescents and parents in our clinic preferred multiple combined visits, as depicted in figure 2a [4].

Efficacy of Transition by Assessing Self-Efficacy

In the Erasmus MC-Sophia, we have started a transitional clinic (TC) in 2006 for IBD patients between ages 14 and 18 years. The TC is located in the adult department, and patients are seen together by both the pediatric and the adult gastroenterologist at the first visit, and once yearly thereafter. At all other visits (at least 4 per year), the pediatric gastroenterologist sees the patients alone. In addition to this, the IBD nurse has scheduled appointments with all patients.

In a recent pilot study, we tested a self-efficacy questionnaire, the 'IBD-yourself', among 50 patients (mean age 15.6 years) and a mirror version in 40 parents [5]. Self-efficacy is a person's belief in his/her capability to organize and execute actions required to deal with prospective situations. For example, if a patient is convinced he/she is capable of talking to his/her doctor about his/her disease, self-efficacy is high in this matter. The items on the self-efficacy questionnaire showed good to excellent internal consistency, as demonstrated by Cronbach's alphas of 0.85, 0.88 and 0.92 for questions relating to independent behavior during outpatient clinic visit, self-efficacy in treatment, and ability to discuss the disease in social environment, respectively.

When patients, parents and doctors were asked to score general self-efficacy on a visual analogue scale (0–100%), no significant differences were found: a mean score of 66, 71 and 66% was given by patients, parents, and doctors, respectively.

A good correlation was found between both the number of visits to the IBD transition clinic and the age of the patient and readiness of the adolescent ($r = 0.37$; $p = 0.02$, and $r = 0.45$; $p = 0.005$, respectively) for transition. Gender differences were not seen, except for knowledge about the disease, which was better in boys.

These results suggest that the self-efficacy questionnaire is a new and valuable tool that deserves further val-

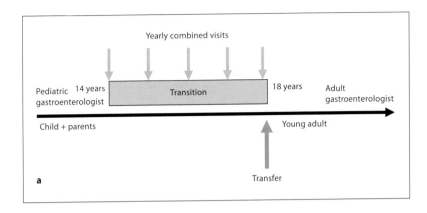

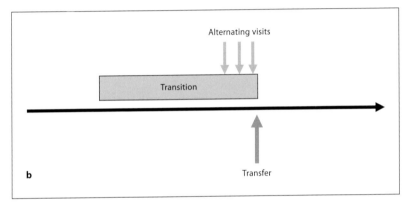

Fig. 2. a Transition protocol with 3–5 combined visits, once a year, to a pediatric and an adult gastroenterologist, both sitting in the room. At the visits in between, the patient is seen by the pediatric gastroenterologist. However, the adult gastroenterologist is involved in the care already at age 14 years. b Transition protocol with 3 alternating visits, once every 2–3 months, to either a pediatric or an adult gastroenterologist. Before this alternating schedule, the patient is enrolled in a transition protocol that involves only the pediatric gastroenterologist. Around age 16 years, the adult gastroenterologist starts to be involved in the care of the patient. c Transition protocol with 1 combined visit with both pediatric and adult gastroenterologist present in the room. Prior to this final visit, the patient is enrolled in a transition protocol that involves only the pediatric gastroenterologist. Only around transfer does the adult gastroenterologist start to be involved in the care of the patient.

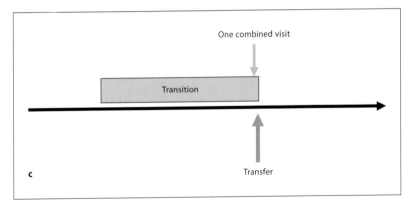

idation by assessment of quality and efficacy of IBD transition programs. Second, the results indicate that our IBD transition program is effective in increasing readiness for transfer to the adult caregivers in adolescent IBD patients.

Disclosure Statement

The author declares that no financial or other conflict of interest exists in relation to the content of the article.

References

1 Medical Position Statement: Transition of the patient with inflammatory bowel disease from pediatric to adult care: recommendations of the North American Society for Pediatric Gastroenterology, Hepatology and Nutrition (NASPGHAN). J Pediatr Gastroenterol Nutr 2002;34:245–248.

2 Hait E, Arnold JH, Fishman LN: Educate, communicate, anticipate-practical recommendations for transitioning adolescents with IBD to adult health care. Inflamm Bowel Dis 2006;12:70–73.

3 Hait EJ, Barendse RM, Arnold JH, Valim C, Sands BE, Korzenik JR, Fishman LN: Transition of adolescents with inflammatory bowel disease from pediatric to adult care: a survey of adult gastroenterologists. J Pediatr Gastroenterol Nutr 2009;48:61–65.

4 Van Pieterson M, van der Toorn P, van der Woude CJ, Escher JC: Transition of care in IBD: expectations and outcome in adolescents and young adults. J Pediatr Gastroenterol Nutr 2007;44:e95.

5 Zijlstra M, Breij L, van der Woude CJ, de Ridder L, van Pieterson M, Escher JC: Assessment of self-efficacy during transition in adolescents with inflammatory bowel disease. Poster (P194) presented at 4th congress of ECCO, Hamburg, February 5–7, 2009. J Crohns Colitis 2009;3:S87.

Dig Dis 2009;27:387–393
DOI: 10.1159/000228579

Fistula Treatment: The Unresolved Challenge

Pierre Michetti

Division of Gastroenterology and Hepatology, Centre Hospitalier Universitaire Vaudois, Lausanne, Switzerland

Key Words

Crohn's disease · Fistulas · Medical management · Anti-TNF therapy

Abstract

Fistulas are common complications in Crohn's disease, as their cumulative prevalence reaches up to two thirds of the patients in the long term. Fistulas worsen the overall patient prognosis, with permanent sphincter and perineal tissue destruction as well as professional and personal disabilities. The importance of healing these fistulas has been less well appreciated than mucosal healing for luminal disease. Management should not be left to any specialty alone, but requires an optimal combination of surgery, infection control, and immunosuppression. Outcome of therapy beyond fistula drainage is unclear and the means of assessing healing over a long time period is poorly characterized. Recent studies suggested that a substantial proportion of patients can achieve fistula healing with surgical and medical therapies. However, studies that measure the benefit of integrated approaches, of early intervention and of precise healing assessment are still missing. Such information is particularly needed in this subset of sick patients that undergo substantial physical and emotional distress because of pain, discharge, incontinence, perineal and genital disfigurement. The advent of adequate pelvic imaging, improved surgical outcomes, and potent biological therapies make it timely to develop best-management strategies and appropriateness of care criteria.   Copyright © 2009 S. Karger AG, Basel

Introduction

The development of fistulas represents a critical complication in the course of Crohn's disease. In population-based cohorts, the cumulative incidence of fistula formation has been evaluated between 17 and 50%, while higher incidences have been observed in referral center patient populations. In a population-based cohort followed between 1970 and 1995, fistulas occurred in 35% of Crohn's patients over time [1]. Of those fistulas, 54% were perianal, 24% enteroenteric, 9% rectovaginal, and 13% involved other locations, including enterocutaneous, enterovesical and intra-abdominal fistulas. A third of these patients experienced fistulas development late in the course of the disease (after the first 10 years of disease evolution) or had to face recurrent fistulas. In a long follow-up study conducted in referral centers, Cosnes et al. [2] observed new cases of fistulas as late as 25 years after the onset of disease reaching a cumulative incidence of 73%, which emphasizes the difficulties of Crohn's disease classification and prognosis evaluation. In approximately 10% of patients, however, fistula formation is the initial feature of the disease, which may precede the onset of other symptoms of Crohn's disease by several years [2, 3]. The risk of fistula development is higher in patients with colonic Crohn's disease, in particular in those with rectal involvement, as compared with patients without colorectal disease.

Fistulas are classified according to their location and to the organs they involve; they can be external or inter-

Prof. Pierre Michetti
Division of Gastroenterology and Hepatology, BH-10N
Centre Hospitalier Universitaire Vaudois, Rue du Bugnon 46
CH–1011 Lausanne (Switzerland)
Tel. +41 21 314 0690, Fax +41 21 314 0707, E-Mail pierre.michetti@chuv.ch

nal. Perianal fistulas, the most common, can be further classified as low (located below the dentate line), high (above the dentate line), simple (low, painless, with a single opening, and no evidence of anal canal stricture or rectovaginal extension) or complex (high, made of multiple tracts and openings, rectovaginal or associated with pain, with anorectal stricture, or with active inflammatory rectal disease) [4].

Diagnosis

The initial diagnosis of external fistula is clinical, while the symptoms associated with internal fistulas may vary greatly according to the location of the tracts and the organs involved. Furthermore, as treatment options evolved, additional diagnosis information became essential for adequate management of the patients. Indeed, several features of the fistulizing disease impact on therapy choices and sequence, namely the precise anatomy of the fistula tracts, their complexity, the presence or absence of abscesses and pelvic sepsis and the presence or absence of rectal inflammatory disease. This information is crucial from the onset of management to avoid adverse clinical outcome of both medical and surgical therapies [5]. For the most common perianal fistulas, proper evaluation may include, in addition to the physical examination, an examination under general anesthesia, pelvic MRI, CT scan imaging, and/or endoscopic or endorectal ultrasound imaging [6]. These techniques help define the precise extension of the disease and are needed to rule out complications such as abscesses. Adequate diagnosis has been obtained in 100% of cases when the evaluation included pelvic MRI and examination under anesthesia, or when either of these techniques was combined to endorectal ultrasounds, underlying that more than one diagnosis modality should be used in each case [7].

Assessment and Scoring of Fistulas in Crohn's Disease
Various definitions of fistula activity and healing have been used in the literature, but none have met general acceptance. The Crohn's Disease Activity Index (CDAI), the most commonly used index in clinical trials to measure symptoms, only attributes 20 points to fistula, regardless of the number or type of fistulas. A score had been proposed by Present et al. [8] to measure fistula progression or healing, but this system has not been sufficiently validated thereafter. The Perianal Disease Activity Index (PDAI), in contrast, has been validated. This score, developed by Irvine, comprises 5 categories (dis-

charge, pain, restriction of sexual activities, type of perianal disease, and degree of induration) each graded on a 5-point scale, from no symptom (0) to severe symptoms (4) [9]. This score has been used to evaluate response to metronidazole [10] but has not been used as primary endpoint for studies testing the outcome of anti-TNF therapies [8, 11]. In these more recent studies, primary efficacy endpoint was defined as a reduction of 50% in the number of draining fistulas observed in 2 or more consecutive visits, as assessed by the study investigator, using gentle finger compression. This finger compression technique has the disadvantage of being investigator dependent. Thus, at this stage, there is no widely accepted and validated scoring system for fistulas in Crohn's disease. Furthermore, there is no consensus on the time at which assessments should be performed and when a fistula can be considered as healed. This point has been highlighted by the observation that fistula tracts persist after fistula closure and that completely healed fistulas can reopen after cessation of therapy [12–14].

Medical Management

The treatment of fistulas in Crohn's disease includes medical and surgical options, which should often be combined. The various therapies will be discussed below. The results of uncontrolled studies should be considered with caution as the natural history of fistulas is sometimes unpredictable. This is illustrated by the relatively high placebo response observed in trials that have included a placebo arm. The importance of such placebo comparators when investigating the potential benefit of therapies in Crohn's disease has been recently confirmed by a meta-analysis of placebo response rates [15]. This analysis confirmed prior observations that about 10% of patients with fistulas will heal spontaneously during a given observation period while receiving a placebo.

Aminosalicylates and Corticosteroids
Mesalamine is no longer recognized as an active therapy for Crohn's disease and no study showed efficacy on fistula healing [16]. Corticosteroids are efficacious in controlling acute flares of Crohn's disease. However, patients with active disease and fistulas enrolled in studies testing the benefit of corticosteroids experienced a worse outcome and increased need for surgery as compared to patients without fistulas or not on steroids [17, 18]. Fistula should thus be considered as a contraindication for the use of steroids in Crohn's disease patients.

Antibiotics

Antibiotics are widely used in the management of Crohn's disease fistulas. They are used both as primary therapies for this condition, despite the lack of high-quality evidence, but also as adjuvant therapy for abscesses and infections associated with the development of fistulas. Metronidazole has been the most studied antibiotic in this indication. In a classical open-label series, Bernstein et al. [19] obtained complete healing of fistulas in 56% of 18 patients after 10 weeks. A follow-up study showed that dose reduction was associated with recurrence in all patients, but that resuming the initial dose was effective [20]. However, persistent healing after cessation of drug therapy occurred in only 28% of patients. In a recent small placebo-controlled trial in which 10 patients were randomized to ciprofloxacin, 7 to metronidazole, and 8 to placebo, remission at week 10 occurred in 3 patients (30%) treated with ciprofloxacin, no patients (0%) treated with metronidazole, and 1 patient (12.5%) treated with placebo, casting doubts on the value of metronidazole alone to treat Crohn's-related fistulas [21].

Ciprofloxacin has also been shown to be effective in small uncontrolled studies. In the small randomized study by Thia et al. [21] described above, this antibiotic was more effective than placebo or metronidazole, but the results were not significantly better than placebo or metronidazole. Clearly, this study lacked the power to determine whether a type 2 statistical error could have taken place. The combination of metronidazole and ciprofloxacine has given better results. In an open-label study that included 52 patients, from which 31 also received azathioprine before or 8 weeks after the start of the antibiotics [10], after 20 weeks of therapy, 48% of patients had a clinical response in the group receiving azathioprine, against 15% of patients on antibiotics alone. These results suggest that antibiotics can be used as a bridge therapy to azathioprine as well as maintenance therapy. Antibiotics, however, can be poorly tolerated and induce serious adverse events when used for long periods of time. In a small but randomized and placebo-controlled trial, the combination of ciprofloxacin and infliximab tended to be better than infliximab alone in 24 patients treated for 6 weeks with antibiotics or placebo before a classical 3-dose regimen of infliximab 5 mg/kg was initiated. In this study, 73% of patients under combined therapy achieved response, as compared to 39% on infliximab alone (OR 2.37; 95% CI 0.94–5.98, p = 0.07) [22]. Taken together, these data indicate that antibiotics are efficacious in the short-term management of fistulas and their associated infections, but the recurrence rate at withdrawal is high and complete healing not frequently achieved with antibiotics alone.

Immunosuppressive Agents

In 1980, Present et al. [8] described the use of 6-mercaptopurine in the treatment of Crohn's disease. In this study 36 patients had 40 fistulas. Thirty-one percent of the fistulas closed on active therapy, while only 6% closed in the placebo group. The onset of response occurred in more than 3 months in 32% of responders. Further uncontrolled studies confirmed these results as well as a meta-analysis in which the OR for response was estimated at 4.44 (CI 1.5–13.2) [23]. The usual dosing of thioguanine analogues is 2.0–2.5 mg/kg for azathioprine and 1.0–1.5 mg/kg for 6-mercaptopurine. The use of erythrocyte levels of 6-thioguanine has been described for the titration of the dose of these agents, but convincing evidence that this tool improves the response rate in patients with fistulas is lacking. These drugs belong to the armamentarium for the treatment of fistulas in Crohn's disease, but their slow onset of action make them good candidates for combination with agents acting faster such as antibiotics.

Calcineurin inhibitors have also been used on fistulas in Crohn's disease. Ciclosporin has been tested in several uncontrolled studies. In these studies response was limited, but occurred within 1–2 weeks [24–26]. In their study, Egan et al. [24] observed, however, that 9 of 10 patients who had failed to respond to thioguanine analogues responded to ciclosporin. These studies, although uncontrolled, suggest that intravenous ciclosporin could have a role in fistulizing Crohn's disease, but more data are needed before a recommendation can be made regarding this therapy. Tacrolimus has been tested in a randomized, placebo-controlled trial in which 48 patients were assigned to either oral tacrolimus 0.2 mg/kg or placebo for 10 weeks [27]. The outcome was an improvement of fistula drainage in 43% of patients in patients on active drug, versus 8% on placebo. However, fistula healing was not different (10 vs. 8%, respectively) and serious adverse event occurred on tacrolimus, which improved after dose reduction. At present, no recommendation can therefore be made regarding tacrolimus in this indication.

Anti-TNF Agents

The development of anti-TNF agents has induced a paradigm shift in the management of Crohn's disease, including of its fistulizing form. Infliximab is the only member agent of this class to have been tested prospectively in a randomized trial primarily designed to test its efficacy in fistulizing Crohn's disease. Present et al. [12] enrolled 85 patients in this landmark study and assigned them to receive 5 or 10 mg/kg infliximab or placebo at baseline, as well as 2 and 6 weeks later. The primary endpoint was a reduction of at least 50% of draining fistulas on two consecutive visits. This outcome was met in 62% of infliximab-treated patients versus 26% in the placebo group (p < 0.002) and complete closure of fistulas occurred in 46% and 13% of the patients, respectively (p = 0.0009). There was no difference between the two infliximab doses tested. The median time to respond was 2 weeks. In a further randomized trial aimed at testing infliximab as maintenance therapy for fistulizing Crohn's disease, Sands et al. [14] confirmed these short-term results with 69% of 306 patients with abdominal or perianal fistulas who responded to an open-label induction therapy with infliximab as an initial part of the ACCENT II trial. The primary endpoint of this study was, however, to determine the time to loss of response in patients who had responded to induction therapy. This time was 40 weeks in patients assigned to infliximab and 14 weeks in patients switched to placebo for maintenance (p < 0.001). At week 54, 19% of patients in the placebo maintenance group had a complete absence of draining fistulas, as compared with 36% of patients in the infliximab maintenance group (p = 0.009). In a post hoc analysis, closure of rectovaginal fistulas occurred in 64% of 25 female patients [14, 28]. Not surprisingly, infliximab also reduced hospitalizations, surgeries and other procedures in this trial [29]. If these results represent the best results to date in fistulizing Crohn's disease therapy, they also indicate that there is still a substantial proportion of patients who are in need of further therapy, either because of primary failure or because of loss of response to infliximab. Whether increasing the dose, as demonstrated for luminal disease, is effective in fistula patients remains to be established.

Adalimumab was tested in two large randomized placebo-controlled trials for its ability to induce remission in Crohn's disease. In the CLASSIC-1 trial, various induction doses were tested in 299 patients [30]. In the GAIN trial, 325 patients with loss of response to infliximab or intolerance to this drug were enrolled to receive the highest dose tested in the CLASSIC-1 study, i.e. 160 mg at baseline and 80 mg 2 weeks later [31]. In these trials, 32 and 45 patients, respectively, had fistulas but adalimumab was not found superior to placebo in controlling this feature of their disease. In a further large randomized trial aimed at evaluating adalimumab as maintenance therapy in patients who had responded to induction therapy with open-label adalimumab induction therapy (80 mg/40 mg at week 0/2), Colombel et al. [32] randomized all patients to receive then double-blind placebo or adalimumab 40 mg every other week or weekly through week 56 (irrespective of fistula status). Patients completing week 56 of therapy were then eligible to enroll in an open-label extension. Of 854 patients enrolled, 117 had draining fistulas at both screening and baseline (70 randomized to adalimumab and 47 randomized to placebo). The mean number of draining fistulas per day was significantly decreased in adalimumab-treated patients (33%) compared with placebo-treated patients (13%, p = 0.016) at week 56 of the double-blind treatment period [32]. Of all patients with healed fistulas at week 56 (both adalimumab and placebo groups), 90% (28 of 31) maintained healing following 1 year of open-label adalimumab therapy (observed analysis) [33]. Although not obtained in a study primarily aimed at testing adalimumab in fistulizing Crohn's disease, these results compare to those obtained with infliximab and further suggest that adalimumab may represent an option for patients who have lost response or who have become intolerant to infliximab.

Certolizumab pegol differ from the two other anti-TNF agents for being a pegylated Fab fragment of a humanized anti-TNF antibody, thus not being able to induce apoptosis of TNF-producing cells. The value of this compound for the treatment of Crohn's disease has been established in two large randomized trials, named PRECiSE 1 and 2. In these two trials, only small numbers of patients with fistulas were included. Of the 662 patients of PRECiSE 1, fistula closure was obtained in 14 of 46 patients treated with certolizumab and in 19 of 61 patients in the placebo group (30 and 31%, respectively) [34]. Of the 425 patients of the 668 who had responded to the open-label induction phase of PRECiSE 2, only 58 had draining fistulas at baseline (28 treated with certolizumab and 30 in the placebo group) [35]. At the end of the randomized 24-week period, 54 and 43% had complete fistula closure, but the difference was not significant. Thus, we still lack convincing data to show the efficacy of this drug in fistulizing Crohn's disease.

Other Medical Therapies

Methotrexate has not been prospectively tested in fistulizing Crohn's disease. In a retrospective chart review, 37 courses of methotrexate therapy were given to 33 patients with luminal and/or fistulizing Crohn's disease who all had failed or were intolerant to 6-mercaptopurine. In 16 patients with fistulas, 4 (25%) had complete closure, 5 (31%) had partial closure [36].

Oral spherical adsorptive carbon (AST-120) has recently been tested in a placebo-controlled randomized trial in Japan. Sixty-two patients were randomized, 57 of whom received AST-120 (n = 27) or placebo (n = 30) [37]. The improvement rate in the AST-120 group (37.0%) was significantly higher than that in the placebo group (10.0%; p = 0.025). The corresponding remission rates were 29.6% and 6.7%, respectively (p = 0.035). This novel compound might, with respect to its low toxicity, represent an option for perianal fistula patients.

Surgical Management

Depending of the populations and length of follow-up, 20–80% of Crohn's disease patients with perianal fistulas will eventually require surgery [1, 38–40] and about 30% of patients with complicated perianal Crohn's disease may eventually require a permanent stoma [41, 42]. Surgical therapy has to be adapted to each case, but the overall goal of surgery should be to cure the fistulas without damaging sphincter function.

Low perianal fistulas in patients without rectal inflammation can be treated by fistulotomy, with reported healing rates of 80% or more [43]. All other fistulas demand a multidisciplinary approach of which surgery is an integral part. Surgeons should be involved in the precise diagnosis of the lesions during examination under anesthesia, with the goal to drain abscesses and to place noncutting setons, to prevent recurrent abscess formation. These steps, however, are unlikely to suffice to induce healing, as shown by the fact that only 20% of fistulas treated by loose setons were healed after 10 years of observation in a series of 20 patients [44].

Further surgical steps may include the advancement flap procedure and/or diverting stomas. In two studies, initial healing rates with advancement flaps were 71–89%, but with recurrence rates of 34–63% during subsequent follow-up [45–47]. Repeat procedure is possible but failure rate increases [48]. Furthermore, if infliximab treatment did not harm the success rate of this surgery, it did not seem to help towards better outcome either [49]. Temporary stoma may then be needed in these patients, either to protect repeated flap procedures during healing, or as an alternative to such repairs. Mueller et al. [41] achieved a healing rate of 47% in 51 patients with temporary stoma placement. However, permanent stomas are not rare in this group of patients. In another series of 356 consecutive Crohn's disease patients, 24% (86) had perianal Crohn's disease and underwent 344 operations [50].

Forty-two patients (49%) ultimately required permanent diversion; among them were 21 of 32 patients (66%) with anal stricture and 12 of 20 women (60%) with rectovaginal fistula. In multivariate logistic regression, the presence of colonic disease and anal canal stricture were predictors of permanent diversion. The OR associated with the risk of permanent diversion in the presence of colonic disease and in the absence of anal stricture was 10 (p = 0.0345). In the presence of both colonic disease and anal canal stenosis, the OR associated with permanent stoma was 33 (p = 0.0023). Permanent ileostomy does not protect against the risk of further fistula recurrence.

Surgical fistula management also includes attempts to close the fistular tracts by fibrin glue or by insertion of bioprosthetic plugs. Fibrin glue has been shown effective in some studies [51–53], but less convincing results have also been reported [54]. The best results, evaluated after a median follow-up of 11.7 months in 30 patients, were obtained after 8 weeks of seton drainage and under general anesthesia (68.4 success vs. 18.2% in local anesthesia, p = 0.02) [51]. This technique compared favorably to conventional surgical management for complex fistulas in a randomized trial [55]. More recently, collagen-based plugs (Cook Surgisis® AFP anal fistula plug) were proposed as an alternative to close perianal fistulas by insertion of the material from the internal opening of the tract. Initial experience with this technique is encouraging, even if most of the reported cases are not Crohn's-related fistulas and results quite uneven across studies, ranging from 14 to 86% of fistula closure [56–58]. In an open-label prospective comparison study, plug insertion was more effective than fibrin glue therapy [59]. At this stage it is too early to make a recommendation, as a variety of issues such as bowel preparation, treatment of fistula tract, closure of the internal opening, and postoperative management have to be further defined, as well as the 'ideal' indication of this technique [60].

Conclusions

The treatment of fistulizing Crohn's disease has evolved considerably, but remains a challenge, as no approach, neither medical nor surgical, leads to reliable success rate. Novel immunosuppressive agents and even more anti-TNFs have remarkably improved the possibilities of medical management, but long-term success is not sufficient for the majority of patients who remained affected in their daily life by their fistular disease. Surgical approaches have progressed just as much as the medical ones. Advancement flaps allowed a substantial proportion of patients to go on with their life, but again, long-term recurrence is the rule rather the exception. Fibrin glue and fistula plugs are promising techniques, but more should be learned about them before they can become main street therapies. Most important, however, is that we need to all work together to study, compare and eventually define integrated treatment medico-surgical strategies that provide patients with the best from all approaches in an organized and synergistic fashion [61]. It is high time for active comparator trials and strategy comparing studies, and time to stop single-component, placebo-controlled trials, as there should nowadays be no patient with fistula to whom an active therapy cannot be given to treat this terrible condition.

Disclosure Statement

Pierre Michetti has served as paid consultant for Abbott, Berlex, Centocor, Ferring, Schering-Plough, and UCB. He received research grants from Berlex and UCB.

References

1 Schwartz DA, Loftus EV Jr, Tremaine WJ, Panaccione R, Harmsen WS, Zinsmeister AR, Sandborn WJ: The natural history of fistulizing Crohn's disease in Olmsted County, Minnesota. Gastroenterology 2002;122: 875–880.

2 Cosnes J, Cattan S, Blain A, Beaugerie L, Carbonnel F, Parc R, Gendre JP: Long-term evolution of disease behavior of Crohn's disease. Inflamm Bowel Dis 2002;8:244–250.

3 Hellers G, Bergstrand O, Ewerth S, Holmstrom B: Occurrence and outcome after primary treatment of anal fistulae in Crohn's disease. Gut 1980;21:525–527.

4 Sandborn WJ, Fazio VW, Feagan BG, Hanauer SB: Aga technical review on perianal Crohn's disease. Gastroenterology 2003;125: 1508–1530.

5 Williamson PR, Hellinger MD, Larach SW, Ferrara A: Twenty-year review of the surgical management of perianal Crohn's disease. Dis Colon Rectum 1995;38:389–392.

6 Spradlin NM, Wise PE, Herline AJ, Muldoon RL, Rosen M, Schwartz DA: A randomized prospective trial of endoscopic ultrasound to guide combination medical and surgical treatment for Crohn's perianal fistulas. Am J Gastroenterol 2008;103:2527–2535.

7 Schwartz DA, Wiersema MJ, Dudiak KM, Fletcher JG, Clain JE, Tremaine WJ, Zinsmeister AR, Norton ID, Boardman LA, Devine RM, Wolff BG, Young-Fadok TM, Diehl NN, Pemberton JH, Sandborn WJ: A comparison of endoscopic ultrasound, magnetic resonance imaging, and exam under anesthesia for evaluation of Crohn's perianal fistulas. Gastroenterology 2001;121:1064–1072.

8 Present DH, Korelitz BI, Wisch N, Glass JL, Sachar DB, Pasternack BS: Treatment of Crohn's disease with 6-mercaptopurine: a long-term, randomized, double-blind study. N Engl J Med 1980;302:981–987.

9 Irvine EJ: Usual therapy improves perianal Crohn's disease as measured by a new disease activity index: McMaster IBD study group. J Clin Gastroenterol 1995;20:27–32.

10 Dejaco C, Harrer M, Waldhoer T, Miehsler W, Vogelsang H, Reinisch W: Antibiotics and azathioprine for the treatment of perianal fistulas in Crohn's disease. Aliment Pharmacol Ther 2003;18:1113–1120.

11 Hinojosa J, Gomollon F, Garcia S, Bastida G, Cabriada JL, Saro C, Ceballos D, Penate M, Gassull MA: Efficacy and safety of short-term adalimumab treatment in patients with active Crohn's disease who lost response or showed intolerance to infliximab: a prospective, open-label, multicentre trial. Aliment Pharmacol Ther 2007;25:409–418.

12 Present DH, Rutgeerts P, Targan S, Hanauer SB, Mayer L, van Hogezand RA, Podolsky DK, Sands BE, Braakman T, DeWoody KL, Schaible TF, van Deventer SJ: Infliximab for the treatment of fistulas in patients with Crohn's disease. N Engl J Med 1999;340: 1398–1405.

13 Ardizzone S, Maconi G, Colombo E, Manzionna G, Bollani S, Bianchi Porro G: Perianal fistulae following infliximab treatment: clinical and endosonographic outcome. Inflamm Bowel Dis 2004;10:91–96.

14 Sands BE, Anderson FH, Bernstein CN, Chey WY, Feagan BG, Fedorak RN, Kamm MA, Korzenik JR, Lashner BA, Onken JE, Rachmilewitz D, Rutgeerts P, Wild G, Wolf DC, Marsters PA, Travers SB, Blank MA, van Deventer SJ: Infliximab maintenance therapy for fistulizing Crohn's disease. N Engl J Med 2004;350:876–885.

15 Pascua M, Su C, Lewis JD, Brensinger C, Lichtenstein GR: Meta-analysis: factors predicting post-operative recurrence with placebo therapy in patients with Crohn's disease. Aliment Pharmacol Ther 2008;28:545–556.

16 Travis SP, Stange EF, Lemann M, Oresland T, Chowers Y, Forbes A, D'Haens G, Kitis G, Cortot A, Prantera C, Marteau P, Colombel JF, Gionchetti P, Bouhnik Y, Tiret E, Kroesen J, Starlinger M, Mortensen NJ: European evidence based consensus on the diagnosis and management of Crohn's disease: current management. Gut 2006;55(suppl 1):i16–i35.

17 Jones JH, Lennard-Jones JE: Corticosteroids and corticotrophin in the treatment of Crohn's disease. Gut 1966;7:181–187.

18 Malchow H, Ewe K, Brandes JW, Goebell H, Ehms H, Sommer H, Jesdinsky H: European Cooperative Crohn's Disease Study (ECCDS): results of drug treatment. Gastroenterology 1984;86:249–266.

19 Bernstein LH, Frank MS, Brandt LJ, Boley SJ: Healing of perineal Crohn's disease with metronidazole. Gastroenterology 1980;79: 357–365.

20 Brandt LJ, Bernstein LH, Boley SJ, Frank MS: Metronidazole therapy for perineal Crohn's disease: a follow-up study. Gastroenterology 1982;83:383–387.

21 Thia KT, Mahadevan U, Feagan BG, Wong C, Cockeram A, Bitton A, Bernstein CN, Sandborn WJ: Ciprofloxacin or metronidazole for the treatment of perianal fistulas in patients with Crohn's disease: a randomized, double-blind, placebo-controlled pilot study. Inflamm Bowel Dis 2009;15:17–24.

22 West RL, van der Woude CJ, Hansen BE, Felt-Bersma RJ, van Tilburg AJ, Drapers JA, Kuipers EJ: Clinical and endosonographic effect of ciprofloxacin on the treatment of perianal fistulae in Crohn's disease with infliximab: a double-blind placebo-controlled study. Aliment Pharmacol Ther 2004;20: 1329–1336.

23 Pearson DC, May GR, Fick GH, Sutherland LR: Azathioprine and 6-mercaptopurine in Crohn disease: a meta-analysis. Ann Intern Med 1995;123:132–142.

24 Egan LJ, Sandborn WJ, Tremaine WJ: Clinical outcome following treatment of refractory inflammatory and fistulizing Crohn's disease with intravenous cyclosporine. Am J Gastroenterol 1998;93:442–448.

25 Hanauer SB, Smith MB: Rapid closure of Crohn's disease fistulas with continuous intravenous cyclosporin A. Am J Gastroenterol 1993;88:646–649.

26 Present DH, Lichtiger S: Efficacy of cyclosporine in treatment of fistula of Crohn's disease. Dig Dis Sci 1994;39:374–380.

27 Sandborn WJ, Present DH, Isaacs KL, Wolf DC, Greenberg E, Hanauer SB, Feagan BG, Mayer L, Johnson T, Galanko J, Martin C, Sandler RS: Tacrolimus for the treatment of fistulas in patients with Crohn's disease: a randomized, placebo-controlled trial. Gastroenterology 2003;125:380–388.

28 Sands BE, Blank MA, Patel K, van Deventer SJ: Long-term treatment of rectovaginal fistulas in Crohn's disease: response to infliximab in the Accent II study. Clin Gastroenterol Hepatol 2004;2:912–920.

29 Lichtenstein GR, Yan S, Bala M, Blank M, Sands BE: Infliximab maintenance treatment reduces hospitalizations, surgeries, and procedures in fistulizing Crohn's disease. Gastroenterology 2005;128:862–869.

30 Hanauer SB, Sandborn WJ, Rutgeerts P, Fedorak RN, Lukas M, MacIntosh D, Panaccione R, Wolf D, Pollack P: Human anti-tumor necrosis factor monoclonal antibody (adalimumab) in Crohn's disease: The Classic-I Trial. Gastroenterology 2006;130:323–333, quiz 591.

31 Sandborn WJ, Rutgeerts P, Enns R, Hanauer SB, Colombel JF, Panaccione R, D'Haens G, Li J, Rosenfeld MR, Kent JD, Pollack PF: Adalimumab induction therapy for Crohn disease previously treated with infliximab: a randomized trial. Ann Intern Med 2007;146:829–838.

32 Colombel JF, Sandborn WJ, Rutgeerts P, Enns R, Hanauer SB, Panaccione R, Schreiber S, Byczkowski D, Li J, Kent JD, Pollack PF: Adalimumab for maintenance of clinical response and remission in patients with Crohn's disease: The CHARM Trial. Gastroenterology 2007;132:52–65.

33 Colombel JF, Schwartz DA, Sandborn WJ, Kamm MA, D'Haens G, Rutgeerts PJ, Enns RA, Panaccione R, Schreiber S, Li J, Kent JD, Lomax KG, Pollack PF: Adalimumab for the treatment of fistulas in patients with Crohn's disease. Gut 2009;58:940–948.

34 Sandborn WJ, Feagan BG, Stoinov S, Honiball PJ, Rutgeerts P, Mason D, Bloomfield R, Schreiber S: Certolizumab pegol for the treatment of Crohn's disease. N Engl J Med 2007;357:228–238.

35 Schreiber S, Khaliq-Kareemi M, Lawrance IC, Thomsen OO, Hanauer SB, McColm J, Bloomfield R, Sandborn WJ: Maintenance therapy with certolizumab pegol for Crohn's disease. N Engl J Med 2007;357:239–250.

36 Mahadevan U, Marion JF, Present DH: Fistula response to methotrexate in Crohn's disease: a case series. Aliment Pharmacol Ther 2003;18:1003–1008.

37 Fukuda Y, Takazoe M, Sugita A, Kosaka T, Kinjo F, Otani Y, Fujii H, Koganei K, Makiyama K, Nakamura T, Suda T, Yamamoto S, Ashida T, Majima A, Morita N, Murakami K, Oshitani N, Takahama K, Tochihara M, Tsujikawa T, Watanabe M: Oral spherical adsorptive carbon for the treatment of intractable anal fistulas in Crohn's disease: a multicenter, randomized, double-blind, placebo-controlled trial. Am J Gastroenterol 2008;103:1721–1729.

38 Ba'ath ME, Mahmalat MW, Kapur P, Smith NP, Dalzell AM, Casson DH, Lamont GL, Baillie CT: Surgical management of inflammatory bowel disease. Arch Dis Child 2007;92:312–316.

39 Fichera A, Michelassi F: Surgical treatment of Crohn's disease. J Gastrointest Surg 2007;11:791–803.

40 Gupta N, Cohen SA, Bostrom AG, Kirschner BS, Baldassano RN, Winter HS, Ferry GD, Smith T, Abramson O, Gold BD, Heyman MB: Risk factors for initial surgery in pediatric patients with Crohn's disease. Gastroenterology 2006;130:1069–1077.

41 Mueller MH, Geis M, Glatzle J, Kasparek M, Meile T, Jehle EC, Kreis ME, Zittel TT: Risk of fecal diversion in complicated perianal Crohn's disease. J Gastrointest Surg 2007;11:529–537.

42 Loffler T, Welsch T, Muhl S, Hinz U, Schmidt J, Kienle P: Long-term success rate after surgical treatment of anorectal and rectovaginal fistulas in Crohn's disease. Int J Colorectal Dis 2009;24:521–526.

43 Williams JG, Rothenberger DA, Nemer FD, Goldberg SM: Fistula-in-ano in Crohn's disease. Results of aggressive surgical treatment. Dis Colon Rectum 1991;34:378–384.

44 Buchanan GN, Owen HA, Torkington J, Lunniss PJ, Nicholls RJ, Cohen CR: Longterm outcome following loose-seton technique for external sphincter preservation in complex anal fistula. Br J Surg 2004;91:476–480.

45 Hyman N: Endoanal advancement flap repair for complex anorectal fistula. Am J Surg 1999;178:337–340.

46 Makowiec F, Jehle EC, Becker HD, Starlinger M: Clinical course after transanal advancement flap repair of perianal fistula in patients with Crohn's disease. Br J Surg 1995;82:603–606.

47 van der Hagen SJ, Baeten CG, Soeters PB, van Gemert WG: Long-term outcome following mucosal advancement flap for high perianal fistulas and fistulotomy for low perianal fistulas. Recurrent perianal fistulas: failure of treatment or recurrent patient disease? Int J Colorectal Dis 2006;21:784–790.

48 Mizrahi N, Wexner SD, Zmora O, Da Silva G, Efron J, Weiss EG, Vernava AM, 3rd, Nogueras JJ: Endorectal advancement flap: are there predictors of failure? Dis Colon Rectum 2002;45:1616–1621.

49 Gaertner WB, Decanini A, Mellgren A, Lowry AC, Goldberg SM, Madoff RD, Spencer MP: Does infliximab infusion impact results of operative treatment for Crohn's perianal fistulas? Dis Colon Rectum 2007;50:1754–1760.

50 Galandiuk S, Kimberling J, Al-Mishlab TG, Stromberg AJ: Perianal Crohn disease: predictors of need for permanent diversion. Ann Surg 2005;241:796–801.

51 de Parades V, Far HS, Etienney I, Zeitoun JD, Atienza P, Bauer P: Seton drainage and fibrin glue injection for complex anal fistulas. Colorectal Dis 2009; Epub ahead of print.

52 Vitton V, Gasmi M, Barthet M, Desjeux A, Orsoni P, Grimaud JC: Long-term healing of Crohn's anal fistulas with fibrin glue injection. Aliment Pharmacol Ther 2005;21:1453–1457.

53 Witte ME, Klaase JM, Gerritsen JJ, Kummer EW: Fibrin glue treatment for simple and complex anal fistulas. Hepatogastroenterology 2007;54:1071–1073.

54 Loungnarath R, Dietz DW, Mutch MG, Birnbaum EH, Kodner IJ, Fleshman JW: Fibrin glue treatment of complex anal fistulas has low success rate. Dis Colon Rectum 2004;47:432–436.

55 Lindsey I, Smilgin-Humphreys MM, Cunningham C, Mortensen NJ, George BD: A randomized, controlled trial of fibrin glue vs. conventional treatment for anal fistula. Dis Colon Rectum 2002;45:1608–1615.

56 O'Connor L, Champagne BJ, Ferguson MA, Orangio GR, Schertzer ME, Armstrong DN: Efficacy of anal fistula plug in closure of Crohn's anorectal fistulas. Dis Colon Rectum 2006;49:1569–1573.

57 Safar B, Jobanputra S, Sands D, Weiss EG, Nogueras JJ, Wexner SD: Anal fistula plug: Initial experience and outcomes. Dis Colon Rectum 2009;52:248–252.

58 Schwandner O, Stadler F, Dietl O, Wirsching RP, Fuerst A: Initial experience on efficacy in closure of cryptoglandular and Crohn's transsphincteric fistulas by the use of the anal fistula plug. Int J Colorectal Dis 2008;23:319–324.

59 Johnson EK, Gaw JU, Armstrong DN: Efficacy of anal fistula plug vs. fibrin glue in closure of anorectal fistulas. Dis Colon Rectum 2006;49:371–376.

60 Schwandner O: Innovative management of anal fistula by the use of the anal fistula plug: hype or help? Minerva Chir 2008;63:413–419.

61 Kamm MA, Ng SC: Perianal fistulizing Crohn's disease: a call to action. Clin Gastroenterol Hepatol 2008;6:7–10.

Dig Dis 2009;27:394–403
DOI: 10.1159/000228580

Drug Monitoring in Inflammatory Bowel Disease: Helpful or Dispensable?

Tony Bruns   Andreas Stallmach

Division of Gastroenterology, Hepatology and Infectious Disease, Department of Internal Medicine II, Friedrich Schiller University of Jena, Jena, Germany

Key Words

Inflammatory bowel disease · Pharmacogenetics · Drug monitoring · Azathioprine · 6-Mercaptopurine · Toxicity

Abstract

Thiopurines, methotrexate and the calcineurin inhibitors cyclosporin A and tacrolimus are classical immunosuppressive treatment modalities for inflammatory bowel disease (IBD). Since a high inter-patient variability exists in drug efficacy and toxicity, their application requires the knowledge of appropriate indications as well as strategies for individualization of dosage and monitoring for adverse events. Results of pharmacogenetic studies that examine the relationship between single-gene polymorphisms and associated effects on the pharmacokinetics and pharmacodynamics may be helpful for the optimization of individualized therapy. Although 85–95% of patients worldwide present with the homozygote thiopurine S-methyltransferase (TPMT) wild-type genotype and a normal enzyme activity, cost-benefit analyses suggest assessment of TPMT enzyme activity prior to thiopurine therapy for IBD to prevent life-threatening toxicity. Monitoring of 6-mercaptopurine metabolites is a helpful, but not an indispensable tool in thiopurine non-responders to discriminate poor adherence and under-dosing from pharmacogenetic thiopurine resistance and thiopurine refractory disease. Response to and adverse events of methotrexate therapy are hard to predict. Pharmacogenetic indices of methotrexate metabolization have been evaluated in rheumatoid arthritis (RA) but not in IBD yet. In contrast to RA, concentration of methotrexate polyglutamates correlates positively with non-response and adverse effects in IBD. Calcineurin inhibitor metabolism is mainly controlled by cytochrome P-450 isoenzymes 3A4/3A5 and P-glycoprotein that underlie a variety of gene polymorphisms and are susceptible to drug interactions. Independent from pharmacokinetic alterations a MDR1 polymorphism may predict cyclosporin failure in severe ulcerative colitis. Frequent monitoring of whole blood levels is required since efficacy and toxicity are dose-dependent.

Copyright © 2009 S. Karger AG, Basel

Introduction

Because of their efficacy, safety profile, and comparatively low cost, conventional immunosuppressants remain the foundation of IBD therapy. Since a great inter-patient variability exists in drug efficacy and drug toxicity, their application requires the knowledge of appropriate indications as well as strategies for individualization of dosage and monitoring for adverse events. Besides the influence of behavioral and environmental factors, genetic differences are estimated to account for 20–95% variability in the therapeutic effects of medications [1]. To optimize therapeutic efforts and minimize side effects, phar-

KARGER

Fax +41 61 306 12 34
E-Mail karger@karger.ch
www.karger.com

© 2009 S. Karger AG, Basel
0257–2753/09/0273–0394$26.00/0

Accessible online at:
www.karger.com/ddi

Andreas Stallmach, Division of Gastroenterology, Hepatology and Infectious Disease
Department of Internal Medicine II, Friedrich Schiller University of Jena
Erlanger Allee 101, DE–07740 Jena (Germany)
Tel. +49 3641 932 4221, Fax +49 3641 932 4222
E-Mail andreas.stallmach@med.uni-jena.de

macogenetic studies currently examine the relationship between single-gene polymorphisms and associated effects on the phamacokinetics and pharmacodynamics of medications. Thus, the question arises how to translate these findings into a clinical practice of monitoring the efficacy and toxicity of azathioprine, 6-mercaptopurine, methotrexate, cyclosporin, and tacrolimus.

Thiopurines

Azathioprine (AZA) and 6-mercaptopurine (6-MP) are a well-established, effective maintenance therapy for moderate and severe Crohn's disease (CD) [2] and for ulcerative colitis (UC) [3]. The use of AZA in CD has constantly increased since its first application in 1969 [4] to a cumulative 5-year probability of more than 50% [5]. Thiopurine-related adverse events occur in 5% up to 40% [6] in both a dose-dependent and a dose-independent idiosyncratic manner and lead to therapy discontinuation in up to 10–26% of treated patients [7, 8]. Whereas myelotoxicity, nausea, and malaise have been proposed as dose-dependent side effects, the exact categorization of rash, flu-like symptoms and pancreatitis is not conclusive, yet [9, 10].

Both thiopurine drugs, AZA and 6-MP, are prodrugs that undergo extensive metabolism: mercaptopurine is metabolized by thiopurine S-methyltransferase (TPMT), hypoxanthine guanine phosphoribosyltransferase (HPGRT), and xanthine oxidase (XO). HPGRT, inosine-5-monophosphate dehydrogenase (IMPDH), and guanidine-5-monophosphate synthetase (GMPS) catalyze the metabolic steps for production of 6-thioguanine nucleotides (6-TGN) – the considered predominantly active metabolites of thiopurines [11]. TPMT competes with HPGRT for its substrate 6-MP to produce 6-methyl-mercaptopurine (6-MMP) that is considered to be responsible for distinct side-effects of thiopurine therapy. So the question arises whether determination of TPMT enzyme activity or measurement of 6-TGN/6-MMP concentration is suitable for adaptation of thiopurine therapy.

TPMT Enzyme Activity

Although 23 genetic variants of TPMT have been described [6], approximately 85–95% of patients worldwide present with the homozygote TPMT*1 wild-type genotype and a normal TPMT activity [12–14]. However, interindividual differences in enzyme activity up to the 50-fold have been described [15]. A retrospective study on more than 3,000 British patients revealed that approximately 80% of individuals present with a normal and 10% with a decreased enzyme activity [16]. Whereas the initially reported prevalence of an absent TPMT enzyme activity was 1:300 (0.3%) [15], this study revealed a higher prevalence of 1:220 (0.45%). 9% of patients have an increased TPMT activity [16] that cannot be detected by TPMT genotype analysis. It is important to note that TPMT phenotyping is susceptible to prior transfusions since enzyme activity is determined in red blood cells [17].

Bone marrow toxicity occurs in 2–12% of patients under thiopurine therapy [18, 19]. 0.3–0.5% of cases are life-threatening [20] and 1 in 1,000 patients treated with AZA or 6-MP will die because of this [21]. The risk of severe thiopurine-related myelotoxicity is increased in patients with TPMT mutations and a few fatal cases have been reported [22, 23]. Priest et al. [20] reported that TPMT analysis may predict 90% of life-threatening episodes and 60% of severe and moderate episodes of neutropenia. However, 73% of patients with severe bone-marrow suppression do not carry a TPMT mutation [24]. Six currently available economic evaluations – three of them in inflammatory bowel disease (IBD) – report that TPMT analysis in patients undergoing thiopurine therapy is a cost-effective use of healthcare resources [25]. The costs to save a life-year by TPMT screening amount to between GBP 347 (30-year-olds) and GBP 817 (60-year-olds) [21].

TPMT mutations are also associated with the development of drug-related adverse events other than myelotoxicity as determined in a current prospective study [26]. 79% of patients carrying heterozygote TPMT mutations did not tolerate 6 months of AZA therapy in standard doses mainly due to nausea and gastric intolerance within 6 weeks. Interestingly, myelotoxicity did not occur before 12 weeks, suggesting an underestimation of the relative risk of TPMT mutations for myelotoxicity in retrospective studies. Since thiopurine-related hepatotoxicity is associated with higher median 6-MMP levels [27] as well as with elevated 6-TGN levels [28, 29], determination of TPMT activity may also predict the susceptibility to thiopurine-induced liver injury. Although a single study reported a possible association of nodular regenerative hyperplasia and heterozygote TPMT mutation [30], several studies failed to prove a correlation of TPMT activity and drug-induced liver damage [31].

Conclusively, we recommend determination of TPMT enzyme activity prior to initiating thiopurine therapy, since several studies indicate that TPMT phenotyping may provide advantages over genotyping in predicting drug-related toxicity [20, 32]. Furthermore, only phenotyping may identify patients with high enzyme activity who are likely to develop thiopurine resistance [33, 34] as well as patients with low enzyme activity despite homozygous TPMT wild type.

Deficiency of inosine triphosphate pyrophosphatase (ITPase), a further enzyme involved in 6-MP metabolism, results in the accumulation of potentially toxic 6-thio inosine triphosphates. In a British study, the ITPA 94C>A deficiency-associated allele was significantly associated with pancreatitis and flu-like symptoms [35] whereas a heterozygous ITPA polymorphism was neither associated with leucopenia [36] nor with other side effects [37].

Metabolite Monitoring

A couple of retrospective [38, 39] and two prospective studies [26, 40] demonstrated a positive correlation of pre-treatment TPMT activity and clinical response to thiopurine therapy. Because decreased TPMT enzyme activity correlates with elevated 6-TGN levels and 6-TGN is considered to be the immunosuppressant metabolite, it appears very likely that 6-TGN concentration may predict drug efficacy. However, many studies [41–43] failed to prove an association between clinical activity scores and 6-TGN concentration. Dubinsky et al. [27] were the first to define the therapeutic range of 6-TGN and to demonstrate a significantly higher response in thiopurine-treated children with 6-TGN levels above 235 pmol per 8×10^8 RBC. These results were subsequently confirmed in adult CD [44] and in adult UC [45]. Despite heterogeneous results, a meta-analysis of 12 studies [46] demonstrated a positive correlation between clinical response and high 6-TGN levels (threshold: 230–260 pmol/ 8×10^8 RBC) with an odds ratio of 3.3.

Whereas low 6-TGN levels correlate with increased disease activity, 6-TGN levels above 450 seem to correlate with an increased risk for myelotoxicity [47]. Furthermore, 6-TGN levels and thiopurine dosage correlate very poorly. Remarkably, standard dosing regimens of 6-MP (≥ 1 mg/kg per day) will result in insufficient 6-TGN levels below 230 pmol/8×10^8 RBC in two thirds of the patients [48].

Thus, individualization of thiopurine therapy by 6-TGN monitoring for optimum efficacy may seem promising but is limited by inconstant 6-TGN levels and broad overlapping ranges of efficacy and toxicity. For instance, 4 weeks of dose-fixed therapy are necessary to achieve a steady state in 6-TGN concentration [26]. Furthermore, in 37 of 51 patients with thiopurine failure AZA/6-MP dose escalation results in minor 6-TGN level changes but in a significant increase of 6-MMP levels [33]. Thiopurine therapy that is solitarily 6-TGN controlled may therefore lead to severe hepatotoxicity [49]. In a recent study, 6-TGN levels above 400 pmol/8×10^8 RBC in patients lacking steroid-free clinical remission was a 100% predictive factor of thiopurine refractoriness [50].

Based on currently available data monitoring of the 6-MP metabolites, 6-TGN and 6-MMP can be recommended in the absence of clinical response after 3–4 months of therapy to discriminate poor adherence and under-dosing (low 6-TGN levels and low 6-MMP levels) from pharmocogenetic thiopurine resistance (low 6-TGN levels and high 6-MMP levels) or thiopurine refractory disease (high 6-TGN levels and high 6-MMP levels) [11].

Routine pretreatment determination of TPMT enzyme activity and determination of 6-TGN levels in absence of clinical response are, however, no substitutes for follow-up laboratory monitoring. Biweekly measurement of full blood count and liver function tests within the first 3 months of therapy and every 3 months thereafter is a common monitoring scheme, although liver function tests may not be required that frequently [51]. Weekly measurements of serum amylase within the first 8 weeks of treatment may be helpful in preventing the clinical development of drug-induced pancreatitis as suggested by a retrospective study [52].

Methotrexate

The application of the folate-analogue methotrexate (MTX) to achieve and maintain remission in IBD is complicated by the difficulty to predict its efficacy and toxicity. Whereas it has been shown to be effective in induction and in maintenance of remission in CD [53– 55] comparable to azathioprine [56], a meta-analysis by the Cochrane Collaboration revealed that there has only been one well-designed, randomized controlled trial assessing methotrexate for induction of remission in UC [57]. In that study no benefit for orally applied low-dose MTX (12.5 mg weekly) over placebo was found [58]. Whether oral application of MTX is pharmacokinetically equivalent to subcutaneous or intramuscular application remains uncertain due to discrepant study results [59, 60]. Because of its serum half-time of 5–8 h [61], blood levels of MTX and its metabolite 7-hydroxymethotrexate are of no diagnostic value to monitor efficacy and toxicity in a low-dose therapeutic scheme [62].

Methotrexate-Related Toxicity

10–18% of patients with IBD discontinue MTX because of the occurrence of adverse effects [63]. Life-threatening toxicity of low-dose MTX is increased in patients with impaired renal function, older age, increasing mean corpuscular volume, and trimethoprim-sulfamethoxazole co-medication [64]. According to a meta-analysis by the Cochrane Collaboration, low-dose administration of folic or folinic acid (≤ 5 mg weekly) in rheumatoid arthritis (RA) prevents 80% of oral and gastrointestinal MTX-related toxicity without altering efficacy [65]. Nausea, stomatitis and diarrhea occur early due to the directly antiproliferative activity of MTX, but later toxicity, such as liver damage, may result from an intracellular accumulation of MTX-PG [66]. Severe fibrosis or cirrhosis occurs in up to 20% of patients treated with low-dose MTX for psoriasis for 3 years [67] and 7% progress at least one histological grade per each gram methotrexate taken [68]. The incidence of MTX-related hepatotoxicity seems to be substantially lower in patients with IBD despite the high incidence of abnormal liver function test. Te et al. [69] reported one case of hepatic fibrosis in 20 IBD patients receiving cumulative methotrexate doses of more than 1,500 mg questioning the usefulness of routine liver biopsies. Neither abnormal liver chemistry tests, which occur in up to one third of patients, nor transient elastography [70] are able to predict MTX-related liver fibrosis reliably [69]. Thus, risk factors for liver disease such as obesity, diabetes mellitus, alcohol consumption or hepatotoxic co-medication have to be taken into account to individually monitor for hepatotoxicity.

The most unpredictable and a possible lethal side effect of MTX is hypersensitivity pneumonitis. These patients present with acute onset of fever, dyspnea, tachypnea, hypoxemia, leukocytosis, and restrictive lung function in absence of positive blood and sputum cultures. Diagnostic criteria have been published to confirm the diagnosis [71]. Very recently, two forms of methotrexate-induced pneumonitis have been suggested: type 1 that occurs early, predominated by neutrophils, lung fibrosis and a high mortality; and type 2 that occurs late, predominated by lymphocytes with less fibrosis and lower mortality [72].

Metabolite Monitoring and Pharmacogenetics

As an antagonist of the enzyme dihydrofolate reductase MTX prevents pyrimidine and purine synthesis and thus inhibits cellular proliferation. Studies indicate that low-dose MTX rather acts through blocking proliferation of lymphocytes and monocytes by promoting apoptosis, inhibiting T_H1 cytokine production (IL-2, IFN-γ, TNF-α), upregulating IL-10, and increasing extracellular adenosine release [73, 74]. For this purpose, MTX is ac-

tively transported into cells and subsequently polyglutamated by the enzyme folyl polyglutamate synthase (FPGS). Intracellular levels of MTX polyglutamates (MTX-PG) in RBC and polymorphonuclear cells have been shown to correlate with clinical efficacy in RA [75]. Interestingly, a pilot study of MTX-PG levels in 18 patients with CD demonstrated a correlation of higher MTX-PG4/5 levels with worse disease activity and frequent adverse effects instead [76]. Further numerous polymorphisms in MTX transporter genes (SLC19A1, ABCB1, ABCC2), in the folate metabolism pathway (MTHFR, MTHFD1, SHMT, TYMS) and in the adenosine pathway (ATIC, AMPD1, ITPA) have been reported to be associated with MTX efficacy and toxicity in RA [77]. A composite pharmacogenetic index comprising low penetrance genetic polymorphisms of a folate carrier (RFC-1), an AICAR transformylase (ATIC), and a thymidylate synthase (TSER) was an independent predictor of high disease activity in a multivariate analysis of 226 patients treated with low-dose MTX for RA [78]. A similar pharmacogenetic index consisting of MTHFR, TSER, ATIC and SHMT polymorphisms was also designed to predict MTX-related side effects in RA [79].

Less and inconclusive data exist for patients with IBD: the methylenetetrahydrofolate reductase (MTHFR) 1298C mutation has been reported to be associated with MTX-related side effects in one [80] of two studies [80, 81]. Basing on these data metabolite monitoring and pharmacogenetic testing in MTX therapy can currently not be recommended for IBD due to the lack of valid data, the lack of standardized methods, and its high costs. Toxicity monitoring in IBD patients treated with MTX should rather be performed by careful physical examination for signs and symptoms of myelotoxicity (incidence: 1–5%), infections (13%) and pneumonitis (<5%) plus surveillance of full blood count, liver tests, and creatinine weekly during the first month, biweekly during months 2–4, and monthly thereafter [82].

Calcineurin Inhibitors

Cyclosporin A (CsA) and tacrolimus (FK506) are effective therapeutic options in selected patients with severe IBD. After forming complexes with their intracellular receptors (cyclophilin and FKBP) both drugs suppress NF-κB and T cell activation by inhibition of calcineurin, a transcription factor regulating protein phosphatase, leading to a decreased production of IL-2 and TNF-α [83, 84].

Efficacy and Safety of CsA

CsA has been introduced for chronic active steroid-resistant CD in 1989 [85] and for severe UC in 1990 [86, 87]. The response rate to CsA in patients with active CD is highly variable, but oral CsA in doses of 5 mg/kg/day has not been effective for the induction and maintenance of remission in at least three controlled large trials [88]. In contrast, early data on CsA application for severe corticosteroid-resistant UC appeared more promising: 82% of treated patients responded and 63% of patients maintained their response at 6 months and could be weaned entirely from steroids and CsA [87, 89]. CsA at 4 mg/kg/day was as effective as methylprednisolone at 40 mg/day for severe flares of UC to achieve response after 8 days (64 vs. 53%) [90]. However, retrospective outcome data question long-term efficacy: 25% of initial responders undergo colectomy after a mean interval of 6 months [91] and 88% of treated patients within 7 years [92]. A multivariate analysis identified the following three predictive factors for avoiding a colectomy under cyclosporin: pulse rate ≤90 bpm, body temperature ≤37.5°C, and CRP level ≤45 mg/l [93]. Basing on current data a Cochrane analysis concluded that short-term CsA therapy may be attempted in cases of severe ulcerative colitis but is not based on strong evidence [94].

The largest series [95] so far reported the following severe adverse events associated with CsA application in 111 IBD patients within a mean duration of 9 months of therapy: serious infection (6%), nephrotoxicity (5%), seizures (4%), anaphylaxis (1%). Toxicity lead to therapy discontinuation in 5% and resulted in the death of 2 (2%) patients. One patient died of infectious complications by *Klebsiella pneumoniae* after acute kidney failure and persistently high CsA levels. Arts et al. [91] reported death from opportunistic infections in 3 of 86 patients under immunosuppressive triple therapy (*Pneumocystis jiroveci* pneumonia, *Aspergillus fumigatus* pneumonia). Therefore, prophylaxis against *Pneumocystis jiroveci* has to be considered in patients treated with CsA immunosuppression [96, 97] despite the lack of recommendation in current ACG practice guidelines [98].

Minor side effects of cyclosporin include paresthesias, hypomagnesemia, hypertension, hypertrichosis, headache, minor nephrotoxicity, abnormal liver function tests, minor infections, elevated serum potassium levels, and gingival swelling when applied intravenously at 4 mg/kg/day for 7–10 days (mean blood level 506 ng/ml) and then switched to oral CsA at 8 mg/kg/day (mean blood level 303 ng/ml) [95]. In order to reduce possible side effects, a randomized, double-blind comparison of 4 and 2 mg/kg/day cyclosporin in 73 patients with severe flares of UC was performed by van Assche et al. [99]. In both groups approximately 85% of patients responded within 8 days after a median of 4 days despite lower mean CsA blood levels in the 2 mg/kg/day group (237 vs. 332 ng/ml). However, differences in the frequency of adverse events were not observed.

Efficacy and Safety of Tacrolimus

Similarly to CsA, tacrolimus has been used to treat patients with flares of UC nonresponding to i.v. corticosteroids. The only double-blind, randomized, placebo-controlled study [100] assessed the efficacy of tacrolimus in 65 patients with moderate-to-severe active UC and compared two target whole blood concentrations (5–10 and 10–15 ng/ml) to placebo. Although remission rates after two weeks of treatment did not statistically differ, clinical improvement was observed significantly more often in the high-target level group (68%) but not in the low-target level group (38%) compared to placebo (10%). These data demonstrate a dose-dependent efficacy with a statistically significant benefit for clinical improvement of tacrolimus in trough levels of 10–15 ng/ml with an odds ratio of 14.63 [101]. The role of tacrolimus in fistulizing CD has been evaluated in one randomized, placebo-controlled trial [102] demonstrating fistula improvement in 43 vs. 8% after 10 weeks at a rather high daily dosage of 0.2 mg/kg/day – but not fistula remission (10 vs. 8%).

Despite the higher immunosuppressant efficacy of FK506 and its higher toxicity in kidney and liver transplant recipients compared to cyclosporin [103, 104], the reported long-time toxicity of tacrolimus in patients with IBD appears to be comparatively low. Over a mean therapy duration of 25 months the following adverse events occurred in 53 patients and led to therapy discontinuation in 4%: tremor and paresthesias (9%), mild nephrotoxicity (8%), opportunistic infections with *Candida albicans* or *CMV* (8%), hypertension (2%), and hyperkalemia (2%) [105]. However, these findings are limited by a retrospective single-center study design and by low-target blood levels of 4–8 ng/ml, which have not been demonstrated to be effective in controlled trials. Until further controlled data on efficacy and safety become available, tacrolimus (like cyclosporin) should be used as a therapeutic bridge to a different maintenance therapy.

Calcineurin Inhibitor Drug Monitoring and Pharmacogenetics

CsA and FK506 are lipophilic molecules with highly interindividually and intraindividually variable absorption kinetics depending on gastrointestinal function and bile secretion [106]. The transport of CsA and tacrolimus is mediated by ATP-dependent cellular efflux by the multidrug resistance-1 (MDR1) gene coded P-glykoprotein sharing the same binding sites with *Vinca* alkaloids and verapamil [107]. It has been demonstrated that 56% of the variability in CsA oral clearance and 32% of the variability in CsA peak blood concentration were accounted for by variation in liver enzyme activity of cytochrome P450 3A4 (CYP3A4) [108]. Thus, cyclosporin blood levels depend on individual expression levels of functional CYP3A4 and P-glykoprotein as well as on concomitant medications. Amiodarone, azole antifungal agents, diltiazem and verapamil, high-dose methylprednisolone, macrolides and metoclopramide increase plasma levels of CsA, whereas carbamazepine, phenobarbital, phenytoin and rifampin decrease it [109].

Furthermore, differences in ethnicity may play a role in the metabolism of calcineurin inhibitors. For instance, the CYP3A4*1B polymorphism, that has been shown to increase CYP3A4 transcription in vitro, is found in <4% of Caucasians and Asians but in 46–66% of people from African descent [106]. Determination of genetic polymorphisms of CYP3A4, CYP3A5 and MDR1 to estimate required doses of CsA and its influence on patients' response has been evaluated in several post-transplantation studies but has not revealed consistent results due to differences in dosing regimens, measurement methods and patient population [106]. Only individuals with the wild-type CYP3A5*1 express CYP3A5 at significant levels [106]. It has been shown that these patients require higher doses to target trough levels of tacrolimus in renal transplant recipients [110]. An observed increase in tacrolimus concentration after the withdrawal of steroids [111] results from a steroid-dependent induction of hepatic CYP3A and P-glycoprotein [112] and may be aggravated in CYP3A5*1 non-carriers [113, 114].

The predictive value of MDR1 polymorphisms on CsA resistance in patients with severe steroid-resistant UC has been investigated by Daniel et al. [115]. The presence of a C3435T polymorphism (TT genotype, 23% prevalence) predicted CsA failure defined as colectomy within 30 days with an odds ratio of 3.77. Interestingly, the presence of the TT genotype was not associated with daily CsA dosage or mean CsA blood levels, suggesting the absence of a pharmacokinetic alteration. These findings are consistent with that of a recent meta-analysis that concluded no definite effect of MDR1 C3435T polymorphism on CsA pharmacokinetics [116].

On the base on these little data pharmacogenetically guided dosing of CsA and tacrolimus is currently not feasible. A 'user's guide' of CsA monitoring has been recommended by Kornbluth et al. [117] in 1997: during intravenous application monitoring for signs of anaphylaxis within the first hour, monitoring blood pressure every 4 h and daily monitoring of disease activity, headache, nausea or paresthesias are recommended. CsA blood levels should be determined daily after a dose titration and every second day when in the therapeutic range. After a clinical response within 4–10 days, i.v. CsA should be continued for at least 7 days before switching to oral CsA in twice daily i.v. dosage. Clinical status as well as CsA blood levels, full blood count, erythrocyte sedimentation rate, creatinine, liver function tests, and electrolytes including magnesium should be assessed weekly within the first month, biweekly within the second month, and every 3–4 weeks thereafter. An analogous recommendation for laboratory monitoring of tacrolimus seems plausible [51].

Conclusion

Despite a variety of genetically determined variations in the metabolism of classical immunosuppressants, only measurement of TPMT enzyme activity prior to thiopurine therapy can be recommended at the present time to prevent life-threatening toxicity. As cyclosporin and tacrolimus blood levels must be monitored regularly anyway, the cost-effectiveness of prior estimation of pharmacokinetic abnormalities has to be proven in large multicenter trials. However, genetic susceptibilities for response to therapeutic efforts may be helpful in selecting the adequate immunosuppressive agent. Methotrexate appears as the niche to translate acquired knowledge into clinical practice to individually predict efficacy and toxicity. Altogether, pharmacogenetically guided dosing is currently not applicable in general clinical practice. Sufficient knowledge of adverse events is required to individualize clinical and laboratory monitoring strategies for immunosuppressant therapy in IBD.

Disclosure Statement

The authors declare that no financial or other conflict of interest exists in relation to the content of the article.

References

1 Evans WE, McLeod HL: Pharmacogenomics: drug disposition, drug targets, and side effects. N Engl J Med 2003;348:538–549.

2 Pearson DC, May GR, Fick G, Sutherland LR: Azathioprine for maintaining remission of Crohn's disease. Cochrane Database Syst Rev 2000;2:CD000067.

3 Ohno K, Masunaga Y, Ogawa R, Hashiguchi M, Ogata H: A systematic review of the clinical effectiveness of azathioprine in patients with ulcerative colitis. Yakugaku Zasshi 2004;124:555–560.

4 Brooke BN, Hoffmann DC, Swarbrick ET: Azathioprine for Crohn's disease. Lancet 1969;ii:612–614.

5 Cosnes J, Nion-Larmurier I, Beaugerie L, Afchain P, Tiret E, Gendre JP: Impact of the increasing use of immunosuppressants in Crohn's disease on the need for intestinal surgery. Gut 2005;54:237–241.

6 Teml A, Schaeffeler E, Herrlinger KR, Klotz U, Schwab M: Thiopurine treatment in inflammatory bowel disease: clinical pharmacology and implication of pharmacogenetically guided dosing. Clin Pharmacokinet 2007;46:187–208.

7 O'Brien JJ, Bayless TM, Bayless JA: Use of azathioprine or 6-mercaptopurine in the treatment of Crohn's disease. Gastroenterology 1991;101:39–46.

8 Gearry RB, Barclay ML, Burt MJ, Collett JA, Chapman BA: Thiopurine drug adverse effects in a population of New Zealand patients with inflammatory bowel disease. Pharmacoepidemiol Drug Saf 2004;13:563–567.

9 de Jong DJ, Derijks LJJ, Naber AHJ, Hooymans PM, Mulder CJJ: Safety of thiopurines in the treatment of inflammatory bowel disease. Scand J Gastroenterol Suppl 2003;239:69–72.

10 Marinaki AM, Duley JA, Arenas M, Ansari A, Sumi S, Lewis CM, Shobowale-Bakre M, Fairbanks LD, Sanderson J: Mutation in the ITPA gene predicts intolerance to azathioprine. Nucleosides Nucleotides Nucleic Acids 2004;23:1393–1397.

11 Gearry RB, Barclay ML: Azathioprine and 6-mercaptopurine pharmacogenetics and metabolite monitoring in inflammatory bowel disease. J Gastroenterol Hepatol 2005;20:1149–1157.

12 Ameyaw MM, Collie-Duguid ES, Powrie RH, Ofori-Adjei D, McLeod HL: Thiopurine methyltransferase alleles in British and Ghanaian populations. Hum Mol Genet 1999;8:367–370.

13 Haglund S, Lindqvist M, Almer S, Peterson C, Taipalensuu J: Pyrosequencing of TPMT alleles in a general Swedish population and in patients with inflammatory bowel disease. Clin Chem 2004;50:288–295.

14 Chang J, Lee L, Chen C, Shih M, Wu M, Tsai F, Liang D: Molecular analysis of thiopurine S-methyltransferase alleles in South-east Asian populations. Pharmacogenetics 2002;12:191–195.

15 Weinshilboum RM, Sladek SL: Mercaptopurine pharmacogenetics: monogenic inheritance of erythrocyte thiopurine methyltransferase activity. Am J Hum Genet 1980;32:651–662.

16 Holme SA, Duley JA, Sanderson J, Routledge PA, Anstey AV: Erythrocyte thiopurine methyl transferase assessment prior to azathioprine use in the UK. QJM 2002;95:439–444.

17 Schwab M, Schaeffeler E, Marx C, Zanger U, Aulitzky W, Eichelbaum M: Shortcoming in the diagnosis of TPMT deficiency in a patient with Crohn's disease using phenotyping only. Gastroenterology 2001;121:498–499.

18 Present DH, Meltzer SJ, Krumholz MP, Wolke A, Korelitz BI: 6-Mercaptopurine in the management of inflammatory bowel disease: short- and long-term toxicity. Ann Intern Med 1989;111:641–649.

19 Warman JI, Korelitz BI, Fleisher MR, Janardhanam R: Cumulative experience with short- and long-term toxicity to 6-mercaptopurine in the treatment of Crohn's disease and ulcerative colitis. J Clin Gastroenterol 2003;37:220–225.

20 Priest VL, Begg EJ, Gardiner SJ, Frampton CMA, Gearry RB, Barclay ML, Clark DWJ, Hansen P: Pharmacoeconomic analyses of azathioprine, methotrexate and prospective pharmacogenetic testing for the management of inflammatory bowel disease. Pharmacoeconomics 2006;24:767–781.

21 Winter JW, Walker A, Shapiro D, Gaffney D, Spooner RJ, Mills PR: Cost-effectiveness of thiopurine methyltransferase genotype screening in patients about to commence azathioprine therapy for treatment of inflammatory bowel disease. Aliment Pharmacol Ther 2004;20:593–599.

22 Slanar O, Chalupná P, Novotný A, Bortlík M, Krska Z, Lukás M: Fatal myelotoxicity after azathioprine treatment. Nucleosides Nucleotides Nucleic Acids 2008;27:661–665.

23 Boonsrirat U, Angsuthum S, Vannaprasaht S, Kongpunvijit J, Hirankarn N, Tassaneeyakul W, Avihingsanon Y: Azathioprine-induced fatal myelosuppression in systemic lupus erythematosus patient carrying TPMT*3C polymorphism. Lupus 2008;17:132–134.

24 Colombel JF, Ferrari N, Debuysere H, Marteau P, Gendre JP, Bonaz B, Soulé JC, Modigliani R, Touze Y, Catala P, Libersa C, Broly F: Genotypic analysis of thiopurine S-methyltransferase in patients with Crohn's disease and severe myelosuppression during azathioprine therapy. Gastroenterology 2000;118:1025–1030.

25 Payne K, Newman WG, Gurwitz D, Ibarreta D, Phillips KA: TPMT Testing in azathioprine: a 'cost-effective use of healthcare resources'? Per Med 2009;6:103–113.

26 Ansari A, Arenas M, Greenfield SM, Morris D, Lindsay J, Gilshenan K, Smith M, Lewis C, Marinaki A, Duley J, Sanderson J: Prospective evaluation of the pharmacogenetics of azathioprine in the treatment of inflammatory bowel disease. Aliment Pharmacol Ther 2008;28:973–983.

27 Dubinsky MC, Lamothe S, Yang HY, Targan SR, Sinnett D, Théorêt Y, Seidman EG: Pharmacogenomics and metabolite measurement for 6-mercaptopurine therapy in inflammatory bowel disease. Gastroenterology 2000;118:705–713.

28 Derijks LJJ, Gilissen LPL, de Boer NKH, Mulder CJJ: 6-Thioguanine-related hepatotoxicity in patients with inflammatory bowel disease: dose or level dependent? J Hepatol 2006;44:821–822.

29 de Boer NK, Mulder CJ, van Bodegraven AA: Nodular regenerative hyperplasia and thiopurines: the case for level-dependent toxicity. Liver Transpl 2005;11:1300–1301.

30 Breen DP, Marinaki AM, Arenas M, Hayes PC: Pharmacogenetic association with adverse drug reactions to azathioprine immunosuppressive therapy following liver transplantation. Liver Transpl 2005;11:826–833.

31 Gisbert JP, González-Lama Y, Maté J: Thiopurine-induced liver injury in patients with inflammatory bowel disease: a systematic review. Am J Gastroenterol 2007;102:1518–1527.

32 Winter JW, Gaffney D, Shapiro D, Spooner RJ, Marinaki AM, Sanderson JD, Mills PR: Assessment of thiopurine methyltransferase enzyme activity is superior to genotype in predicting myelosuppression following azathioprine therapy in patients with inflammatory bowel disease. Aliment Pharmacol Ther 2007;25:1069–1077.

33 Dubinsky MC, Yang H, Hassard PV, Seidman EG, Kam LY, Abreu MT, Targan SR, Vasiliauskas EA: 6-MP metabolite profiles provide a biochemical explanation for 6-MP resistance in patients with inflammatory bowel disease. Gastroenterology 2002;122:904–915.

34 Ansari, AR, Soon, SY, Arenas, M: Thiopurine methyltransferase activity predicts both toxicity and clinical response to azathioprine in inflammatory bowel disease: the London IBD Forum prospective study. Gastroenterology 2004;126(suppl 2):A1293.

35 Marinaki AM, Duley JA, Arenas M, Ansari A, Sumi S, Lewis CM, Shobowale-Bakre M, Fairbanks LD, Sanderson J: Mutation in the ITPA gene predicts intolerance to azathioprine. Nucleosides Nucleotides Nucleic Acids 2004;23:1393–1397.

36 Allorge D, Hamdan R, Broly F, Libersa C, Colombel J: ITPA genotyping test does not improve detection of Crohn's disease patients at risk of azathioprine/6-mercaptopurine induced myelosuppression. Gut 2005; 54:565.

37 Dieren JMV, Vuuren AJV, Kusters JG, Nieuwenhuis EES, Kuipers EJ, Woude CJVD: ITPA genotyping is not predictive for the development of side effects in AZA treated inflammatory bowel disease patients. Gut 2005;54:1664.

38 Ansari A, Hassan C, Duley J, Marinaki A, Shobowale-Bakre E, Seed P, Meenan J, Yim A, Sanderson J: Thiopurine methyltransferase activity and the use of azathioprine in inflammatory bowel disease. Aliment Pharmacol Ther 2002;16:1743–1750.

39 Cuffari C, Dassopoulos T, Turnbough L, Thompson RE, Bayless TM: Thiopurine methyltransferase activity influences clinical response to azathioprine in inflammatory bowel disease. Clin Gastroenterol Hepatol 2004;2:410–417.

40 Kwan LY, Devlin SM, Mirocha JM, Papadakis KA: Thiopurine methyltransferase activity combined with 6-thioguanine metabolite levels predicts clinical response to thiopurines in patients with inflammatory bowel disease. Dig Liver Dis 2008;40:425–532.

41 Cuffari C, Theoret Y, Latour S, Seidman G: 6-Mercaptopurine metabolism in Crohn's disease: correlation with efficacy and toxicity. Gut 1996;39:401–406.

42 Lowry PW, Franklin CL, Weaver AL, Pike MG, Mays DC, Tremaine WJ, Lipsky JJ, Sandborn WJ: Measurement of thiopurine methyltransferase activity and azathioprine metabolites in patients with inflammatory bowel disease. Gut 2001;49:665–670.

43 Reuther LO, Sonne J, Larsen NE, Larsen B, Christensen S, Rasmussen SN, Tofteng F, Haaber A, Johansen N, Kjeldsen J, Schmiegelow K: Pharmacological monitoring of azathioprine therapy. Scand J Gastroenterol 2003;38:972–977.

44 Cuffari C, Hunt S, Bayless T: Utilisation of erythrocyte 6-thioguanine metabolite levels to optimise azathioprine therapy in patients with inflammatory bowel disease. Gut 2001; 48:642–646.

45 Seidman EG, Theoret Y, Fisher R, Seidman J, Amre O: Thiopurine drug metabolite levels guide treatment in ulcerative colitis. Gastroenterology 2004;126:A209.

46 Osterman MT, Kundu R, Lichtenstein GR, Lewis JD: Association of 6-thioguanine nucleotide levels and inflammatory bowel disease activity: a meta-analysis. Gastroenterology 2006;130:1047–1053.

47 Wright S, Sanders DS, Lobo AJ, Lennard L: Clinical significance of azathioprine active metabolite concentrations in inflammatory bowel disease. Gut 2004;53:1123–1128.

48 Morales A, Salguti S, Miao CL, Lewis JD: Relationship between 6-mercaptopurine dose and 6-thioguanine nucleotide levels in patients with inflammatory bowel disease. Inflamm Bowel Dis 2007;13:380–385.

49 Gardiner SJ, Gearry RB, Burt MJ, Ding SL, Barclay ML: Severe hepatotoxicity with high 6-methylmercaptopurine nucleotide concentrations after thiopurine dose escalation due to low 6-thioguanine nucleotides. Eur J Gastroenterol Hepatol 2008;20:1238–1242.

50 Roblin X, Biroulet LP, Phelip JM, Nancey S, Flourie B: A 6-thioguanine nucleotide threshold level of 400 pmol/8 × 10 erythrocytes predicts azathioprine refractoriness in patients with inflammatory bowel disease and normal TPMT activity. Am J Gastroenterol 2008;103:3115–3122.

51 Siegel CA, Sands BE: Review article: practical management of inflammatory bowel disease patients taking immunomodulators. Aliment Pharmacol Ther 2005;22:1–16.

52 Castiglione F, Del Vecchio Blanco G, Rispo A, Mazzacca G: Prevention of pancreatitis by weekly amylase assay in patients with Crohn's disease treated with azathioprine. Am J Gastroenterol 2000;95:2394–2395.

53 Feagan BG, Rochon J, Fedorak RN, Irvine EJ, Wild G, Sutherland L, Steinhart AH, Greenberg GR, Gillies R, Hopkins M: Methotrexate for the treatment of Crohn's disease. The North American Crohn's Study Group Investigators. N Engl J Med 1995;332:292–297.

54 Feagan BG, Fedorak RN, Irvine EJ, Wild G, Sutherland L, Steinhart AH, Greenberg GR, Koval J, Wong CJ, Hopkins M, Hanauer SB, McDonald JW: A comparison of methotrexate with placebo for the maintenance of remission in Crohn's disease. North American Crohn's Study Group Investigators. N Engl J Med 2000;342:1627–1632.

55 Alfadhli AAF, McDonald JWD, Feagan BG: Methotrexate for induction of remission in refractory Crohn's disease. Cochrane Database Syst Rev 2005;1:CD003459.

56 Ardizzone S, Bollani S, Manzionna G, Imbesi V, Colombo E, Bianchi Porro G: Comparison between methotrexate and azathioprine in the treatment of chronic active Crohn's disease: a randomised, investigator-blind study. Dig Liver Dis 2003;35:619–627.

57 Chande N, MacDonald JK, McDonald JWD: Methotrexate for induction of remission in ulcerative colitis. Cochrane Database Syst Rev 2007;4:CD006618.

58 Oren R, Arber N, Odes S, Moshkowitz M, Keter D, Pomeranz I, Ron Y, Reisfeld I, Broide E, Lavy A, Fich A, Eliakim R, Patz J, Bardan E, Villa Y, Gilat T: Methotrexate in chronic active ulcerative colitis: a double-blind, randomized, Israeli multicenter trial. Gastroenterology 1996;110:1416–1421.

59 Moshkowitz M, Oren R, Tishler M, Konikoff FM, Graff E, Brill S, Yaron M, Gilat T: The absorption of low-dose methotrexate in patients with inflammatory bowel disease. Aliment Pharmacol Ther 1997;11:569–573.

60 Kurnik D, Loebstein R, Fishbein E, Almog S, Halkin H, Bar-Meir S, Chowers Y: Bioavailability of oral vs. subcutaneous low-dose methotrexate in patients with Crohn's disease. Aliment Pharmacol Ther 2003;18:57–63.

61 Bannwarth B, Péhourcq F, Schaeverbeke T, Dehais J: Clinical pharmacokinetics of low-dose pulse methotrexate in rheumatoid arthritis. Clin Pharmacokinet 1996;30:194–210.

62 Egan LJ, Sandborn WJ, Tremaine WJ, Leighton JA, Mays DC, Pike MG, Zinsmeister AR, Lipsky JJ: A randomized dose-response and pharmacokinetic study of methotrexate for refractory inflammatory Crohn's disease and ulcerative colitis. Aliment Pharmacol Ther 1999;13:1597–1604.

63 Fraser AG, Morton D, McGovern D, Travis S, Jewell DP: The efficacy of methotrexate for maintaining remission in inflammatory bowel disease. Aliment Pharmacol Ther 2002;16:693–697.

64 al-Awadhi A, Dale P, McKendry RJ: Pancytopenia associated with low dose methotrexate therapy: a regional survey. J Rheumatol 1993;20:1121–1125.

65 Ortiz Z, Shea B, Suarez Almazor M, Moher D, Wells G, Tugwell P: Folic acid and folinic acid for reducing side effects in patients receiving methotrexate for rheumatoid arthritis. Cochrane Database Syst Rev 2000;2: CD000951.

66 Fraser AG: Methotrexate: first-line or second-line immunomodulator? Eur J Gastroenterol Hepatol 2003;15:225–231.

67 Malatjalian DA, Ross JB, Williams CN, Colwell SJ, Eastwood BJ: Methotrexate hepatotoxicity in psoriatics: report of 104 patients from Nova Scotia, with analysis of risks from obesity, diabetes and alcohol consumption during long term follow-up. Can J Gastroenterol 1996;10:369–375.

68 Whiting-O'Keefe QE, Fye KH, Sack KD: Methotrexate and histologic hepatic abnormalities: a meta-analysis. Am J Med 1991;90: 711–716.

69 Te HS, Schiano TD, Kuan SF, Hanauer SB, Conjeevaram HS, Baker AL: Hepatic effects of long-term methotrexate use in the treatment of inflammatory bowel disease. Am J Gastroenterol 2000;95:3150–3156.

70 Laharie D, Zerbib F, Adhoute X, Boué-Lahorgue X, Foucher J, Castéra L, Rullier A, Bertet J, Couzigou P, Amouretti M, de Lédinghen V: Diagnosis of liver fibrosis by transient elastography (FibroScan) and noninvasive methods in Crohn's disease patients treated with methotrexate. Aliment Pharmacol Ther 2006;23:1621–1628.

71 Searles G, McKendry RJ: Methotrexate pneumonitis in rheumatoid arthritis: potential risk factors: 4 four case reports and a review of the literature. J Rheumatol 1987;14:1164–1171.

72 Chikura B, Sathi N, Lane S, Dawson JK: Variation of immunological response in methotrexate-induced pneumonitis. Rheumatology 2008;47:1647–1650.

73 Wessels JAM, Huizinga TWJ, Guchelaar H: Recent insights in the pharmacological actions of methotrexate in the treatment of rheumatoid arthritis. Rheumatology 2008; 47:249–255.

74 van Dieren JM, Kuipers EJ, Samsom JN, Nieuwenhuis EE, van der Woude CJ: Revisiting the immunomodulators tacrolimus, methotrexate, and mycophenolate mofetil: their mechanisms of action and role in the treatment of IBD. Inflamm Bowel Dis 2006; 12:311–327.

75 Angelis-Stoforidis P, Vajda FJ, Christophidis N: Methotrexate polyglutamate levels in circulating erythrocytes and polymorphs correlate with clinical efficacy in rheumatoid arthritis. Clin Exp Rheumatol 1999;17:313–320.

76 Brooks AJ, Begg EJ, Zhang M, Frampton CM, Barclay ML: Red blood cell methotrexate polyglutamate concentrations in inflammatory bowel disease. Ther Drug Monit 2007; 29:619–625.

77 Ranganathan P: An update on methotrexate pharmacogenetics in rheumatoid arthritis. Pharmacogenomics 2008;9:439–451.

78 Dervieux T, Furst D, Lein DO, Capps R, Smith K, Caldwell J, Kremer J: Pharmacogenetic and metabolite measurements are associated with clinical status in patients with rheumatoid arthritis treated with methotrexate: results of a multicentred cross sectional observational study. Ann Rheum Dis 2005;64:1180–1185.

79 Weisman MH, Furst DE, Park GS, Kremer JM, Smith KM, Wallace DJ, Caldwell JR, Dervieux T: Risk genotypes in folate-dependent enzymes and their association with methotrexate-related side effects in rheumatoid arthritis. Arthritis Rheum 2006;54:607–612.

80 Herrlinger KR, Cummings JRF, Barnardo MCNM, Schwab M, Ahmad T, Jewell DP: The pharmacogenetics of methotrexate in inflammatory bowel disease. Pharmacogenet Genomics 2005;15:705–711.

81 Soon S, Ansari A, Marinaki T, Arenas M, Magdalinou K, Sanderson J: C677T and A1298C methylenetetrahydrofolate reductase (MTHFR) gene polymorphisms does not predict toxicity or efficacy of methotrexate in patients with inflammatory bowel disease. Gastroenterology 2004;126: A210.

82 Schröder O, Stein J: Low dose methotrexate in inflammatory bowel disease: current status and future directions. Am J Gastroenterol 2003;98:530–537.

83 Liu J, Farmer JD, Lane WS, Friedman J, Weissman I, Schreiber SL: Calcineurin is a common target of cyclophilin-cyclosporin A and FKBP-FK506 complexes. Cell 1991;66: 807–815.

84 Frantz B, Nordby EC, Bren G, Steffan N, Paya CV, Kincaid RL, Tocci MJ, O'Keefe SJ, O'Neill EA: Calcineurin acts in synergy with PMA to inactivate I kappa B/MAD3, an inhibitor of NF-kappa B. EMBO J 1994;13:861–870.

85 Brynskov J, Freund L, Rasmussen SN, et al: A placebo-controlled, double-blind, randomized trial of cyclosporine therapy in active chronic Crohn's disease. N Engl J Med 1989;321:845–850.

86 Lichtiger S, Present DH: Preliminary report: cyclosporin in treatment of severe active ulcerative colitis. Lancet 1990;336:16–19.

87 Lichtiger S, Present DH, Kornbluth A, Gelernt I, Bauer J, Galler G, Michelassi F, Hanauer S: Cyclosporine in severe ulcerative colitis refractory to steroid therapy. N Engl J Med 1994;330:1841–1845.

88 McDonald JWD, Feagan BG, Jewell D, Brynskov J, Stange EF, Macdonald JK: Cyclosporine for induction of remission in Crohn's disease. Cochrane Database Syst Rev 2005;2: CD000297.

89 Kornbluth A, Lichtiger S, Present D, Hanauer S: Long-term results of oral cyclosporin in patients with severe ulcerative colitis: a double-blind randomized multicenter trial. Gastroenterology 1994;106:A714.

90 D'Haens G, Lemmens L, Geboes K, Vandeputte L, Van Acker F, Mortelmans L, Peeters M, Vermeire S, Penninckx F, Nevens F, Hiele M, Rutgeerts P: Intravenous cyclosporine versus intravenous corticosteroids as single therapy for severe attacks of ulcerative colitis. Gastroenterology 2001;120: 1323–1329.

91 Arts J, D'Haens G, Zeegers M, Van Assche G, Hiele M, D'Hoore A, Penninckx F, Vermeire S, Rutgeerts P: Long-term outcome of treatment with intravenous cyclosporin in patients with severe ulcerative colitis. Inflamm Bowel Dis 2004;10:73–78.

92 Moskovitz DN, Van Assche G, Maenhout B, Arts J, Ferrante M, Vermeire S, Rutgeerts P: Incidence of colectomy during long-term follow-up after cyclosporine-induced remission of severe ulcerative colitis. Clin Gastroenterol Hepatol 2006;4:760–765.

93 Cacheux W, Seksik P, Lemann M, Marteau P, Nion-Larmurier I, Afchain P, Daniel F, Beaugerie L, Cosnes J: Predictive factors of response to cyclosporine in steroid-refractory ulcerative colitis. Am J Gastroenterol 2008;103:637–642.

94 Shibolet O, Regushevskaya E, Brezis M, Soares-Weiser K: Cyclosporine A for induction of remission in severe ulcerative colitis. Cochrane Database Syst Rev 2005;1: CD004277.

95 Sternthal MB, Murphy SJ, George J, Kornbluth A, Lichtiger S, Present DH: Adverse events associated with the use of cyclosporine in patients with inflammatory bowel disease. Am J Gastroenterol 2008;103:937–943.

96 Poppers DM, Scherl EJ: Prophylaxis against Pneumocystis pneumonia in patients with inflammatory bowel disease: toward a standard of care. Inflamm Bowel Dis 2008;14: 106–113.

97 Hoffmann JC, Schwandner O, Bruch H: Ulcerative colitis: fulminant disease. Z Gastroenterol 2004;42:1002–1006.

98 Kornbluth A, Sachar DB: Ulcerative colitis practice guidelines in adults (update): American College of Gastroenterology, Practice Parameters Committee. Am J Gastroenterol 2004;99:1371–1385.

99 van Assche G, D'Haens G, Noman M, Vermeire S, Hiele M, Asnong K, Arts J, D'Hoore A, Penninckx F, Rutgeerts P: Randomized, double-blind comparison of 4 mg/kg versus 2 mg/kg intravenous cyclosporine in severe ulcerative colitis. Gastroenterology 2003; 125:1025–1031.

100 Ogata H, Matsui T, Nakamura M, Iida M, Takazoe M, Suzuki Y, Hibi T: A randomised dose finding study of oral tacrolimus (FK506) therapy in refractory ulcerative colitis. Gut 2006;55:1255–1262.

101 Baumgart DC, Macdonald JK, Feagan B: Tacrolimus (FK506) for induction of remission in refractory ulcerative colitis. Cochrane Database Syst Rev 2008;3: CD007216.

102 Sandborn WJ, Present DH, Isaacs KL, Wolf DC, Greenberg E, Hanauer SB, Feagan BG, Mayer L, Johnson T, Galanko J, Martin C, Sandler RS: Tacrolimus for the treatment of fistulas in patients with Crohn's disease: a randomized, placebo-controlled trial. Gastroenterology 2003;125:380–388.

103 Webster A, Woodroffe RC, Taylor RS, Chapman JR, Craig JC: Tacrolimus versus cyclosporin as primary immunosuppression for kidney transplant recipients. Cochrane Database Syst Rev 2005;4: CD003961.

104 Haddad EM, McAlister VC, Renouf E, Malthaner R, Kjaer MS, Gluud LL: Cyclosporin versus tacrolimus for liver transplanted patients. Cochrane Database Syst Rev 2006;4:CD005161.

105 Baumgart DC, Pintoffl JP, Sturm A, Wiedenmann B, Dignass AU: Tacrolimus is safe and effective in patients with severe steroid-refractory or steroid-dependent inflammatory bowel disease: a long-term follow-up. Am J Gastroenterol 2006;101: 1048–1056.

106 Utecht KN, Hiles JJ, Kolesar J: Effects of genetic polymorphisms on the pharmacokinetics of calcineurin inhibitors. Am J Health Syst Pharm 2006;63:2340–2348.

107 Saeki T, Ueda K, Tanigawara Y, Hori R, Komano T: Human P-glycoprotein transports cyclosporin A and FK506. J Biol Chem 1993;268:6077–6080.

108 Lown KS, Mayo RR, Leichtman AB, Hsiao HL, Turgeon DK, Schmiedlin-Ren P, Brown MB, Guo W, Rossi SJ, Benet LZ, Watkins PB: Role of intestinal P-glycoprotein (mdr1) in interpatient variation in the oral bioavailability of cyclosporine. Clin Pharmacol Ther 1997;62:248–260.

109 Hebert MF: Contributions of hepatic and intestinal metabolism and P-glycoprotein to cyclosporine and tacrolimus oral drug delivery. Adv Drug Deliv Rev 1997;27:201–214.

110 Tsuchiya N, Satoh S, Tada H, Li Z, Ohyama C, Sato K, Suzuki T, Habuchi T, Kato T: Influence of CYP3A5 and MDR1 (ABCB1) polymorphisms on the pharmacokinetics of tacrolimus in renal transplant recipients. Transplantation 2004;78:1182–1187.

111 van Duijnhoven EM, Boots JMM, Christiaans MHL, Stolk LML, Undre NA, van Hooff JP: Increase in tacrolimus trough levels after steroid withdrawal. Transpl Int 2003;16:721–725.

112 Shimada T, Terada A, Yokogawa K, Kaneko H, Nomura M, Kaji K, Kaneko S, Kobayashi K, Miyamoto K: Lowered blood concentration of tacrolimus and its recovery with changes in expression of CYP3A and P-glycoprotein after high-dose steroid therapy. Transplantation 2002;74:1419–1424.

113 Roberts PJ, Rollins KD, Kashuba ADM, Paine MF, Nelsen AC, Williams EE, Moran C, Lamba JK, Schuetz EG, Hawke RL: The influence of CYP3A5 genotype on dexamethasone induction of CYP3A activity in African Americans. Drug Metab Dispos 2008;36:1465–1469.

114 Kuypers DR: Influence of interactions between immunosuppressive drugs on therapeutic drug monitoring. Ann Transplant 2008;13:11–18.

115 Daniel F, Loriot M, Seksik P, Cosnes J, Gornet J, Lémann M, Fein F, Vernier-Massouille G, De Vos M, Boureille A, Treton X, Flourié B, Roblin X, Louis E, Zerbib F, Beaune P, Marteau P: Multidrug resistance gene-1 polymorphisms and resistance to cyclosporine A in patients with steroid resistant ulcerative colitis. Inflamm Bowel Dis 2007;13:19–23.

116 Jiang Z, Wang Y, Xu P, Liu R, Zhao X, Chen F: Meta-analysis of the effect of MDR1 C3435T polymorphism on cyclosporine pharmacokinetics. Basic Clin Pharmacol Toxicol 2008;103:433–444.

117 Kornbluth A, Present DH, Lichtiger S, Hanauer S: Cyclosporin for severe ulcerative colitis: a user's guide. Am J Gastroenterol 1997;92:1424–1428.

Dig Dis 2009;27:404–411
DOI: 10.1159/000228581

Growth Retardation in Early-Onset Inflammatory Bowel Disease: Should We Monitor and Treat These Patients Differently?

Anne M. Griffiths

Division of Gastroenterology/Nutrition, The Hospital for Sick Children, Toronto, Ont., Canada

Key Words

Inflammatory bowel disease · Chronic undernutrition · Pro-inflammatory cytokines

Abstract

Growth impairment and associated pubertal delay are common complications of pediatric inflammatory bowel disease (IBD), particularly Crohn's disease (CD). Chronic undernutrition (related primarily to inadequate intake) and pro-inflammatory cytokines are the two major and interrelated contributory factors. Pathogenic mechanisms include interference with growth hormone/insulin-like growth factor-1 axis, with gonadotropin-releasing hormone secretion patterns, and direct cytokine effects on growing bone. Chronic corticosteroid therapy compounds disease-related causes of growth impairment. The influence on growth of polymorphisms in IBD susceptibility or modifier genes is under study. Accurate recognition of impaired growth requires appreciation of normal growth. Pre-illness standard deviation scores (SDS) for height should be obtained and compared with height SDS at diagnosis, so that the impact of disease on growth can be fully appreciated. The greater the deficit prior to recognition of IBD, the greater is the demand for catch-up growth. Height velocity should be regularly monitored and its adequacy for age and pubertal stage assessed. Restoration and maintenance of pre-illness growth pattern indicate success of therapy. Current treatment regimens limit use of corticosteroids, via optimization of immunomodulatory drugs, use of enteral nutrition in CD, and, if necessary, surgery for ulcerative colitis and for intestinal complications of localized CD. Biologic agents with the potential for mucosal healing hold promise of growth enhancement even among children, whose growth with previously available therapies remained compromised. For all therapies, there is a window of opportunity to achieve normal growth before puberty is too advanced.

Copyright © 2009 S. Karger AG, Basel

Introduction

Inflammatory bowel disease (IBD) manifests during childhood or adolescence in up to 25% of patients. Unique to pediatric patient populations is the potential for linear growth impairment as a complication of chronic intestinal inflammation. The challenge in treating each child is to employ pharmacologic, nutritional, and, where appropriate surgical interventions to not only decrease mucosal inflammation and thereby alleviate symptoms, but also to optimize growth and normalize associated pubertal development. Normal growth is a marker of therapy success. While older cohort studies provide a benchmark for linear growth outcomes with traditional therapies, there is reason for optimism that the more recent biologic agents, which more often lead to mucosal healing, will reduce the prevalence of this otherwise common complication.

Anne M. Griffiths, MD
Division of Gastroenterology/Nutrition, The Hospital for Sick Children
555 University Avenue
Toronto, Ont. M5G 1X8 (Canada)
Tel. +1 416 813 7734, Fax +1 416 813 6531, E-Mail anne.griffiths@sickkids.ca

This paper will review the core knowledge essential for the recognition of growth retardation, highlight the pathogenic factors involved, and propose management strategies for young patients in the current era, incorporating the observed growth patterns into treatment algorithms.

Patterns of Normal Growth and Pubertal Development

An appreciation of the variation in normal growth patterns is essential to the recognition of abnormal growth. 'Normal' children grow at very different rates. A child's growth is dependent on both genes and the environment; it appears to be principally mediated by hormones and nutrition. Linear growth can be represented by stature (attained height) or by the rate of growth (height velocity). A child's attained height represents the culmination of growth in all preceding years; height velocity reflects growth status at a particular point in time.

Linear growth velocity decreases from birth onwards, punctuated by a short period of growth acceleration (the 'adolescent growth spurt') just prior to completion of growth. Healthy children grow at a consistent rate in the range of 4–6 cm annually from 6 years of age until the onset of puberty. At puberty there is a rapid alteration in body size and shape; height velocity approximately doubles for a year or more. The age of onset of puberty, and of the pubertal growth spurt, varies among normal individuals and between ethnic populations. It begins earlier in girls than in boys; moreover, the pubertal growth spurt occurs in mid-puberty (prior to menarche) in girls but in late puberty (after Tanner stage 4) in boys [1]. There is hence quite consistently a 2-year difference in the timing of peak height velocity (PHV) in girls compared to boys. In North American females PHV occurs at a mean age of 11.5 years, but in males not until 13.5 years (2 SD = 1.8 years). The occurrence of menarche is an indication that linear growth is nearing completion; usually, girls gain only 5–8 cm more in height within the two subsequent years [1].

Monitoring and Assessment of Growth

Standardized charts are available for graphically recording height, weight and height velocity such that an individual child's growth can be compared to normative values. Reference data most appropriate to the child being monitored should be utilized. An individual child's growth measurement can be represented as a percentile or as a standard deviation score, a quantitative expression of distance from the reference population mean (50th percentile) for the same age and gender. Healthy children grow steadily along the same height percentile and hence maintain the same standard deviation score for height from early childhood through until adulthood. Combined parental heights can be used to estimate a child's potential height. Some temporary deviation from the usual growth channel may occur if the pubertal growth spurt occurs particularly early (temporary increase in height velocity and height centile) or late (temporary decrease in height velocity and height centile).

Definitions of Impaired Growth

Within a large patient group, skewing of SDS for height below population reference values is evidence of disease-associated growth impairment. Mean height SDS of a population characterized by normal growth approximates zero. Growth disturbance in an individual child is indicated by an abnormal growth rate. A definition in terms of static height measurement, although sometimes used, may be misleading, since it is so influenced by parental heights. An individual child may be normally short; conversely a previously tall child may not have increased his height in 2 years, but still be of average stature. A shift from higher to lower centiles on a growth chart of height attained more sensibly signifies growth faltering. Height velocity expressed either as a centile or as a standard deviation score for age and gender is the most sensitive parameter by which to recognize impaired growth.

Prevalence of Growth Impairment in Pediatric IBD

Inflammatory disease occurring during early adolescence is likely to have a major impact on nutritional status and growth because of the very rapid accumulation of lean body mass that normally occurs at this time. Further, boys are more vulnerable to disturbances in growth than girls because their growth spurt comes later and is ultimately longer and greater.

The percentage of patients with IBD, whose growth is adversely affected, varies with the type of IBD (CD vs. ulcerative colitis [UC]), the time of assessment (at diagnosis versus during treatment versus at attainment of final height); the definition of growth impairment; and with the nature of the population under study (tertiary referral center versus population-based) [2–9]. It has nevertheless been consistently observed that impairment of linear growth is common prior to recognition of

Table 1. Prevalence of linear growth impairment in pediatric IBD at time of diagnosis: data from the Hospital for Sick Children, Toronto, during three decades

Time period	Time of assessment	Patients studied	Height SDS	Percentage with height <3rd centile (<–2 SDS)
1980–1986	at diagnosis	pre-pubertal (Tanner I or II) CD patients (n = 100)	–1.1 ± 1.3	21
1990–1996	at diagnosis	pre-pubertal (Tanner I or II) CD patients (n = 161)	–0.74 ± 1.2	22
2001–2006	at diagnosis	pre-pubertal (Tanner I or II) CD patients (n = 120)	–0.50 ± 1.1	7
2001–2006	at diagnosis	pre-pubertal (Tanner I or II) UC patients (n = 85)	+0.04 ± 0.9	2

Table 2. Factors contributing to growth impairment in children with CD

Factor	Explanation
Pro-inflammatory cytokines	direct interference with IGF-1 mediation of linear growth
Decreased food intake	cytokine-mediated anorexia, fear of worsening gastrointestinal symptoms
Stool losses	mucosal damage leading to protein-losing enteropathy; diffuse small intestinal disease or resection leading to steatorrhea
Increased nutritional needs	fever; energy required catch-up growth
Corticosteroid treatment	interference with growth hormone and IGF-1

CD and may even dominate the clinical presentation. As shown in table 1, at diagnosis mean standard deviation score (SDS) for height is reduced among children with CD as a group compared to reference populations, whereas no significant reduction is observed in height-for-age SDSs among young patients with UC. The greater the height deficit at diagnosis, the greater the catch-up growth required. Why linear growth impairment is less common in UC than in CD is not entirely clear. The usual colitic symptom of bloody diarrhea is more promptly investigated than the often subtle presenting symptoms of CD, accounting at least in part for the lesser effect on growth prior to diagnosis.

Delay in epiphyseal closure allows growth to continue longer than normal. Hence mean SDS for height may improve over the course of treatment, when the chronic inflammation can be controlled. With traditional treatments during subsequent years, growth impairment continued to complicate CD, particularly. In spite of gains, mean adult height of patients with pre-pubertal onset of disease remained reduced compared to population reference data. The limited data concerning final height in UC suggest less frequent reduction in height velocity and mean final attained height comparable to reference population data.

Older studies are important as a benchmark of outcomes with traditional therapy in pediatric IBD. It is to be hoped that the now better understanding of the pathogenesis of growth impairment, together with the greater efficacy of current therapeutic regimens in healing intestinal inflammation, may lead to enhanced growth of young patients, particularly those with CD, diagnosed in the present decade.

Pathophysiology of Growth Impairment in IBD

The multiple factors potentially contributing to growth impairment in IBD are summarized in table 2. The precise mechanisms by which growth is inhibited have been the subject of recent detailed reviews [10, 11]. Basic to understanding pathophysiology is an appreciation of the normal physiology and regulation of growth. The growth hormone/insulin-like growth factor-1 (GH/IGF-1) axis plays a pivotal role in normal postnatal growth [11]. Thyroxine, cortisol and the sex steroids are also implicated in its maintenance. IGF-1 is produced predominantly in the liver under the influence of GH and is the key mediator of GH effects at the growth plate of bones. The bio-availability of IGF-1 depends on its unbound or 'free' fraction.

IGF-1-binding protein-3 (IGFBP-3) potentiates the action of IGF-1 by 'loosely' binding to it, thus prolonging the time it is available within the circulation to interact with its receptor [12]. Caloric and protein restriction can cause a reduction in the levels of IGFBP-3 [12]. The pubertal growth spurt is primarily induced by estrogen, which acts to increase the activity of the GH/IGF-1 axis. In addition, the sex steroids, especially the androgens, appear to stimulate growth by a direct effect on growth plate chondrocytes. Estrogen is known to be the key hormone that promotes epiphyseal fusion.

An association between low IGF-1 levels and impaired linear growth in children with chronic inflammatory conditions, including IBD, is well recognized. However, GH production has been shown to be normal, suggesting that a significant degree of 'GH resistance' is operative. Chronic undernutrition and inflammatory cytokines are the principal and interrelated determinants of this resistance, to which may be added the effects of chronic corticosteroid therapy [13].

Chronic Caloric Insufficiency

Growth requires energy. Multiple factors contribute to undernutrition in IBD. However, reduced intake, rather than excessive losses or increased needs, is generally the major cause.

Caloric intakes of growth-impaired CD patients have been reported to average 54% of that recommended for children of similar height for age [14]. Deliberate food restriction avoids symptoms. More importantly, cytokine-mediated disease-related anorexia can be profound. Work in a rat model suggests that TNF-α plays a prominent role through an interaction with the hypothalamic appetite pathways [15]. While clinical studies have demonstrated that significant intestinal fat malabsorption is uncommon in CD, leakage of protein is frequent. In general, resting energy expenditure (REE) does not differ from normal in CD patients with inactive disease; however, it can exceed predicted rates in the presence of fever and sepsis. Moreover, malnourished adolescents with CD fail to reduce their REE as efficiently as comparably malnourished patients with anorexia nervosa [16]. This relative failure of a compensatory mechanism has been attributed to effects of pro-inflammatory cytokines.

Direct Cytokine Effects

A simple nutritional hypothesis fails to explain all the observations related to growth patterns among children with IBD. Multiple cytokines contribute to the inflammation in IBD including tumor necrosis factor-α (TNF-α), interferon-γ (IFN-γ), and multiple interleukins (including IL-6, IL-12, IL-17 and IL-23). These inflammatory cytokines inhibit linear growth through pathways that involve IGF-1 as well as through other pathways [11]. Data from both animal models and/or human studies support potential mechanisms involving the GH/IGF-1 pathways, including downregulation of the growth hormone receptor, upregulation of post-receptor inhibitory proteins, reduced protein synthesis and/or increased protein degradation [11]. Animal experiments have shown that TNF-α and IL-1 increase chondrocyte death, and thus may have a deleterious effect on growth [17]. In an organ culture model of fetal rat parietal bone, marked impairment in osteoblast function and bone growth was observed with the addition of serum from children with CD, but not from children with UC, nor from healthy controls [18]. These and other experimental data suggest that increased IL-6 may represent a major generalized mechanism by which chronic inflammation affects the developing skeleton. Finally, cytokines appear to alter gonadotropin-releasing hormone (GnRH) secretion patterns and impair end-organ responsiveness to circulating testosterone, thereby compounding the effects of undernutrition in delaying progression through puberty [19].

The Interplay between Nutrition and Cytokines

The relative contributions of malnutrition and inflammation to linear growth delay were explored by Ballinger et al. [20] using a rat model of TNBS colitis. Two control groups were used: healthy controls with free access to food, and a pair-fed group comprised of healthy animals with daily food intake restricted to match that of colitic rats. In the colitic rats IGF-1 levels were reduced to 35% of control values. Comparison with the healthy but undernourished pair-fed rats suggested that malnutrition accounted for 53% of the total depression of IGF-1 in colitic rats, with the remaining 47% attributable to inflammation [20].

Corticosteroid-Induced Suppression of Linear Growth

The growth-suppressive effects of glucocorticoids are multifactorial, and include central suppression of GH release, decreased hepatic transcription of GH receptor, such that production of IGF-1 is decreased, and decreased IGF-1 binding in cartilage [12]. Hence exogenous corticosteroids create a state of functional GH deficiency. Dose, preparation and timing of glucocorticoids all influence the degree of growth suppression observed. It appears that concentrations of glucocorticoids required to

Table 3. Techniques to assess and monitor linear growth in children with CD

Initial evaluation

Accurate measurement of the patient's height and weight by trained staff using reliable equipment

Accurate pubertal assessment

Accurate measurement of the biological parents' heights and calculation of mid-parental height (MPH). Formula to estimate a subject's potential adult height: male: MPH +6.5 cm; female: MPH –6.5 cm

Obtain pre-illness anthropologic (height, weight) data on the patient

Radiological bone age estimation in patients with suspected growth delay

Dietetic assessment of caloric, Ca, vitamin D and micronutrient intake

Ongoing monitoring

Accurate height and weight measurements by trained staff using reliable equipment

Calculate height velocity

Calculate z-score for height, weight and height velocity data and/or plot sequentially on gender specific, ethnically appropriate reference curve

Accurate pubertal assessment

Consider bone age estimation if linear growth delay persists or develops

Endeavour to follow until adult height achieved (i.e. attainment of Tanner stage 5 and <0.5 cm linear growth annually)

exert direct suppression on the growth plate may be lower than those required to suppress GH secretion. Growth, particularly in pre-pubertal children, can be impaired by relatively modest daily doses of prednisone (3–5 mg/m^2) [21]. This effect may be reduced, but is not necessarily eliminated, by alternate-day therapy. Selectively eliminating evening administration may avoid blunting of both nocturnal GH secretion and/or ACTH-induced adrenal androgen production [21]. Catch-up growth, following the cessation of glucocorticoid therapy, does not always fully compensate for growth deficits. Although chronic daily dosing and frequent induction courses of steroids have been shown to lead to bone demineralization; at present there is no good evidence that short-term use of steroids for the induction of remission in CD is detrimental to long-term growth.

Influence of Genetic Factors

At times the severity of growth impairment in individual patients seems out of keeping with the perceived level of intestinal inflammation as judged by symptoms,

raising the speculation that genetic polymorphisms might influence growth patterns. The very complex genetic basis of susceptibility to IBD is being unraveled through genome-wide association studies. The difficulty and lack of consistency in defining growth impairment, however, makes analysis of correlation with genotype almost impossible in large scale studies. It remains feasible, however, that common genetic polymorphisms which alter cytokine expression may contribute to growth impairment, although not influence overall susceptibility to CD. A recent study of Israeli patients suggests that relatively common variations in the promoter region for TNF-α may have an independent effect on linear growth outcomes [22]. Similarly, data from Sawczenko et al. [23] demonstrate a potential causal relationship between variation in the promoter region for Il-6, subsequent IL-6 expression, and a differential in linear growth impairment during active inflammation.

Management and Prevention of Growth Impairment

The Importance of Monitoring Growth

Recommendations for accurately appraising and monitoring growth are summarized in table 3. In caring for children with IBD, it is important to obtain pre-illness heights, so that the impact of the chronic intestinal inflammation can be fully appreciated. Part of the assessment of response to therapy in children with IBD is a regular analysis of whether rate of growth is normal for age and pubertal stage and whether catch-up growth to pre-illness centiles is being achieved. A properly calibrated wall-mounted stadiometer is required for accurate and reproducible serial measurements. Height velocity must be appraised in the context of current pubertal stage, because of the variation in normal rates of growth before puberty, during puberty and near the end of puberty. If growth and puberty appear either delayed or very advanced, radiologic determination of bone age can be used to indicate the remaining growth potential.

One of the difficulties in evaluating growth in response to a therapy is the relatively long interval of time required for valid assessment. Published normal standards for height velocity throughout childhood are based on height increments during 12-month periods [24]. When growth velocity is calculated over short time periods, small errors in individual measurements are significantly magnified, and the normal seasonal variation in growth is overlooked. The consensus from pediatric endocrinologists is that height velocity should be calculated over intervals no shorter than 6 months [24]. A valid indicator of anticipated linear growth would allow a more timely change in therapy.

Psychosocial Impact of Impaired Growth

Growth impairment and accompanying pubertal delay have a significant psychosocial impact on adolescents, as the physical differences between them and healthy peers become progressively more obvious. In the development process of a disease-specific health related quality of life instrument for pediatric IBD, body image issues including height and weight were among the concerns most frequently cited by adolescents with CD [25].

Treating to Facilitate Growth

Traditionally, the key differences in management of IBD in children and young adolescents compared to adults have included greater attention to avoidance of long-term corticosteroid therapy, more frequent use of enteral nutrition as an alternate primary therapy in CD, and earlier consideration of resection of localized CD and steroid-dependent UC [26]. These strategies are all aimed at optimizing growth prior to completion of puberty. New biologic therapies, particularly anti- TNF-α, have brought the management of IBD into a new era. Children whose disease remains chronically active despite use of immunomodulatory drugs now benefit from such therapy. Ongoing monitoring of long-term safety issues is required, but these biologic agents hold the promise of improving disease-related outcomes including growth in pediatric IBD [27].

The efficacy of specific medical therapies may be extrapolated from randomized controlled trial data accrued in adults. Evidence of efficacy in enhancing linear growth, however, requires pediatric studies. The importance of persistent inflammation in the pathogenesis of growth impairment makes it intuitive that therapies which achieve mucosal healing are more likely to facilitate normal growth.

Enteral Nutrition. Administration of formulated food as the sole-source nutrition has been an important alternative to conventional corticosteroids in the treatment of active pediatric CD. Such exclusive enteral nutrition (EEN) has been shown to decrease mucosal cytokine production and induce endoscopic healing [28]. Changes in IGF-1 levels occur within 14 days; not surprisingly, EEN is associated with improved height velocity in comparison to steroid therapy [29]. One of the limitations of EEN has been the tendency for symptoms to recur promptly following its cessation. Both 'cyclical EEN' (elemental diet 1 month out of 4) and 'nocturnal supplemental EEN' (EEN 4 nights per week with unrestricted daytime diet) have been associated with disease control and improved growth [30, 31]. However, a subset of patients fail to grow despite nutritional repletion, presumably because intestinal inflammation remains chronically active.

Corticosteroids. Conventional corticosteroids are still commonly used as initial therapy for active pediatric CD. Chronic daily administration and frequent induction courses directly inhibit growth through mechanisms discussed above and must be avoided. Moreover, clinical response to corticosteroids in CD is often not associated with mucosal healing [32], leading to continued cytokine interference with linear growth. Similarly, limited reported experience with controlled ileal release budesonide in children with CD involving the ileum ± right colon suggests that height velocity is impaired despite control of symptoms [33].

Immunomodulatory Drugs. The steroid-sparing roles of immunomodulatory drugs, azathioprine, 6-mercaptopurine and methotrexate, are well documented. Sustained clinical remission and decreased steroid requirement were, however, not associated with improved linear growth in a randomized placebo controlled trial of 6-mercaptopurine in children and adolescents newly diagnosed with CD [34]. Recent retrospective data showed enhancement of linear growth, when methotrexate was given to young patients intolerant of or refractory to thiopurine therapy [35].

Anti-TNF-α. The efficacy of anti-TNF agents in pediatric patients is well established. Considering the role cytokines, including TNF-α, play in growth impairment, and the ability of anti-TNF-α antibodies to achieve mucosal healing, it is of little surprise that both observational and clinical trial data demonstrate a beneficial effect on linear growth, as long as treatment is undertaken early enough prior to or during puberty [27, 36].

Surgical Treatment. Sustained steroid-dependency and associated impairment of linear growth should not be tolerated in children with UC, where colectomy cures the disease and restores growth. Timely surgical intervention may be the optimal management for some young patients with CD, notably those with localized internal penetrating or stricturing disease. Despite the almost inevitable endoscopic and subsequent clinical recurrence of CD, the period of postoperative remission allows important catch-up growth in patients appropriately selected for surgery and undergoing operation prior to or during early puberty [37, 38].

Hormonal Interventions. Treatment of intestinal inflammation and assurance of adequate nutrition are of paramount importance in facilitating linear growth. The role of hormonal therapy in promoting growth has been extremely limited. Mauras et al. [39] reported improvement in IGF-1 levels and height velocity in a pilot study of 10 children with CD, whose growth was impaired in the context of ongoing steroid dependency. Given the variety of potential risks and complications, GHT should be considered experimental in the setting of IBD, and is still best limited to formal investigative study settings. Three to six months of testosterone therapy, carefully supervised by pediatric endocrinologists, has been used in boys with extreme delay of puberty and its associated growth spurt [20].

Adjustments in Treatment Algorithms for the Growth-Impaired Child

All of the foregoing discussion applies to the management of any child with IBD. All young patients should have linear growth regularly monitored, and assessed in the context of pre-illness heights, stature of family members, and their own pubertal stage. Pediatric IBD treatment algorithms recognize the need for effective therapy to control inflammation without chronic corticosteroids, and thereby to facilitate growth. It can be argued that mucosal healing, increasingly the therapeutic goal in IBD, is particularly important in children. The recent top-down versus step-up study of infliximab in adults with CD demonstrated a substantially greater likelihood of mucosal healing with earlier treatment [40]. At the very least, it is time for a similar randomized controlled pediatric trial of traditional versus emerging strategies, but including linear growth along with mucosal healing as an outcome.

The child with significant growth retardation prior to recognition of IBD poses a particular challenge. Greater awareness of CD in children likely accounts for fewer extreme delays in diagnosis. As is evident in the most recent data in table 1, children with CD are still shorter at time of diagnosis as a group than healthy peers, but the discrepancy has lessened in comparison to previous decades. When encountered, children with marked delay in growth prior to diagnosis should be treated more aggressively by whatever means is most suitable for their type, localization, and extent of CD. Rapid healing of diseased bowel with effective medical treatment (or segmental resection if CD is localized and complicated by stricture and/or internal penetration) offers the best chance of catch-up growth.

Disclosure Statement

The author receives research support for investigator-initiated research from Schering Canada, has been a consultant for UCB Pharma, Abbott, Schering Canada, Centocor, and Schering-Plough, and has been an investigator in clinical trials sponsored by Centocor and Abbott.

References

1 Rogol AD, Roemmich JN, Clark PA: Growth at puberty. J Adolesc Health 2002;31:192–200.
2 Griffiths AM, Nguyen P, Smith C, MacMillan H, Sherman PM: Growth and clinical course of children with Crohn's disease. Gut 1993; 34: 939–943.
3 Pfefferkorn M, Burke G, Griffiths A, et al: Growth abnormalities persist in newly diagnosed children with Crohn disease despite current treatment paradigms. J Pediatr Gastroenterol Nutr 2009;48:168–174.
4 Kirschner BS: Growth and development in chronic inflammatory bowel disease. Acta Paediatr Scand Suppl 1990;366:98–104.
5 Kanof ME, Lake AM, Bayless TM: Decreased height velocity in children and adolescents before the diagnosis of Crohn's disease. Gastroenterology 1988;95:1523–1527.

6 Hildebrand H, Karlberg J, Kristiansson B: Longitudinal growth in children and adolescents with inflammatory bowel disease. J Pediatr Gastroenterol Nutr 1994;18:165–173.
7 Markowitz J, Grancher K, Rosa J, Aiges H, Daum F: Growth failure in pediatric inflammatory bowel disease. J Pediatr Gastroenterol Nutr 1993;16:373–380.
8 Sawczenko A, Sandhu BK: Presenting features of inflammatory bowel disease in Great Britain and Ireland. Arch Dis Child 2003;88:995–1000.
9 Wine E, Reif SS, Leshinsky-Silver E, et al: Pediatric Crohn's disease and growth retardation: the role of genotype, phenotype, and disease severity. Pediatrics 2004;114:1281–1286.
10 Ballinger A: Fundamental mechanisms of growth failure in inflammatory bowel disease. Horm Res 2002;58(suppl 1):7–10.
11 Walters TD, Griffiths AM: Mechanisms of growth impairment in Crohn's disease. Nat Pract Clin Gastroenterol, in press.

12 De Benedetti F, Meazza C, Oliveri M, et al: Effect of IL-6 on IGF binding protein-3:a study in IL-6 transgenic mice and in patients with systemic juvenile idiopathic arthritis. Endocrinology 2001;142:4818–4826.
13 De Benedetti F, Alonzi T, Moretta A, et al: Interleukin 6 causes growth impairment in transgenic mice through a decrease in insulin-like growth factor-I: a model for stunted growth in children with chronic inflammation. J Clin Invest 1997;99:643–650.
14 Kelts DG, Grand FJ, Shen G, Watkins JB, Werlin SL, Boehme C: Nutritional basis of grwoth failure in children and adolescents with Crohn's disease. Gastroenterology 1979;76:720–727.
15 Ballinger A, Elh-Haj T, Perrett, et al: The role of the medial hypothalamic serotonin in the suppression of feeding in a rat model of colitis. Gastroenterology 2000;118:544–553.

16 Azcue M, Rashid M, Griffiths A, Pencharz PB: Energy expenditure and body composition in children with Crohn's disease: effect of enteral nutrition and treatment with prednisolone. Gut 1997;41:203–208.

17 Martensson K, Chrysis D, Savendahl L: Interleukin-1beta and TNF-alpha act in synergy to inhibit longitudinal growth in fetal rat metatarsal bones. J Bone Miner Res 2004; 19:1805–1812.

18 Varghese S, Wyzga N, Griffiths AM, Sylvester FA: Effects of serum from children with newly diagnosed Crohn disease on primary cultures of rat osteoblasts. J Pediatr Gastroenterol Nutr 2002;35:641–648.

19 Ballinger AB, Savage MO, Sanderson I: Delayed puberty associated with inflammatory bowel disease. Pediatr Res 2003;53:205–210.

20 Ballinger AB, Azooz O, El-Haj T, Poole S, Farthing MJ: Growth failure occurs through a decrease in insulin-like growth factor 1 which is independent of undernutrition in a rat model of colitis. Gut 2000;46:694–700.

21 Allen DB: Influence of inhaled corticosteroids on growth: a pediatric endocrinologist's perspective. Acta Paediatr 1998;87: 123–129.

22 Levine A, Shamir R, Wine E, et al: TNF promoter polymorphisms and modulation of growth retardation and disease severity in pediatric Crohn's disease. Am J Gastroenterol 2005;100:1598–1604.

23 Sawczenko A, Azooz O, Paraszczuk J, et al: Intestinal inflammation-induced growth retardation acts through IL-6 in rats and depends on the -174 IL-6 G/C polymorphism in children. Proc Natl Acad Sci USA 2005;102: 13260–13265.

24 Griffiths AM, Otley AR, Hyams J, et al: A review of activity indices and end points for clinical trials in children with Crohn's disease. Inflamm Bowel Dis 2005;11:185–196.

25 Griffiths AM, Nicholas D, Smith C, et al: Development of a quality-of-life index for pediatric inflammatory bowel disease: dealing with differences related to age and IBD type. J Pediatr Gastroenterol Nutr 1999;28:S46–S52.

26 Walker-Smith JA: Management of growth failure in Crohn's disease. Arch Dis Child 1996;75:351–354.

27 Hyams JS, Crandall W, Kugathasan S, Griffiths AM, Olson A, Baldassano R, and the REACH Study Group: Induction and maintenance infliximab therapy for the treatment of moderate-to-severe Crohn's disease in children. Gastroenterology 2007; 132:863–873.

28 Fell JM, Paintin M, Arnaud-Battandier F, et al: Mucosal healing and a fall in mucosal pro-inflammatory cytokine mRNA induced by a specific oral polymeric diet in paediatric Crohn's disease. Aliment Pharmacol Ther 2000;14:281–289.

29 Heuschkel RB, Menache CC, Megerian JT, Baird AE: Enteral nutrition and corticosteroids in the treatment of acute Crohn's disease in children. J Pediatr Gastroenterol Nutr 2000;31:8–15.

30 Belli DC, Seidman E, Bouthillier L, et al: Chronic intermittent elemental diet improves growth failure in children with Crohn's disease. Gastroenterology 1988;94: 603–610.

31 Wilschanski M, Sherman P, Pencharz P, Davis L, Corey M, Griffiths A: Supplementary enteral nutrition maintains remission in paediatric Crohn's disease. Gut 1996;38: 543–548.

32 Seidman E, Jones A, Issenman R: Cyclical exclusive enteral nutrition versus alternate day prednisone in maintaining remission of pediatric Crohn's disease. J Pediatr Gastroenterol Nutr 1996;23:A344.

33 Kundhal P, Zachos M, Holmes JL, Griffiths AM: Controlled ileal release budesonide in pediatric Crohn disease: efficacy and effect on growth. J Pediatr Gastroenterol Nutr 2001;33:75–80.

34 Markowitz J, Grancher K, Kohn N, Lesser M, Daum F: A multicenter trial of 6-mercaptopurine and prednisone in children with newly diagnosed Crohn's disease. Gastroenterology 2000;119:895–902.

35 Turner D, Grossman A, Rosh J, Kugathasan S, Gilman AR, Baladassano R, Griffiths AM: Methotrexate following unsuccessful thiopurine therapy in pediatric Crohn's disease. Am J Gastroenterol 2007;102:2804–2812.

36 Walters TD, Gilman AR, Griffiths AM: Linear growth improves during infliximab therapy in children with chronically active severe Crohn disease. Inflamm Bowel Dis 2007;13:424–430.

37 Griffiths AM, Wesson DE, Shandling B, Corey M, Sherman PM: Factors influencing postoperative recurrence of Crohn's disease in childhood. Gut 1991;32:491–495.

38 Baldassano RN, Han PD, Jeshion WC, et al: Pediatric Crohn's disease: risk factors for postoperative recurrence. Am J Gastroenterol 2001;96:2169–2176.

39 Mauras N, George D, Evans J, et al: Growth hormone has anabolic effects in glucocorticosteroid-dependent children with inflammatory bowel disease: a pilot study. Metabolism 2002; 51: 127–135.

40 D'Haens D, Baert F, van Aasche G, et al: Early combined immunosuppression or conventional management in patients with newly diagnosed Crohn's disease: an open randomized trial. Lancet 2008;371:660–667.

Dig Dis 2009;27:412–417
DOI: 10.1159/000228582

Prebiotics, Probiotics and Helminths: The 'Natural' Solution?

Francisco Guarner

Digestive System Research Unit, Centro de Investigación Biomédica en Red de Enfermedades Hepáticas y Digestivas (CIBEREHD), University Hospital Vall d'Hebron, Barcelona, Spain

Key Words
Microbiota · Mucosal immunity · Regulatory T cells · Immunotolerance · Dysbiosis

Abstract

Background: The pathophysiological mechanisms that generate chronic inflammatory lesions in inflammatory bowel disease (IBD) have, at least in part, been unveiled. Abnormal communication between gut microbial communities and the mucosal immune system is being incriminated as the core defect leading to intestinal injury in genetically susceptible individuals. The therapeutic manipulation of gut microecology has attracted high expectation as a strategic area for the control and prevention of IBD. *Method:* Literature review. *Results:* The gut is the major site for induction of regulatory T cells, which secrete immunoregulatory cytokines such as IL-10 and TGF-β and can regulate both Th1 and Th2 responses. Recent findings suggest that some gut commensals, including lactobacilli, bifidobacteria and helminths, play a major role in the induction of regulatory T cells in gut lymphoid follicles. Such T cell-mediated regulatory pathways are essential homeostatic mechanisms by which the host can tolerate the massive burden of innocuous antigens within the gut without responding through inflammation. In clinical practice, the evidence for the use of probiotics or prebiotics is strongest in the case of pouchitis. In addition, one probiotic strain appears to be equivalent to mesalazine in maintaining remission of ulcerative colitis. However, studies of probiotics in Crohn's disease have been disappointing. *Conclusions:* Further research is needed to optimize the use of probiotics, prebiotics or helminths for these indications.

Introduction

Inflammatory bowel diseases (IBD) typically exhibit undulating activity with bouts of uncontrolled, chronic mucosal inflammation, followed by remodeling processes that occur during periods of remission [1]. The precise etiologies of these chronic inflammatory conditions remain to be elucidated and, therefore, the available medical therapies can only to some extent control the eruptions of disease activity, but fail completely regarding the eradication or permanent cure of such diseases.

During the past few years, the pathophysiological mechanisms that lead to the mucosal injury have been unveiled to a large extent. These mechanisms result from a complex interaction of environmental, genetic and immunoregulatory factors. Two broad hypotheses have arisen regarding the fundamental nature of the pathogenesis of IBD [2]. The first argues that primary dysregulation of the mucosal immune system leads to excessive

KARGER

Fax +41 61 306 12 34
E-Mail karger@karger.ch
www.karger.com

© 2009 S. Karger AG, Basel
0257–2753/09/0273–0412$26.00/0

Accessible online at:
www.karger.com/ddi

Francisco Guarner
Digestive System Research Unit, CIBEREHD
University Hospital Vall d'Hebron, Passeig Vall d'Hebron, 119–129
ES–08035 Barcelona (Spain)
E-Mail fguarner@vhebron.net

immunologic responses to normal microbiota. The second suggests that changes in the composition of gut microbiota and/or deranged epithelial barrier function elicit pathologic responses from the normal mucosal immune system (fig. 1). In either case, abnormal communication between gut microbial communities and the mucosal immune system is being incriminated as the core defect leading to IBD in genetically susceptible individuals.

Bacteria and IBD

Infectious diseases are produced by specific microbial agents that possess the capacity of transmitting the disease to susceptible individuals. An infectious origin of Crohn's disease or ulcerative colitis is not supported by such criterion since transmission of these diseases has never been documented. However, there is a substantial body of evidence implicating the enteric bacteria in the pathogenesis of both Crohn's disease and ulcerative colitis. Luminal bacteria appear to provide the stimulus for immuno-inflammatory responses leading to mucosal injury. In Crohn's disease, fecal stream diversion reduces inflammation and induces mucosal healing in the excluded intestinal segment, whereas infusion of intestinal contents quickly reactivates the disease [3]. In ulcerative colitis, short-term treatment with an enteric-coated preparation of broad-spectrum antibiotics rapidly reduced metabolic activity of the flora and mucosal inflammation [4]. The presence of bacteria within the intestinal lumen is the critical condition that triggers mucosal inflammation in IBD.

However, the inflammatory capacity of bacteria is varied. Some resident bacteria activate the inflammatory cascade, whereas some other bacteria have been shown to possess anti-inflammatory properties [5–7]. A microbial imbalance in the gut ecosystem could explain the abnormal reactivity of the mucosal immune system against enteric bacteria.

Intestinal Microbial Ecosystem

The human gut is the natural habitat for a large, diverse and dynamic population of micro-organisms which over millennia have adapted to live on the mucosal surfaces or in the lumen [8]. Our current knowledge about the microbial composition of the intestinal ecosystem is still very limited. Studies using classical tech-

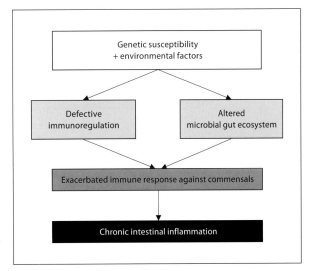

Fig. 1. Genetic susceptibility in combination with a series of environmental factors leads to chronic inflammatory lesions in patients with IBD. The most recent hypothesis suggests that either defects in immunoregulation or altered structure-function of the gut microbiota would trigger exaggerated immune responses against some of the commensal bacteria, leading to chronic intestinal inflammation.

niques of microbiological culture can only recover a minor fraction of fecal bacteria. Over 60% of bacteria cells that are observed by microscopic examination of fecal specimens cannot be grown in culture [9]. Molecular biological techniques based on the sequence diversity of the bacterial genome are being used to characterize noncultivable bacteria. Molecular studies on the fecal microbiota have highlighted that only 7 of the 55 known divisions or superkingdoms of the domain 'bacteria' are detected in the human gut ecosystem, and of these, 3 bacterial divisions dominate, i.e. *Bacteroidetes, Firmicutes* and *Actinobacteria* [10]. However, at species and strain level, microbial diversity between individuals is highly remarkable up to the point that each individual harbors his or her own distinctive pattern of bacterial composition [10]. This pattern appears to be determined at least in part by the host genotype, because similarity in fecal bacterial species is much higher within twins than genetically unrelated couples that share environment and dietary habits [11]. In healthy adults, the fecal composition is host-specific and stable over time, but temporal fluctuations due to environmental factors can be detected and may involve up to 20% of

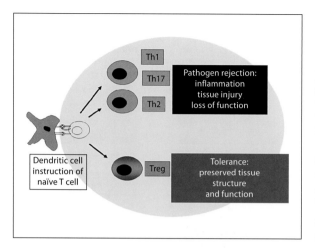

Fig. 2. The specialized lymphoid follicles of the gut mucosa are the major sites for induction and regulation of immune responses [14]. Antigens processed by dendritic cells are presented to naïve lymphocytes in lymphoid follicles. Instruction of these naïve cells by co-stimulatory molecules and cytokines secreted by dendritic cells polarizes phenotypic differentiation to either T helper (Th1, Th17 or Th2) or regulatory T cells (Treg). Proliferation of Th1, Th17 or Th2 cells results in antigen rejection with concomitant inflammation, tissue injury and variable degree of loss of function. In contrast, proliferation of Treg cells is associated with tolerance of the antigen (no rejection) and there is no inflammatory response.

the strains. Bacterial composition in the lumen varies from cecum to rectum, and fecal samples do not reflect luminal contents at proximal segments. However, the community of mucosa-associated bacteria is highly stable from terminal ileum to the large bowel in a given individual [12].

On the other hand, studies comparing animals bred under germ-free conditions with their conventionally raised counterparts have clearly demonstrated the important impact of resident bacteria on host physiology. The interaction between gut bacteria and their host is a symbiotic relationship mutually beneficial for both partners. The host provides a nutrient-rich habitat and the bacteria confer important benefits to the host. Functions of the microbiota include nutrition (fermentation of nondigestible substrates that results in production of short chain fatty acids, absorption of ions, production of amino acids and vitamins), protection (the barrier effect that prevents invasion by alien microbes), and trophic effects on the intestinal epithelium and the immune system (development and homeostasis of local and systemic immunity) [8].

Animals bred in a germ-free environment show low densities of lymphoid cells in the gut mucosa and low levels of serum immunoglobulins. Exposure to commensal microbes rapidly expands the number of mucosal lymphocytes and increases the size of germinal centers in lymphoid follicles [13]. Immunoglobulin-producing cells appear in the lamina propria, and there is a significant increase in serum immunoglobulin levels.

Most interestingly, studies on the mucosal immune system suggest that the gut is the major site for induction of regulatory T cells, which secrete immunoregulatory cytokines such as IL-10 and TGF-β and can regulate both Th1 and Th2 responses [14]. Regulatory pathways mediated by regulatory T cells are essential homeostatic mechanisms by which the host can tolerate the massive burden of innocuous antigens within the gut or on other body surfaces without responding through inflammation (fig. 2). Commensal microbia seem to play a major role in the induction of regulatory T cells in lymphoid follicles. A significant number of experimental studies have shown that some nonpathogenic micro-organisms, including lactobacilli, bifidobacteria and helminths, are particularly effective for the induction of regulatory cytokines and pathways [14].

The Gut Microbiota in IBD

Studies have shown that the composition of the fecal microbiota differs between subjects with IBD and healthy controls [15]. An interesting observation of these studies is that subjects with either ulcerative colitis or Crohn's disease have reduced diversity of bacteria species in both fecal and mucosa-associated communities as compared with healthy subjects [16, 17]. Manichanh et al. [17] employed a metagenomic approach for exhaustive investigation of bacterial diversity in Crohn's disease and found a striking reduction of *Firmicutes* in patients in remission as compared to healthy controls (fig. 3). Reduction in bacterial diversity has also been documented in ulcerative colitis patients [16, 18]. In addition, a recent study in individuals with quiescent ulcerative colitis followed during 1 year observed that the composition of the microbiota was highly variable over time [18]. Temporal instability in the microbiota may be a consequence of low biodiversity and suggests that the intestinal ecosystem in IBD may be more susceptible to environmental influence.

Episodes of altered composition and/or structure of the gut microbiota could represent a major environmental factor triggering immunoinflammatory responses in individuals with genetic susceptibility, and may explain or account for the undulating course of these inflammatory conditions. Prebiotics, probiotics and antibiotics can be used to influence the composition of the gut microbiota, their metabolic activities and their interactions with the mucosal immune system. Therefore, manipulation of microbial ecology in the gut has been the principal target of a series of studies aiming at the prevention and control of inflammatory bowel disorders.

Prebiotics, Probiotics and Helminths

Prebiotics such as inulin and oligofructose can improve the microbial balance in the human intestinal ecosystem by increasing the number and activity of bacteria associated with health benefits [19]. Hypothetically, by increasing the number of 'friendly' bacteria in the gut, prebiotics could prevent mucosal colonization by aerobic enterobacteria able to invade and to induce strong inflammatory responses. This hypothesis has been tested in several experimental studies using different animal models of IBD [20–26]. The experimental data obtained in these studies have consistently demonstrated the anti-inflammatory effects of prebiotics in a wide range of animal models of IBD. Inulin, oligofructose and lactulose can induce changes in the gut microbiota, reduce the release or expression of inflammatory mediators, decrease bacterial translocation, attenuate disease activity indexes and improve mucosal lesions associated with intestinal inflammation. Evidence gained in such studies shows promise for prebiotics as adjuvant therapy for human chronic inflammatory bowel diseases. In fact, the clinical studies published so far suggest efficacy of inulin in mildly active pouchitis [27], as well as in mildly active ulcerative colitis [28, 29]. Inulin has also been tested in a small open-label trial with Crohn's disease patients [30]. However, large controlled studies are still needed to confirm clinical efficacy of inulin for these indications.

The therapeutic efficacy of manipulation of the luminal microecology with probiotics has been extensively tested in animal models of IBD with considerable success [31]. Therefore, probiotic therapy has attracted high expectation as a strategic area for the control and prevention of IBD. Unfortunately, the clinical studies have only shown modest effects at best [32]. The evidence for the clinical use of probiotics in IBD is strongest in the case of pouchitis and, in particular, for the use of the probiotic

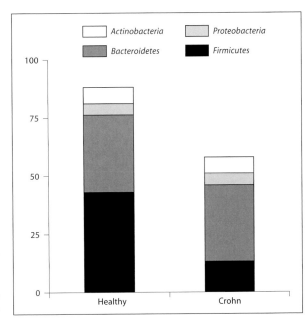

Fig. 3. The fecal microbiota of patients with Crohn's disease contains a markedly reduced diversity of *Firmicutes*. The graph shows data from Manichanh et al. [17] and represents the number of phylotypes per division in 6 healthy persons and 6 patients in clinical remission.

mixture VSL#3. In addition, the *Escherichia coli Nissle* strain appears to be equivalent to mesalazine in maintaining remission of ulcerative colitis. Currently, there are no other recommendations for the clinical use of probiotics in IBD [33]. Further research is needed to optimize the choice of probiotic strains, doses and disease status susceptible to benefit.

Helminths interact with both host innate and adaptive immunity to stimulate immune regulatory pathways and to dampen effector responses that drive host tissue injury [34]. These properties have been investigated for their applicability to treatment of chronic intestinal inflammation in animal models. In addition, there have been several clinical trials using helminths to treat human IBD. Results from these trials suggest that infection with at least some human or animal helminths improves clinical outcome [34]. There was clinical improvement in a double-blind clinical study in ulcerative colitis and an open-label study in Crohn's disease. Worm-based therapies are currently under development, but further evidence is needed before they can be applied in clinical practice.

Conclusions

An altered and exaggerated immune response against some commensal bacteria of the gut ecosystem appears to be the principal mechanism that causes mucosal inflammation and intestinal lesions in IBD. The information currently available does not provide an exact explanation about the origin of this important dysfunction of the interaction between host and commensal bacteria, but an altered microbial composition has been detected in the gut ecosystem of patients with Crohn's disease or ulcerative colitis. Bacteria can influence locally mucosal immune responses and cytokine signaling in different ways. Some bacteria have been shown to down-regulate mucosal inflammation.

Strong experimental evidence supports the hypothesis that therapeutic manipulation of gut microbiota with prebiotics, probiotics or helminths can offer an opportunity to prevent or mitigate intestinal inflammatory lesions in human Crohn's disease, ulcerative colitis, and pouchitis. Encouraging results have been obtained in some clinical trials, but the field needs additional clinical studies in order to confirm their usefulness in routine clinical practice.

Acknowledgements

CIBEREHD is funded by the Instituto de Salud Carlos III (Madrid, Spain). The author is recipient of research grant SAF 2007-64411 from Ministerio de Innovación y Ciencia (Madrid, Spain).

Disclosure Statement

The author declares that no financial or other conflict of interest exists in relation to the content of the article.

References

1 O'Hara AM, Shanahan F: Gut microbiota: mining for therapeutic potential. Clin Gastroenterol Hepatol 2007;5:274–284.

2 Strober W, Fuss I, Mannon P: The fundamental basis of inflammatory bowel disease. J Clin Invest 2007;117:514–521.

3 D'Haens GR, Geboes K, Peeters M, Baert F, Penninckx F, Rutgeerts P: Early lesions of recurrent Crohn's disease caused by infusion of intestinal contents in excluded ileum. Gastroenterology 1998;114:262–267.

4 Casellas F, Borruel N, Papo M, Guarner F, Antolín M, Videla S, Malagelada JR: Antiinflammatory effects of enterically coated amoxicillin-clavulanic acid in active ulcerative colitis. Inflamm Bowel Dis 1998;4:1–5.

5 García-Lafuente A, Antolín M, Guarner F, Crespo E, Salas A, Forcada P, Laguarda M, Gavaldá J, Baena JA, Vilaseca J, Malagelada JR: Incrimination of anaerobic bacteria in the induction of experimental colitis. Am J Physiol 1997;272:G10–G15.

6 Borruel N, Casellas F, Antolín M, Carol M, Llopis M, Espín E, Naval J, Guarner F, Malagelada JR: Effects of nonpathogenic bacteria on cytokine secretion by human intestinal mucosa. Am J Gastroenterol 2003;98: 865–870.

7 O'Hara AM, O'Regan P, Fanning A, O'Mahony C, Macsharry J, Lyons A, Bienenstock J, O'Mahony L, Shanahan F: Functional modulation of human intestinal epithelial cell responses by *Bifidobacterium infantis* and *Lactobacillus salivarius*. Immunology 2006;118:202–215.

8 Guarner F, Malagelada JR: Gut flora in health and disease. Lancet 2003;361:512–519.

9 Suau A, Bonnet R, Sutren M, Godon JJ, Gibson G, Collins MD, Dore J: Direct analysis of genes encoding 16S rRNA from complex communities reveals many novel molecular species within the human gut. Appl Environ Microbiol 1999;65:4799–4807.

10 Eckburg PB, Bik EM, Bernstein CN, Purdom E, Dethlefsen L, Sargent M, Gill SR, Nelson KE, Relman DA: Diversity of the human intestinal microbial flora. Science 2005;308: 1635–1638.

11 Zoetendal E, Akkermans A, Akkermans-van Vliet W, Visser J, de Vos W: The host genotype affects the bacterial community in the human gastrointestinal tract. Microb Ecol Health Dis 2001;13:129–134.

12 Zoetendal EG, von Wright A, Vilpponen-Salmela T, Ben-Amor K, Akkermans AD, de Vos WM: Mucosa-associated bacteria in the human gastrointestinal tract are uniformly distributed along the colon and differ from the community recovered from feces. Appl Environ Microbiol 2002;68:3401–3407.

13 Bouskra D, Brézillon C, Bérard M, Werts C, Varona R, Boneca IG, Eberl G: Lymphoid tissue genesis induced by commensals through NOD1 regulates intestinal homeostasis. Nature 2008;456:507–510.

14 Guarner F, Bourdet-Sicard R, Brandtzaeg P, Gill HS, McGuirk P, van Eden W, Versalovic J, Weinstock JV, Rook GA: Mechanisms of disease: the hygiene hypothesis revisited. Nat Clin Pract Gastroenterol Hepatol 2006; 3:275–284.

15 Guarner F: The intestinal flora in inflammatory bowel disease: normal or abnormal? Curr Opin Gastroenterol 2005;21:414–418.

16 Ott SJ, Musfeldt M, Wenderoth DF, Hampe J, Brant O, Folsch UR, Timmis KN, Schreiber S: Reduction in diversity of the colonic mucosa associated bacterial microflora in patients with active inflammatory bowel disease. Gut 2004;53:685–693.

17 Manichanh C, Rigottier-Gois L, Bonnaud E, Gloux K, Pelletier E, Frangeul L, Nalin R, Jarrin C, Chardon P, Marteau P, Roca J, Dore J: Reduced diversity of faecal microbiota in Crohn's disease revealed by a metagenomic approach. Gut 2006;55:205–211.

18 Martinez C, Antolin M, Santos J, Torrejon A, Casellas F, Borruel N, Guarner F, Malagelada JR: Unstable composition of the fecal microbiota in ulcerative colitis during clinical remission. Am J Gastroenterol 2008;103:643–648.

19 Macfarlane S, Macfarlane GT, Cummings JH: Review article: prebiotics in the gastrointestinal tract. Aliment Pharmacol Ther 2006;24:701–714.

20 Videla S, Vilaseca J, Antolín M, García-Lafuente A, Guarner F, Crespo E, Casalots J, Salas A, Malagelada JR: Dietary inulin improves distal colitis induced by dextran sodium sulfate in the rat. Am J Gastroenterol 2001;96:1486–1493.

21 Osman N, Adawi D, Molin G, Ahrne S, Berggren A, Jeppsson B: Bifidobacterium infantis strains with and without a combination of oligofructose and inulin (OFI) attenuate inflammation in DSS-induced colitis in rats. BMC Gastroenterol 2006;6:31.

22 Cherbut C, Michel C, Lecannu G: The prebiotic characteristics of fructooligosaccharides are necessary for reduction of TNBS-induced colitis in rats. J Nutr 2003;133:21–27.

23 Schultz M, Munro K, Tannock GW, Melchner I, Gottl C, Schwietz H, Scholmerich J, Rath HC: Effects of feeding a probiotic preparation (SIM) containing inulin on the severity of colitis and on the composition of the intestinal microflora in HLA-B27 transgenic rats. Clin Diagn Lab Immunol 2004;11:581–587.

24 Hoentjen F, Welling GW, Harmsen HJM, Zhang XY, Snart J, Tannock GW, Lien K, Churchill TA, Lupicki M, Dieleman LA: Reduction of colitis by prebiotics in HLA-B27 transgenic rats is associated with microflora changes and immunomodulation. Inflamm Bowel Dis 2005;11:977–985.

25 Rumi G, Tsubouchi R, Okayama M, Kato S, Mozsik G, Takeuchi K: Protective effect of lactulose on dextran sulphate sodium-induced colonic inflammation in rats. Dig Dis Sci 2004;49:1466–1472.

26 Camuesco D, Peran L, Comalada M, Nieto A, Di Stasi LC, Rodriguez-Cabezas ME, Concha A, Zarzuelo A, Galvez J: Preventative effects of lactulose in the trinitrobenzenesulphonic acid model of rat colitis. Inflamm Bowel Dis 2005;11:265–271.

27 Welters CFM, Heineman E, Thunnissen BJM, van den Bogaard AEJM, Soeters PB, Baeten CGMI: Effect of dietary inulin supplementation on inflammation of pouch mucosa in patients with an ileal pouch-anal anastomosis. Dis Colon Rectum 2002;45:621–627.

28 Furrie E, Macfarlane S, Kennedy A, Cummings JH, Walsh SV, O'Neil DA, Macfarlane GT: Synbiotic therapy (*Bifidobacterium longum*/Synergy 1) initiates resolution of inflammation in patients with active ulcerative colitis: a randomized controlled pilot trial. Gut 2005;54:242–249.

29 Casellas F, Borruel N, Torrejon A, Varela E, Antolin M, Guarner F, Malagelada JR: Oral oligofructose-enriched inulin supplementation in acute ulcerative colitis is well tolerated and associated with lowered faecal calprotectin. Aliment Pharmacol Ther 2007;25:1061–1067.

30 Lindsay JO, Whelan K, Stagg AJ, Gobin P, Al-Hassi HO, Rayment N, Kamm MA, Knight SC, Forbes A: Clinical, microbiological, and immunological effects of fructo-oligosaccharide in patients with Crohn's disease. Gut 2006;55:348–355.

31 Sartor RB: Probiotic therapy of intestinal inflammation and infections. Curr Opin Gastroenterol 2005;21:44–50.

32 Isaacs K, Herfarth H: Role of probiotic therapy in IBD. Inflamm Bowel Dis 2008;14:1597–1605.

33 World Gastroenterology Organisation Practice Guideline: Probiotics and prebiotics. http://www.worldgastroenterology.org/probiotics-prebiotics.html.

34 Weinstock JV, Elliott DE: Helminths and the IBD hygiene hypothesis. Inflamm Bowel Dis 2009;15:128–133.

Dig Dis 2009;27:418–420
DOI: 10.1159/000235586

Falk Symposium Series

130. Holtmann G, Talley NJ, eds. Gastrointestinal Inflammation and Disturbed Gut Function: The Challenge of New Concepts. Falk Symposium 130. 2003
ISBN 0–7923–8783–X

131. Herfarth H, Feagan BJ, Folsch UR, Schölmerich J, Vatn MH, Zeitz M, eds. Targets of Treatment in Chronic Inflammatory Bowel Diseases. Falk Symposium 131. 2003
ISBN 0–7923–8784–8

132. Galle PR, Gerken G, Schmidt WE, Wiedenmann B, eds. Disease Progression and Carcinogenesis in the Gastrointestinal Tract. Falk Symposium 132. 2003
ISBN 0–7923–8785–6

132A. Staritz M, Adler G, Knuth A, Schmiegel W, Schmoll HJ, eds. Side-effects of Chemotherapy on the Gastrointestinal Tract. Falk Workshop. 2003
ISBN 0–7923–8791–0

132B. Reutter W, Schuppan D, Tauber R, Zeitz M, eds. Cell Adhesion Molecules in Health and Disease. Falk Workshop. 2003   ISBN 0–7923–8786–4

133. Duchmann R, Blumberg R, Neurath M, Schölmerich J, Strober W, Zeitz M. Mechanisms of Intestinal Inflammation: Implications for Therapeutic Intervention in IBD. Falk Symposium 133. 2004   ISBN 0–7923–8787–2

134. Dignass A, Lochs H, Stange E. Trends and Controversies in IBD – Evidence-Based Approach or Individual Management? Falk Symposium 134. 2004
ISBN 0–7923–8788–0

134A. Dignass A, Gross HJ, Buhr V, James OFW. Topical Steroids in Gastroenterology and Hepatology. Falk Workshop. 2004   ISBN 0–7923–8789–9

135. Lukáš M, Manns MP, Špičćák J, Stange EF, eds. Immunological Diseases of Liver and Gut. Falk Symposium 135. 2004   ISBN 0–7923–8792–9

136. Leuschner U, Broomé U, Stiehl A, eds. Cholestatic Liver Diseases: Therapeutic Options and Perspectives. Falk Symposium 136. 2004   ISBN 0–7923–8793–7

137. Blum HE, Maier KP, Rodés J, Sauerbruch T, eds. Liver Diseases: Advances in Treatment and Prevention. Falk Symposium 137. 2004   ISBN 0–7923–8794–5

138. Blum HE, Manns MP, eds. State of the Art of Hepatology: Molecular and Cell Biology. Falk Symposium 138. 2004   ISBN 0–7923–8795–3

138A. Hayashi N, Manns MP, eds. Prevention of Progression in Chronic Liver Disease: An Update on SNMC (Stronger Neo-Minophagen C). Falk Workshop. 2004
ISBN 0–7923–8796–1

139. Adler G, Blum HE, Fuchs M, Stange EF, eds. Gallstones: Pathogenesis and Treatment. Falk Symposium 139. 2004   ISBN 0–7923–8798–8

KARGER

Fax +41 61 306 12 34
E-Mail karger@karger.ch
www.karger.com

© 2009 S. Karger AG, Basel
0257–2753/09/0273–0418$26.00/0

Accessible online at:
www.karger.com/ddi

140. Colombel JF, Gasché C, Schölmerich J, Vucelic C, eds. Inflammatory Bowel Disease: Translation from Basic Research to Clinical Practice. Falk Symposium 140. 2005. ISBN 1–4020–2847–4

141. Paumgartner G, Keppler D, Leuschner U, Stiehl A, eds. Bile Acid Biology and Its Therapeutic Implications. Falk Symposium 141. 2005 ISBN 1–4020–2893–8

142. Dienes HP, Leuschner U, Lohse AW, Manns MP, eds. Autoimmune Liver Disease. Falk Symposium 142. 2005 ISBN 1–4020–2894–6

143. Ammann RW, Büchler MW, Adler G, DiMagno EP, Sarner M, eds. Pancreatitis: Advances in Pathobiology, Diagnosis and Treatment. Falk Symposium 143. 2005 ISBN 1–4020–2895–4

144. Adler G, Blum AL, Blum HE, Leuschner U, Manns MP, Mössner J, Sartor RB, Schölmerich J, eds. Gastroenterology Yesterday – Today – Tomorrow: A Review and Preview. Falk Symposium 144. 2005 ISBN 1–4020–2896–2

145. Henne-Bruns D, Buttenschön K, Fuchs M, Lohse AW, eds. Artificial Liver Support. Falk Symposium 145. 2005 ISBN 1–4020–3239–0

146. Blumberg RS, Gangl A, Manns MP, Tilg H, Zeitz M, eds. Gut–Liver Interactions: Basic and Clinical Concepts. Falk Symposium 146. 2005 ISBN 1–4020–4143–8

147. Jewell DP, Colombel JF, Peña AS, Tromm A, Warren BS, eds. Colitis: Diagnosis and Therapeutic Strategies. Falk Symposium 147. 2006 ISBN 1–4020–4315–5

148. Kruis W, Forbes A, Jauch KW, Kreis ME, Wexner SD, eds. Diverticular Disease: Emerging Evidence in a Common Condition. Falk Symposium 148. 2006 ISBN 1–4020- 4317–1

149. van Cutsem E, Rustgi AK, Schmiegel W, Zeitz M, eds. Highlights in Gastrointestinal Oncology. Falk Symposium 149. 2006 ISBN 1–4020–5108–5

150. Galle PR, Gerken G, Schmidt WE, Wiedenmann B, eds. Disease Progression and Disease Prevention in Hepatology and Gastroenterology. Falk Symposium 150. 2006 ISBN 1–4020–5109–3

151. Fraser A, Gibson PR, Hibi T, Qian JM, Schölmerich J, eds. Emerging Issues in Inflammatory Bowel Disease. Falk Symposium 151. 2006 ISBN 978–1–4020–5701–4

152. Fockens P, Schulz H-J, Rösch T, Špičcák J, eds. Endoscopy 2006 – Update and Live Demonstration. Falk Symposium 152. 2008 ISBN 978–1–4020–9147–6

153. Dignass A, Rachmilewitz D, Stange E-F, Weinstock JV, eds. Immunoregulation in Inflammatory Bowel Diseases – Current Understanding and Innovation. Falk Symposium 153. 2007 ISBN 978–1–4020–5888–2

154. Adler G, Fiocchi C, Lazebnik LB, Vorobiev GI, eds. Inflammatory Bowel Disease – Diagnostic and Therapeutic Strategies. Falk Symposium 154. 2007 ISBN 978–1–4020–6115–8

155. Keppler D, Beuers U, Leuschner U, Stiehl A, Trauner M, Paumgartner G, eds. Bile Acids: Biological Actions and Clinical Relevance. Falk Symposium 155. 2007 ISBN 978–1–4020–6251–3

156. Blum HE, Cox DW, Häussinger D, Jansen PLM, Kullak-Ublick GA, eds. Genetics in Liver Diseases. Falk Symposium 156. 2007 ISBN 978–1–4020–6393–0

157. Diehl AM, Hayashi N, Manns MP, Sauerbruch T, eds. Chronic Hepatitis: Metabolic, Cholestatic, Viral and Autoimmune. Falk Symposium 157. 2007 ISBN 978–1–4020–6522–4

158. Gasche G, Herrerías Gutiérrez JM, Gassull M, Monterio E, eds. Intestinal Inflammation and Colorectal Cancer. Falk Symposium 158. 2007 ISBN 978–1–4020–6825–6

159. Tözün N, Mantzaris G, Dağlı, Schölmerich J, eds. IBD 2007 – Achievements in Research and Clinical Practice. Falk Symposium 159. 2008 ISBN 978–1–4020–6986–4

160. Ferkolj I, Gangl A, Galle PR, Vucelic B, eds. Pathogenesis and Clinical Practice in Gastroenterology. Falk Symposium 160. 2008   ISBN 978–1–4020–8766–0

161. Carey MC, Gabryelewicz A, Díte P, Keim V, Mössner J, eds. Future Perspectives in Gastroenterology. Falk Symposium 161. 2008   ISBN 978–1–4020–8832–2

162. Bosch J, Lammert F, Burroughs AK, Lebrec D, Sauerbruch T, eds. Liver Cirrhosis: From Pathophysiology to Disease Management. Falk Symposium 162. 2008
    ISBN 978–1–4020–8655–7

163. Adler G, Fan DM, Jia JD, LaRusso NF, Owyang, C, eds. Chronic Inflammation of Liver and Gut. Falk Symposium 163. 2008   ISBN 978–1–4020–9352–4

164. Tulassay Z, Dítě P, Krejs GJ, Schölmerich J, Schultz HJ, eds. Intestinal Disorders. Falk Symposium 164. 2009   ISBN 978–1–4020–9590–0

165. Keppler D, Beuers U, Stiehl A, Trauner M, eds. Bile Acid Biology and Therapeutic Actions. Falk Symposium 165. 2009   ISBN 978–1–4020–9643–3

165A. Lieberman DA, Malfertheiner P, Riemann JF, Spechler SJ, eds. Strategies of Cancer Prevention in Gastroenterology. Falk Workshop. 2009
    ISBN 978–90–481–2628–6

166. Ell C, Ponchon T, Riemann JF, Sakai P, Yamamoto H, eds. GI Endoscopy – Standards and Innovations. Falk Symposium 166. 2009   ISBN 978–90–481–2748–1

167. Day CP, Galle PR, Lohse AW, Thorgeirsson SS, eds. Liver under Constant Attack – From Fat to Viruses. Falk Symposium 167. 2009
    ISBN 978–90–481–2758–0

Author Index

Subject Index